MEDICARE

A Strategy for Quality Assurance

VOLUME II Sources and Methods

Committee to Design a Strategy for
Quality Review and Assurance in Medicare

Division of Health Care Services

INSTITUTE OF MEDICINE

Kathleen N. Lohr, editor

NATIONAL ACADEMY PRESS
Washington D.C.   1990

NOTICE: The project that is the subject of this report and its technical appendices was approved by the Governing Board of the National Research Council, whose members are drawn from the councils of the National Academy of Sciences, the National Academy of Engineering, and the Institute of Medicine. The members of the committee responsible for this report were chosen for their special competencies and with regard for appropriate balance.

Volume I of the report has been reviewed by a group other than the authors according to procedures approved by a Report Review Committee consisting of members of the National Academy of Sciences, the National Academy of Engineering, and the Institute of Medicine.

The Institute of Medicine was chartered in 1970 by the National Academy of Sciences to enlist distinguished members of the appropriate professions in the examination of policy matters pertaining to the health of the public. In this, the Institute acts under both the Academy's 1863 congressional charter responsibility to be an adviser to the federal government and its own initiative in identifying issues of medical care, research, and education.

This study was supported by the Health Care Financing Administration, U.S. Department of Health and Human Services, under Cooperative Agreement No. 17-C-99170/3.

Publication IOM-90-02

Library of Congress Cataloging-in-Publication Data

Institute of Medicine (U.S.). Division of Health Care
    Services.
    Medicare : a strategy for quality assurance.

    (Publication IOM ; 90-02)
    "Committee to Design a Strategy for Qualtiy Review
and Assurance in Medicare"—P. following t.p. verso.
    "This study was supported by the Health Care Financing
Administration, U.S. Dept. of Health and Human Services,
under cooperative agreement no. 17-C-991/3"—T.p. verso.
    Includes bibliographical references and indexes.
    1. Medical care—United States—Quality control.
2. Medicare. I. Lohr, Kathleen N., 1941-
II. Institute of Medicine (U.S.) Committee to Design a
Strategy for Quality Review and Assurance in Medicare.
III. United States. Health Care Financing Administration.
IV. Title. V. Series: IOM publication : 90-02
[DNLM: 1. Health Insurance for Aged and Disabled, Title 18.
2. Quality Assurance, Health Care—United States.
WT 30 I591m]
RA395.A3I56 1990   362.1'0973   90-5787
ISBN 0-309-04230-5 (v.1)
ISBN 0-309-04238-0 (v.2)

Volumes I and II of this report *Medicare: A Strategy for Quality Assurance* are available from the National Academy Press, 2101 Constitution Avenue, N.W., Washington, D.C. 20418.

An Executive Summary of Volume I of the report is available from the Institute of Medicine, Division of Health Care Services, 2101 Constitution Avenue, N.W. Washington, D.C. 20418.

Committee to Design a Strategy for Quality Review and Assurance in Medicare

---

*Institute of Medicine Member

Contents

The contents of Volume I are listed below

MEDICARE

1

Overview of the Study to Design a Strategy for Quality Review and Assurance in Medicare

Kathleen N. Lohr

The United States has a high level of quality in much of its health care. As individuals, people (especially the elderly) are usually satisfied with their own medical care and providers. Despite these positive impressions of the overall quality of care in the nation, a large literature documents areas of deficiencies in all parts of the health sector. Some of these problems relate to the overuse of unnecessary and inappropriate services, some to underuse of needed services, and some to poor skills or judgment in the delivery of appropriate services.

Furthermore, recurring crises involving malpractice litigation reflect an undercurrent of quality problems exacerbated by a deteriorating patient-physician relationship. Great variations in rates of use of services in the population are not satisfactorily explained by variations in health needs or resources. Moreover, the growth of for-profit enterprises and of commercialism is seen as leading to possible conflict between physicians and patients. Finally, and perhaps most germane, continuing increases in health expenditures and in the rate at which they rise have led to momentous changes in the health care environment, and these changes have conflicting implications for quality of care and quality assurance.

Given this environment, the Congress of the United States had considerable concerns about the quality of care for the elderly. To address these concerns, they commissioned a study through the Omnibus Budget Reconciliation Act of 1986 (OBRA 1986) to "design a strategy for quality review and assurance in Medicare." Section 9313 of OBRA 1986 called for the Secretary of the U.S. Department of Health and Human Services (DHHS) to solicit a proposal from the National Academy of Sciences (NAS) to conduct the study, and it specified eight legislative charges. These were, "among other items," to:

(A) identify the appropriate considerations which should be used in defining 'quality of care';

(B) evaluate the relative roles of structure, process, and outcome standards in assuring quality of care;

(C) develop prototype criteria and standards for defining and measuring quality of care;

(D) evaluate the adequacy and focus of the current methods for measuring, reviewing, and assuring quality of care;

(E) evaluate the current research on methodologies for measuring quality of care, and suggest areas of research needed for further progress;

(F) evaluate the adequacy and range of methods available to correct or prevent identified problems with quality of care;

(G) review mechanisms available for promoting, coordinating, and supervising at the national level quality review and assurance activities;

(H) develop general criteria which may be used in establishing priorities in the allocation of funds and personnel in reviewing and assuring quality of care.

STUDY COMMITTEE AND TECHNICAL ADVISORY PANEL

Studies undertaken by NAS and the Institute of Medicine (IOM) are conducted by expert committees. These committees comprise individuals selected for their expertise who can provide information and insights from all disciplines and social sectors that are important to the topic of the study. The IOM committee for this study, which was established in the fall of 1987, consisted of 17 individuals and included experts in medicine, nursing, home health and social services, law, economics, epidemiology and statistics, decision analysis, and quality assessment and assurance. Committee members also represented major consumer, purchaser, and business interests. The committee had a broad representation by age, sex, and geographic location.

The OBRA 1986 legislation specified that the IOM should consult with specific organizations and with representatives of major groups that have interests in this issue. To this end, a Technical Advisory Panel (TAP) was appointed early in the study, with representatives from the following groups: American Health Care Association; American Hospital Association; American Medical Association; American Medical Review Research Center; American Nurses Association; Blue Cross and Blue Shield Association; Group Health Association of America; Health Insurance Association of America; Joint Commission on Accreditation of Healthcare Organizations; National Association for Home Care; National Association of Quality Assurance Professionals; National Governors Association; National Medical Association; and Older Women's League.

CONDUCT OF THE STUDY

Phases of the Study

The study was conducted in several phases. A planning phase lasted from summer 1987 through January 1988. During this time, a preliminary and then a final proposal were prepared for the Health Care Financing Administration (HCFA), the study committee was appointed, and IOM staff were hired. The major part of the data collection (described below) was performed between February 1988 and July 1989. Preparation of the IOM committee report (both Volume I and Volume II) was concentrated in the period from August 1989 through February 1990. The report was published and distributed and other dissemination activities (including a conference) were conducted between February and the end of the study in mid-1990.

The work was financed by two grants from the Health Care Financing Administration (HCFA), one for the planning phase and one for the remainder of the study.

Data Collection and Other Study Activities

Main Study Tasks

The committee and IOM staff carried out several major activities during this study; they fall into the general categories of convening meetings, gathering background information, consulting broadly with groups across the country, and acquiring or producing technical documents. First, the committee met nine times for two-to-three-day meetings; the TAP was independently convened twice. Second, a total of 10 background papers were commissioned; Table 1.1 shows the authors and titles of the papers.

Several papers and reports were produced by IOM staff or consultants on various specific aspects of the study. These constitute the main portion of this volume of the report.

A complex public hearing process was started in the early months of the study and continued for about six months (see Chapter 2). It featured two formal public hearings—one in San Francisco and one in Washington, D.C.— at which a total of 42 groups gave oral testimony before the entire committee. Written testimony was received from nearly 140 groups (of nearly 575 contacted), including those that were represented in person.

The study committee placed considerable importance on developing a definition of "quality of care" that would guide their thinking about a Medicare quality assurance program. Testimony from the public hearings, among other sources, provided many ideas and proposals for such a definition.

TABLE 1.1 Commissioned Papers

Title of Paper	Authors
Medicare Quality Assurance Mechanisms and the Law	Andrew Heath Smith
	Maxwell Mehlman
PRO[a] Review of Medicare Health Maintenance Organizations and Competitive Medical Plans	Margaret O'Kane
Quality of Health Care for the Older People in America	Norma Lang
	Janet Kraegel
Strengths and Weaknesses of Health Insurance Data Systems for Assessing Quality	Leslie L. Roos
	Noralou Roos
	Elliot S. Fisher
	Thomas A. Bubolz
Reflections on the Effectiveness of Quality Assurance	Avedis Donabedian
Quality Assurance: Ethical Considerations	Gail Povar
Issues Related to Quality Review and Assurance in Home Health Care	Catherine Hawes
	Robert L. Kane
Study on International Aspects of Quality Assurance	Evert Reerink
Considerations in Defining Quality in Health Care	R. Heather Palmer
	Miriam E. Adams
Quality of Care for Older People in America	Laurence Z. Rubenstein
	Lisa V. Rubenstein
	Karen Josephson

[a]PRO, Peer Review Organization.

Chapter 5 presents the analysis and interpretation of that material and the committee's final definition of quality of care.

Early in the study two sets of focus groups were conducted. Eight focus groups were held among elderly Medicare beneficiaries in four cities (Miami, New York City, Minneapolis, and San Francisco), and an additional eight groups were done among practicing physicians in five cities (Philadelphia, Chicago, New Orleans, Albuquerque, and Los Angeles). Chapter 3 discusses the issues raised through the focus groups.

The most extensive study task was a series of nine major site visits and several smaller site visits to states and cities across the country; these are described in Chapter 4. In the major site visits—two-to-three-day trips to the states of California, Georgia, Illinois, Iowa, Minnesota, New York (two separate site visits), Pennsylvania, Texas, Virginia, and Washington—committee members and staff visited hospitals and hospital associations, home health agencies, health maintenance organizations (HMOs), state departments of health, and other organizations. In addition, meetings were organized with practicing physicians, hospital administrators, representatives of aging, consumer, and community groups, and with other individuals. A major effort was made to visit a representative set of Medicare Peer Review Organizations (PROs). The shorter site visits were to specific organizations (e.g., multispecialty clinics or HMOs) that appeared to offer particular insights into approaches for quality assurance. Altogether, site visitors spoke with over 650 individuals.

Much of the value of the site visits was in learning about and being able to document the wide variety of quality assessment and quality assurance activities being conducted throughout the country. To give a sense of the richness of the efforts beyond the Medicare program, Chapter 6 presents an extensive sampler of methods, instruments, and tools drawn from the site visits, the published literature, and other sources.

Study staff and the committee also carried out several other activities. To address the congressional charge of developing prototypical criteria and standards for defining and measuring quality of care, a special expert panel was convened late in the study to develop recommendations concerning the attributes and standards by which quality-of-care criteria and appropriateness or practice guidelines might be evaluated. This was reported in Chapter 10 of Volume I. Consultants were used to advise on different study topics, such as legal and regulatory issues. We also acquired data on staffing and costs of quality assurance programs from a survey that was being conducted at the same time by a large multihospital system. Additionally, at several of its meetings, the committee heard from a range of experts on quality assurance and related topics. Finally, the committee and staff consulted with staff at HCFA and at several federal and congressional agencies with interests in the Medicare quality assurance program.

Hospital Conditions of Participation

HCFA requested the IOM to conduct a second study, which had been mandated in Section 9305 of OBRA 1986, that would examine whether standards used for hospitals to meet the Conditions of Participation for Medicare could assure the quality of hospital care. The IOM folded this study into the larger effort, and that review is reported mainly in Chapter 7 of this volume.

Medicare Peer Review Organizations

The existing program in Medicare for quality assurance is the PRO program. It, together with predecessor programs (Experimental Medical Care Review Organizations and Professional Standards Review Organizations), was described and discussed in Chapter 6 of Volume I. Much important information about the PRO program, some of which relates directly to evaluative comments in Volume I, could not be retained in that chapter because of space considerations. Thus, a more complete and detailed history and description of the program and its many complex activities are given in Chapter 8 of this volume.

CONCLUDING REMARKS

This volume of source materials is intended to provide documentation of the diverse activities carried out over the two years of this project. The complexities of quality assessment and quality assurance—in conceptualization and in practical application—are such that much of the study committee's final report (Volume I) was oriented to those issues. This volume, therefore, provides much of the "raw material" that underlay the committee's deliberations, findings, conclusions, and recommendations, with the intent that it be a useful reference book well beyond the study's conclusion.

2

Oral and Written Testimony from the Public Hearings

Jo Harris-Wehling

The Institute of Medicine (IOM) committee for the Study to Design a Strategy for Quality Review and Assurance in Medicare convened two public hearings and sought additional written testimony from a large and diverse group of interested organizations. The two public hearing forums provided opportunities for dialogue between the committee and the presenters; the format also allowed several panel members to respond to common questions of relevance for which consensus was questionable or unknown. Groups were able to use the written testimony procedure to provide details on their concerns about and experiences with quality assurance. Having this information during the early phase of the study was helpful for guiding the committee's activities as the study progressed. Because of the diversity and breadth of the information, staff prepared several working papers on the submissions for the committee. This chapter describes the public hearing process used for this study and summarizes the main themes raised by the written submissions.

METHODS

Invitations to Submit Testimony

The invitational package included a transmittal letter, a set of guidelines for written testimony (see Appendix A), and general information items about the IOM and the study. The guidelines asked the submitting groups to respond to 12 key questions about: (1) their definition of quality of care; (2) their views on who should be responsible for quality of care and quality assurance; (3) their own activities as sponsors or subjects of quality assurance programs; and (4) their recommendations about strengthening quality assurance, including research and development.

The 574 groups or individuals invited to testify fell into 10 broadly defined categories. Table 2.1 identifies, by category, the number asked to provide testimony and the number and percentage of those responding. By far the greatest number of invitations was sent to professional associations (238); about one-quarter responded.

Respondents to the Invitations

We convened two formal public hearings. The first was in San Francisco, California, on June 23, 1988; the second was in the Washington, D.C. area on October 21, 1988. We asked 59 groups to appear at one or the other of these hearings. Sixteen groups participated with oral and written statements for the first hearing, and 26 groups participated for the second. Appendix B identifies these organizations and an additional 97 groups that provided only written testimonial documents.

About 30 groups that received an invitational package informed the study office they would not be submitting testimony. Among the reasons given for declining were the following: (1) lack of staff resources to develop a response; (2) internal policies not to take positions on the types of issues the study addressed; and (3) lack of expertise on the subject despite interest in the issues. Some groups asked to receive the committee's final report.

Types of Documents Submitted

The documents submitted by the 139 respondents to our inquiry varied greatly in size and content. They ranged from a one-page letter with no attachments to a three-ring $1^1/_4$-inch notebook accompanied by 3 inches of publications. A typical document was about 10 single-spaced pages. About one-quarter of the submissions were accompanied by some type of publication, such as a set of clinical guidelines or a brochure about the organization.

The information contained in these documents was quite diverse. Some of this diversity relates to the varying interests and experiences of the groups submitting testimony; a state peer review organization of Medicare's Utilization and Quality Control Peer Review Organization (PRO) program, for instance, would be expected to provide different information than a consumer advocacy group. Furthermore, even though the guidelines were sent to all invitees, invitees were free to address any quality issues they wished, not just the topics identified in the guidelines.

About one-quarter of the respondents organized their submissions around the key questions in the guidelines. Some in this group elected to respond in a question-by-question format and others focused on one or two of the key questions without making any comments on the others. The remaining

TABLE 2.1 Number and Percentages of Invitees and Respondents for the
Public Hearing Process Classified by Type of Interest Group

Type of Interest Group	Number Invited	Number Submitting Testimony	Percentage Submitting Testimony
Professional associations	238	61	26
Provider groups	54	19	35
Peer review organizations (PROs)	47	9	19
Business groups and unions	40	8	20
Elderly and consumer interest groups	33	11	33
Disease-specific voluntary and professional groups	30	6	20
Foundations and research groups	30	8	27
Government agencies	23	9	39
Insurers	15	4	27
All other	64	4	6
Total	574	139	24

three-quarters of the submissions varied widely in content and format. In some cases, respondents provided information only on research studies under way or completed; some studies are in the quality assessment and assurance field and others are not. Some respondents addressed only the broad issue of access to health care. Some took up the majority of key questions but confined their comments to only one area of health care (such as home health care) or to only one particular professional practice (such as critical care nursing, enterostomal therapy, or occupational therapy).

Development and Testing of Abstract Form

Staff developed a form to record key information abstracted from each testimonial document. An extensive amount of time was spent in developing the abstract form and building a high level of inter-abstractor reliability. Four drafts were tested by staff before the final version of the form was adopted.

Three staff members were involved in reading the documents and abstracting the information. One staff member reviewed about 75 percent of the documents; a second staff member reviewed the remaining 25 percent. The third staff member participated in the joint review of six documents and also monitored about 20 additional reviews for consistency and thoroughness.

Data Base System

Both hardcopy and database management procedures were set up within the study office to log in basic information as documents arrived. Each testimonial document was assigned a number to facilitate the tracking of documents, the storage of data, software report generation, and the reporting of findings in staff reports.

Data on the abstract forms were entered into two database management files to facilitate the analysis. WordPerfect's secondary file was used for most text-type items on the abstract form. The Paradox database management system was used for the checklist-type sections on the abstract form.

Limitations of the Analysis

Efforts were made to build a high level of inter-abstractor and intra-abstractor reliability. Given the diversity of the documents, however, some errors in abstracting the information undoubtedly have occurred. The major errors are likely to be ones of omission or interpretation. For example, abstractors may have missed some of the "primary concerns about health care" that a respondent addressed or alluded to in the testimony because the respondent may have dispersed comments throughout the document that related to concerns about health care rather than stating them in one identifiable section of the document.

Many respondents have both a parochial interest and a societal interest in quality assessment and assurance of health care; views on specific issues in quality assurance may differ depending on which perspective is being taken at any one time by a given organization. This chapter makes no attempt to differentiate between these interests.

FINDINGS

This section summarizes the content of the testimony received through the public hearing process. The first part comments on major themes that emerged through our analysis of the testimony. Following that are brief synopses of findings keyed to the main topic areas highlighted in the guidelines. In addition to the information summarized in this chapter, many groups provided descriptive information on tools for quality assessment or assurance (such as manuals and guides), on research projects under way, and on leads for additional follow-up. In some cases this information was used to plan the study committee's site visits and as input into the sampler of quality assessment and assurance methods reported in Chapter 6 of this volume.

Main Themes

Several themes or topics appeared in many of the documents, although we did not tally the precise frequency the subjects were mentioned. This section briefly reviews these themes. Later sections elaborate on these topics as they relate to the key questions from the guidelines.

Gaps in Information

The majority of respondents believed that gaps exist in the knowledge base for effective quality assessment and assurance. A few respondents, however, were adamant in stating that no gaps exist in quality assessment. They acknowledged that the quality of health care is less than desired but attributed this to problems with attitudes, implementation, and communication rather than to a lack of specific instruments to measure quality.

Peer Review

The term "peer review" was used by a large percentage of respondents, most of whom indicated their support for the concept. However, the reported effectiveness of peer review differed, depending in part on the type of sponsor for peer review, such as Medicare's PRO program, specialty practices, and internal institutional review committees. Some respondents consider peer review to be a formal process and others view it as a very informal process. Some respondents were adamant about the ineffectiveness of peer review as practiced by PROs, but some of these same respondents stated that the most effective mechanism for assuring quality is peer review.

Access Issues

Access was mentioned frequently as a concern at the San Francisco hearing. It was also mentioned in many of the written documents as a necessary condition for improving the quality of care.

Patient-Physician Relationship

Many respondents noted that the relationship between the patient and the physician is a significant element of the quality of health care. They rarely elaborated the point, however. A few respondents implied that the quality of care would be high if only the patient and physician dyad were not subject to outside influences.

Role of the Elderly in Quality Assessment and Assurance and Health Care Decision Making

There seemed to be general agreement that the elderly consumer does not have a significant role in existing quality assessment and assurance systems. Many respondents indicated the need for more participation of the elderly in health care decision making. They also expressed concern about how to involve the more-frail, the less-informed, and those having multiple psychosocial problems.

Interrelationship of Quality, Costs, and Financing

According to many respondents, a relationship exists between the cost of health care and its quality. Respondents expressed concern that pressure to contain costs results in pressure to provide lower-quality health care. Some respondents stated that, given the limitations of the Medicare financing structure, the elderly do not receive quality care because they cannot afford to purchase needed health care. The major barriers identified were services that are presently not covered and the Medicare beneficiary's out-of-pocket expenditures for charges in excess of the amount reimbursed by Medicare.

Patient-Centered Quality Assurance System

Some respondents believed that an effective quality assessment and assurance system must be structured in a manner that follows the patient through episodes of illness across the multiple settings and providers of care.

Clinical Guidelines, Specialty Board Certification, and Credentialing

Views varied among the respondents as to the value and effectiveness of existing clinical guidelines, board certification and recertification, and credentialing by hospital-based medical staffs as quality assurance methods. Some professional groups emphasized their professional guidelines, certification requirements, and procedure manuals and claimed or implied that these are adequate to assure high-quality care. Other groups pointed out limitations of existing standards, measurement tools, and the like.

Need to Measure, Demonstrate, and Prove Performance Competency

A few practitioner groups explicitly cited the need for new methods to assess competency using performance measures such as chart audits or observations rather than simply fulfilling continuing medical education requirements. Two respondents implied that new, reliable, and visible performance measures are needed to reassure the more sophisticated, inquisitive, and educated consumer or purchaser.

Assessing the Needs of the Elderly

Five respondents, in their discussion on the needs of the elderly, tended not to distinguish any differences in the methods and purposes of quality assessment from those of needs assessment and health status assessment. Other respondents, however, logically linked the process of assessing the needs of the elderly (medical, social, economical, and functional) with the process of assessing quality of service and quality of care. Some respondents discussed the uniqueness of elderly individuals, the importance of the quality of life, the limitations of the Medicare reimbursement system for a population that experiences chronic illnesses, and the need for tools that measure the health status of an individual beyond the scope of the medical model.

Continuous Quality Improvement

A few respondents wrote about the effectiveness of the continuous quality improvement model, and some incorporated its concepts in their definitions of quality. Continuous quality improvement was explicitly mentioned more frequently by researchers and by the Colleges, Academies, and Boards of specialty practices.

Responses to Specific Questions

Defining Quality of Care

In response to key question no. 1, we received about 55 statements (40 percent of all respondents) explicitly defining quality of care. In about 25 additional submissions, the respondents offered parameters by which quality might be defined or evaluated but did not give a definition per se.

Many respondents included structure, process, and outcome dimensions in their definitions. Several definitions included an active role for the patient in decision making, an emphasis on health care beyond the medical model, and a focus on the patient-physician relationship. Some definitions mentioned resource availability as a consideration for defining quality. Chapter 5 of this volume gives a more detailed discussion of the dimensions used by the respondents to define quality of care.

Assessment of Contemporary Health Care

Key question nos. 2 and 3 sought information on respondents' views about the level of quality of care now provided. Most of the concerns expressed were about costs, access, and quality-of-life factors.

About 25 percent of all respondents (32 of 139) believed that health care is good to excellent. Within this subgroup of respondents, however, a large percentage indicated some concern about the quality of health care for a particular subpopulation, such as the rural elderly, poor elderly, elderly women, minority elderly, or nursing home patients. Some respondents addressed quality of health care only from their own perspective as providers.

Examples (paraphrased in some instances) of comments relating to this topic are as follows:

. . . is the best health care system in the world.

If there is a quality problem, the elderly are at greatest risk.

. . . excellent. Physicians are delivering quality care with excellent outcome and patient satisfaction, despite HCFA's administratively burdensome and primitive system.

Serious deficiencies exist in the quality of health care available to the Medicare consumer.

The quality of care provided through the state's hospital systems has never been better.

Cost containment and quality health care. Most respondents identified more than one concern about the quality of health care today. For many the major issue is the perceived inverse relationship between cost containment measures and quality of care. Nearly 50 percent of the respondents (68) expressed uneasiness that the quality of health care would decrease as a result of cost containment efforts. Premature discharges, utilization review, financial incentives for underuse, and health care decisions being made by the (alleged) wrong people (fiscal intermediaries, PROs, utilization review staff of third-party payers) are examples of the cost containment concerns mentioned. Only 11 percent of the respondents identified overuse as a quality-of-care issue.

Medicare benefits. Over 37 percent of the respondents (52) believed that the quality of care for the elderly is less than desired because Medicare does not cover several health services needed by the elderly population. Access to a broader range of services was seen as necessary to improve the quality of care now provided. The most frequently mentioned problem with access to benefits was the lack of coverage of services needed by the chronically ill elderly. Some respondents asserted that a higher quantity of a covered service, such as home health care, is needed to improve quality. Other respondents stressed that the Medicare reimbursement system does not take into account the health needs of the elderly that relate to their quality of life.

Supply and training of health care practitioners. About 40 percent of the respondents (57) were concerned about the availability and supply of health care practitioners. The nursing shortage was mentioned frequently, as was the shortage in specific subspecialties. Concern was also expressed about the need for health care providers to be better trained in aging-specific issues. Training and supervision was a concern of about 25 percent of the respondents (34).

Related to the general issue of the supply of certain health professionals is a question of geographic distribution. About 15 percent (20 respondents) believed that lower-quality care is provided in some geographic locations such as inner cities and rural areas.

Humaneness and continuity. Among those respondents who thought that the health care system is not responsive to the unique characteristics of the elderly population, many cited the need for a more humane relationship between the elderly consumer and the provider. Some comments focused on the fragmentation of the health care system, the increase in subspecialty practices, and a decrease in the role of the primary physician. Over 25 percent called for increased continuity of care among delivery settings as well as among various providers within a given setting; some proposed case management as a solution to the lack of continuity. About 16 percent (22) perceived a current or emerging decrease in the humane aspects of health care. Eight respondents explicitly distinguished quality of service from quality of care; for example, one respondent stated that the elderly ". . . want to be cared about, not just cared for."

Ethical dimensions. Seven respondents explicitly voiced a concern about the ethical implications of the health care system and the Medicare program in particular. Equity issues within the context of rationing health care and the prolongation of life through technology without consideration for the quality of the extended life are examples mentioned by these respondents.

Strengths and weaknesses of Medicare. Responses to key question no. 3 varied, depending in part on the respondent's perception of the meaning of the term "Medicare." Some respondents (within the context of their testimony) treated Medicare as equivalent to the PRO system. Others viewed Medicare as a system for financing and reimbursing specific health care expenditures of beneficiaries. Still others saw Medicare as a public commitment or responsibility to provide high-quality health care to the elderly in accordance with all health care needs, where health is defined broadly. Responses that relate to assessing the adequacy of quality assessment and assurance of the Medicare program are summarized in a later section.

The following comments (paraphrased) summarize the strengths of the Medicare program mentioned by the respondents.

Medicare's emphasis on cost containment and access stimulates an open dialogue between the patient and provider in decision making. A better informed consumer is taking a more active role in making decisions.

Medicare's emphasis on quality has served as a catalyst and an incentive to other payers as well as to hospitals to accept the need for quality assessment and assurance. There is also an increased awareness among health professionals of the need for developing performance standards. Private sector funding of quality assessment and assurance research has increased. Quality of care has improved overall because of the sentinel effect of the PRO system.

Medicare is a statement of a national commitment to provide quality health care for all elderly; it is non-stigmatizing for the consumer and the provider.

Data collection efforts have stimulated advanced computer technology. The data bases create a potential for further advancement in assessment tools such as small area analysis and risk adjustments that are acceptable to physicians.

Respondents identified the following (paraphrased) as weaknesses of the Medicare program:

The program provides inadequate reimbursement, creates disincentives to physicians to care for Medicare beneficiaries, and places limitations on providing marginal or experimental procedures and services.

Medicare does not promote quality nor is it the best buy.

Medicare's cost containment emphasis has shifted the power from the physician to employers and businesses who are ill equipped to ask the right kinds of questions about quality.

Costs of Quality Assessment and Assurance Activities

Very few respondents provided information on the costs of their quality assessment and assurance activities. When information was provided, variations in the cost units used by the respondents limited generalization. The following give a sense of the way various groups describe their costs.
Professional associations:

"100 percent of annual budget"
"not less than 50 percent of annual budget"
"significant resources"

Provider groups:

"six staff members at an annual cost of approximately $155,000"
"$2-$5 per case per reviewer or $20-$30 an hour"
"approximately 2 percent of annual budget"
"the amount indicated in the budget is a small portion of the total amount spent"

PROs:

"$103 per review, the equivalent of 38 percent of total annual budget"
"$38-$39 per case reviewed"
"sixty percent of budget"

Assessment of Adequacy of Quality Assessment and Assurance

The responses to key question no. 4 on the adequacy of the current quality assessment and assurance programs reflected a broad mix of experiences and roles. A few direct health care providers, such as health maintenance organizations (HMOs), described the effectiveness of their internal quality assessment and assurance system and provided comments on the external quality assessment and assurance systems to which they are subject. The nine PROs and two SuperPRO contractors (National Medical Audit; SysteMetrics) that submitted testimony and 16 other respondents (e.g., the Joint Commission, American Psychiatric Association, Aetna, American Association of Homes for the Aging, and Paralyzed Veterans of America) have either major or limited roles in conducting external quality assessment and assurance activities. Other respondents are actively developing tools for assessment and assurance processes; examples included the American College of Physicians through their Clinical Privileges Project and the National Association of Boards of Examiners for Nursing Home Administrators through their national examination for nursing home administrators.

Comments of PROs. Five of the nine PROs submitting testimony identified some problems they have encountered in quality assessment and assurance. Their comments are paraphrased as follows:

> The use of generic screens results in too many false-positives and misses a lot of problems. Generic screens applied across the board are not cost-effective. A better method to focus reviews should be found.

> The lack of clearly defined standards for judging quality of care creates problems, in particular, inconsistency among the physician advisor reviewers. Even though it is difficult to have uniform standards for judging quality, the lack of a clear understanding and agreement about national standards creates a disadvantage for the SuperPRO program.

> It is difficult to institute corrective action plans, improve clinical performance, and resolve existing quality problems because of the limited information available about linking the process of therapy to outcomes.

> No mechanism is available to monitor the performance of providers of services covered under Part B Medicare who "go underground" and cannot be monitored through Part A claims.

It is difficult at times to determine if care provided outside the hospital setting contributed to the quality problems identified during the reviews of inpatient admissions or readmissions. There is a need for comprehensive and coordinated review of care across the continuum of settings.

The complexities and ineffectiveness of the sanction process in combination with due process promote adopting the bottom, minimal level of care as acceptable. This level is clearly not a "standard of excellence" or high quality care. The weakening of the sanction process and the lack of adequate funds for review hinder the effectiveness of the PRO process.

The Medicare system (PRO review and reimbursement) requires a massive amount of paper work.

Poor documentation in medical records by practitioners is a frequent problem. Confidentiality concerns are excessive among practitioners; the result is incomplete data, in particular in psychiatric and social areas.

The SuperPRO lacks knowledgeable and experienced reviewers and is not sensitive to local constraints of personnel and technological resources.

Comments of SuperPRO.

The current system (PRO) is not adequately identifying the worst problems and dealing with them. Some PROs have never found (nor submitted to the DHHS Office of Inspector General) "gross and negligent situations." Their function is to find problems and to correct them but this is not happening to the degree it could. Some PROs are incapable of or unwilling to identify problems or to push findings to a sanction level. Consequently, there is wide variation in performance among the PROs.

Problems exist because of the lack of uniformity in the use and validation of the generic screening process.

Although it is not a problem today, in the future physicians will make wrong decisions based upon the "dollar." This will become a serious problem someday.

Most quality problems do not result in bad outcomes.

There is a lack of consensus in defining quality and defining the magnitude of a given quality problem.

Unnecessary care or care provided in the wrong setting is a frequent problem because of poor judgment, lack of competence, or lack of conscientiousness.

Comments of other groups conducting external quality reviews.

The "only way to win" is to use quality improvement as a positive internal driving force rather than relying on the feared weapon of outside evaluators.

Practitioners and hospitals resist providing clinical information, giving confidentiality as the reason.

Retrospective review cannot ensure quality.

The criteria used are overly subjective and need complete revision. The need for statistically valid outcome indicators and the high cost of survey activities are major concerns. Problems in assuring quality care are due in part to the lack of effective follow-up on initial site visits.

Comments of third-party payers and purchasers.

Current quality assurance programs focus on appropriateness and medical necessity. A standard measurement system may be needed. Good quality assurance is too resource intensive to be practical for payers and plan administrators. The least sensitive but most practical method for payers and plan administrators is claims review, which is however of little value for assessing outpatient care.

It is not possible to disassociate quality considerations and ethics. Quality depends on societal values.

Due process under Medicare is no process. Providers are "entitled" to participate in Medicare. They have to kill someone to get kicked out of the program.

Physicians are being "forced" to miscode their documents or billings to make up for discrepancies in benefit packages.

Comments of direct care providers.

It is difficult to find physicians willing to participate in quality assessment activities. A good data base and acceptable measurement tools are lacking. The patient-specific nature of treatment plan goals makes it difficult to generalize about standards of care.

Resources are being drained to respond to external reviews. In some cases, individual practitioners are not convinced of the value of quality assurance.

Resources for quality assurance are limited. External reviews are mired in structure and process elements. The effectiveness of expensive interventions and low-utility services needs to receive greater emphasis.

Problems occur during assessment with illegible medical records. External reviews by the state are too rigid. Private review organizations using claims-based information are more effective.

External reviewers (e.g., the Joint Commission, HCFA, coalitions, and private payers) give inconsistent messages about quality assessment. Adequate legal protection is not available for physicians participating in quality assessment and assurance activities. Payers do not provide incentives for high quality. The software support for quality assessment is inadequate. Physician and hospital staff need training on how to improve quality.

Problems include the lack of (1) recognized standards to evaluate care, (2) staff time, (3) reliable audit tools to measure particular areas of care, and (4) information systems to retrieve and process quality assurance data. External reviewers do not adequately monitor providers, in particular in the training requirements for home health aides and the quality of services provided by the aides, the accessibility to and quality of home medical equipment, and the administering of procedures such as IV therapy and parenteral nutrition.

Uniform medical information systems for in- and out-patient electronic medical records are lacking. Some health personnel view documentation as an added and unnecessary burden.

External reviews are too stringent, inflexible, and punitive. Quality assessment has created an environment of increased vulnerability in an ever-more-litigious society.

Most Effective and Least Effective Activities

Key question no. 9 in the guidelines asked respondents for their views on the most effective and least effective types of activities in improving quality of health care. Forty-eight respondents listed a total of about 75 activities. The two broad activities identified most frequently as the most effective are first, education, training, and certification and second, peer interaction and adoption of an attitude of self-improvement. The most frequently mentioned activities seen as least effective are those that are punitive and those based on trivial and inflexible practice prescriptions.

The broadly defined activities or approaches reported as the most effective (and the respective number of respondents mentioning it) are listed below.

- education, training, and certification approaches (16)
- peer interaction, existence of overall improvement incentives, adoption of an attitude of self-monitoring, and desire for improvement (15)
- system-directed activities that build communication and improve program structure (8)
- activities that focused primarily on process and outcome (8)
- quality assurance systems based on reliable data and consensus-developed standards (7)
- competitive markets and a range of choices for educated consumers (3)
- corrective actions (2)
- activities like those of the Joint Commission (2)
- qualified personnel and staff in quality assurance (2)
- activities that assure access to care at all levels (2)

The least effective activities or approaches (and the respective number of respondents) are as follows:

• approaches that are punitive, inflexible, nonsubstantiated, or based on trivia (15)
   • retrospective reviews, checkoff lists (9)
   • activities that are based upon regulations (6)
   • approaches that focus on structure (5)
   • assessments that are conducted by poorly qualified individuals (3)
• risk management and cost containment efforts that are presented as quality assessment programs (2)

Adequacy of Current Level of Quality Assessment

Five respondents believed that the current level of quality assessment is adequate. Nine respondents stated that quality assessment and assurance activities are too extensive, but most qualified their responses to indicate one or more areas where the level of activities are inadequate. Ambulatory care was the area most frequently identified as having too little monitoring. Thirty-five respondents, or about 25 percent of all those submitting testimony, judged the level of current activities to be too low.

Adequacy of Current Quality Assessment and Assurance Tools or Methods

Ninety-five respondents identified particular elements of the quality assessment and assurance system they found inadequate. The weaknesses of the system and the number of respondents who identify each as being inadequate are as follows:

   • tools for outcome measurement (49)
   • undemonstrated relationship between process and outcome (49)
   • choice of outcome measures (47)
   • tools for process assessment (validation, consistency in applying) (36)
   • documentation of care (24)
   • funding for review and for monitoring (22)
   • severity or case-mix adjustments (18)
   • commitment of management and providers to quality assurance (18)
   • tools for surveys and accreditation (12)

Seventeen respondents claimed that the data-gathering burden on providers is excessive. They noted duplication of effort and asserted that the return does not equal the time and cost expended. Four respondents expressed concern about the excessive monitoring needed to develop documentation for justifying corrective actions. Ten respondents believed the liability exposure of reviewers is too high.

Respondents provided less specific reactions about the adequacy of quality assurance mechanisms. Of the 38 respondents providing some information on this subject, 15 believed the PRO system was ineffective. Fourteen respondents commented positively on the effectiveness of corrective action plans, informal feedback, restricting privileges, and credentialing; about the same number claimed these assurance mechanisms were ineffective.

A few examples (paraphrased) illustrate the responses about the adequacy of the quality assurance and assessment activities.

Too little monitoring . . . based only on obsolete biomedical model.

Resources being spent are adequate but the emphasis is wrong.

A major need exists for analyzed, comparative data and information about the outcomes and implications of PRO review activities.

Present system is merely "paper reviews" that focus primarily on utilization review.

Quality monitoring as it is currently practiced is woefully inadequate to protect the Medicare patients now and into the immediate future.

Coordinating Quality Assessment and Assurance Activities

The need for more efficient and effective coordination of quality assurance efforts was a concern addressed by about half of the respondents. Many respondents suggested dividing roles and responsibilities among the governmental bodies, the provider facilities, peers of the provider, and patients and consumers. These suggestions were broad in nature and did not focus on the mechanisms of coordination per se.

Fifteen respondents suggested that voluntary accreditation systems have a primary role in quality assessment and assurance programs. No respondent suggested that voluntary systems of accreditation be eliminated.

The greatest area of disagreement among the 70 respondents who commented on coordinating quality assessment and assurance efforts was in defining the role of governmental agencies. About two in three contended that the appropriate role of government should be somewhat passive (e.g., funding research, assuring adequate information is made available to the public, and maintaining data bases). The remainder indicated that the federal and state governments should have a more aggressive role in quality assessment and assurance efforts, but many qualified their statements with concerns about duplication.

About 33 percent of the respondents emphasized that the primary responsibility for quality assessment and assurance lies with the provider and the institution or facility in which care is delivered. Locally based peer review and accrediting boards were mentioned as responsive quality assurance entities. Some respondents indicated that professional groups should develop standards and criteria.

Some examples (paraphrased) of the type of suggestions made are as follows:

Quality assurance activities should be left to the licensing, certification and tort systems that have traditionally performed them.

The federal government should take the lead in developing standards and should work with state governments. Professionals and institutions should have the primary responsibility for quality assurance. Unions, payers, consumers, and employers should have oversight responsibilities and some sanction-type authorities. The individual is responsible for electing healthier life styles. Consumer and purchaser groups have become involved in assessing quality in health care because too often providers and government have not done an adequate job of assuring that all segments of our society have access to and receive high quality care.

Fragmentation of effort among multiple public agencies squanders resources and imposes a critical burden on providers. The principles for greater coordination are (1) appropriate local autonomy; (2) minimization of duplication of research and implementation efforts; and (3) coordination of data acquisition and utilization.

Recommendations

Not all recommendations provided in answer to key question no. 11 were directly relevant to quality assessment and assurance activities. Some respondents suggested more general improvements in the Medicare program or the quality of health care. The typical number of recommendations per respondent was four to five, and just under one-fifth of the respondents gave no recommendation.

The recommendations presented by our respondents are summarized below. They are grouped into five categories relating to health care, broad quality-of-care topics, quality assessment methods, specific quality assurance activities, and research and development. The figures in parentheses are the numbers of respondents giving similar suggestions.

Recommendations for improving the quality of health care generally.
1. Expand financing (19).
   a. Change the Medicare program by expanding coverage and level of benefits.
   b. Eliminate financial barriers such as co-pays and deductibles.
   c. Require physicians to accept Medicare payments as full reimbursement (or, equivalently, to accept assignment) .
   d. Implement fair wages and wage pass-throughs for nurses.

   e. Increase Medicare reimbursement levels.

   f. Establish equal pay scales.

2. Increase the competitive environment (4).

3. Promote greater attention to geriatrics (10).

   a. Implement a nationwide geriatric evaluation unit, provide incentives or require practitioners to have geriatric or gerontology training, and require case management in managed care.

4. Develop strategies to prevent unnecessary transfers to and from skilled nursing facilities at the end of life (1).

5. Provide incentives to practice in rural areas (1).

Recommendations concerning broad quality-of-care topics.

1. Broaden the scope of quality assessment and assurance activities.

   a. Expand the efforts to other settings and services (22).

   b. Include nonmedical disciplines that affect the health of the elderly (12).

   c. Increase the attention given to system and program factors (7).

   d. Promote or require continuing education for all health care providers (4).

   e. Address underutilization (3).

   f. Examine the bioethical issues involved in decisions about the allocation of resources (2).

2. Improve the accountability to the elderly population.

   a. Include consumer (elderly and nonelderly; users and nonusers) interests in quality assurance systems (27).

   b. Make the system more accountable to the elderly consumer, involve the elderly in decision making, and provide more information to the public to allow for informed decision making (17).

3. Promote increased support for quality assurance among practitioners (12).

4. Increase coordination of quality assurance efforts.

   a. Improve coordination among assessors, eliminate duplication, and promote sharing of information (12).

   b. Require PROs to work more closely with hospital medical staff and professional associations and shift corrective action responsibility away from PROs to local groups such as medical staff (8).

   c. Establish a national organization to work with professional societies in developing their own quality assurance activities or systems (3).

   d. Standardize quality assurance activities among PROs (2).

   e. Promote more interactive relationships of the research community with PROs and with providers (1).

5. Maintain flexibility and plurality of approaches (7).

6. Increase the financing for monitoring and review activities (6).

7. Conduct reviews in an open atmosphere with due process, provide legal protection to whistle blowers, and increase legal protection to those involved in the peer review process (4) .

8. Improve the record keeping and documentation of care (4).

9. Implement widescale consumer education programs on consumer responsibility for self-care, on consumer's rights in the health care system, and on the Medicare program (3).

Recommendations concerning quality assessment methods.

1. Establish concrete, precise, acceptable, and standardized definitions of terms (10).

2. Define and refine norms, criteria, and standards.

a. Develop explicit and uniform national standards and criteria (9).

b. Establish routine procedures for updating norms, criteria, and standards (2).

3. Focus on significant deviations from norms or criteria and standards (6).

4. Use peers who (8)

a. Are trained in specialties.

b. Are treating minority and poor elderly.

c. Are practicing in rural areas.

5. Require better trained and experienced surveyors, auditors, reviewers, and physician advisors (7).

6. Conduct retrospective reviews of patterns of care (14).

7. Conduct timely reviews, that is, closer to the time the service is delivered (2).

Recommendations concerning specific quality assurance activities.

1. Provide financial incentives to reward providers for achieving standards of excellence (12).

2. Improve the approaches to staffing and training.

a. Establish minimal staffing levels in care settings such as nursing homes and hospitals, require more certification for home care technicians, and require career ladders in the nursing field (10).

3. Maintain and improve the quality of home health care.

a. Prohibit contracting with individuals directly (rather than agencies) for home health care if public monies are involved and regulate nursing registries (2).

b. Develop a model state licensure law and a single set of conditions of participation for home health care (4).

c. Support deemed status for home health agencies (and nursing homes) (2).

4. Retain strong regulatory activities (4).

   a. Maintain a strong sanction process for PROs.

   b. Be more aggressive in enforcing current survey standards and conditions of participation.

5. Increase the use of remedial medical education (2).

Recommendations for research and development.

1. Research in quality assessment.

   a. Develop national and specialized data bases, improve the analyses of existing data, and determine future data base needs (27).

   b. Conduct consensus development activities on standards of care (case-mix and severity of illness were mentioned frequently) (22).

   c. Develop elderly-specific quality assessment concepts and instruments (e.g., norms, intervention protocols, outcome measures, needs assessment instruments) (18).

   d. Assess the relationship between quality and
      —different delivery settings (14)
      —access to care (both covered and non-covered services) (13)
      —cost containment efforts (8)
      —Medicare payment levels (7)
      —patient-provider relationship (2).

   e. Examine and clarify process-outcome relationships (11).

   f. Improve measurement tools to make them more reliable, valid, and practical (11).

   g. Conduct research on disease-specific quality of care concepts and tools (9).

   h. Develop methods for measuring and assessing performance competency (6).

   i. Increase resources for developing outcome measures (5).

   j. Develop standards of excellence (4).

   k. Define rural-specific quality assessment measures (2).

2. Research in quality assurance.

   a. Evaluate current quality assurance programs including both the PRO program and other efforts (12).

   b. Investigate effective approaches for changing behavior, such as continuing and remedial medical education (7).

   c. Examine the cost-benefit ratios of different quality assurance methods (4).

3. Develop methods to assist the elderly to participate in the health care delivery system (10).

4. Increase research on technology development and assessment (8), including cost-benefit of health care interventions (2).

5. Examine methods to synthesize, transmit, and motivate timely utilization of new information (7).

6. Increase involvement of specialties in quality-of-care research (4) .
7. Increase research in the decision-making process (3).
8. Fund PRO-sponsored research (3).
9. Increase research on the aging process, causes of disability, and early detection and prevention of occupational diseases (3).
10. Study the impact of the current legal system on cost, quality, and appropriateness of care (3).

CONCLUDING REMARKS

The information provided by the participants in the public hearings vastly enriched this study, particularly given the diversity of the groups and the wide range of roles and responsibilities in quality assessment and assurance they reflected. Respondents—who in many cases were constrained in staff resources and time limitations—generously provided thoughtful recommendations for improving the health care system, the Medicare program, and the Medicare quality assurance system.

Testimony varied by source (from, for example, a statewide advocacy group operating with only volunteers to a national health care professional membership organization) and by length and complexity (from the single-page document to the testimony that arrived at the study office in two boxes). The contributions of the participants at the two formal public hearings who gave willingly of their time at their own expense and of the groups that generously provided publications filled with methods and ideas on quality assessment and assurance were especially valuable.

Conflicting views and contradictory recommendations were heard throughout the public hearings. One theme prevailed, however: No one method or group can assure the quality of health care and a cooperative effort toward improving quality is desired by all.

APPENDIX A

GUIDELINES FOR WRITTEN TESTIMONY
A STUDY TO DESIGN A STRATEGY FOR QUALITY REVIEW AND ASSURANCE IN MEDICARE

PART A. BACKGROUND

The IOM Study Committee is interested in a broad set of issues relating to the quality of health care delivered in all major settings in which the elderly receive care, for instance, hospitals, free-standing clinics, physicians' offices, and health maintenance organizations. We are also interested in the quality of home health care and medical or hospital care received by residents of nursing homes. In line with our Congressional mandate to "design a strategy," we are particularly interested in your judgment of the crucial elements of a successful quality review and assurance system.

Among the topics the Study Committee will address during the project are the following:

- different perspectives and definitions of quality of care;
- the current levels of quality of health care;
- potential or emerging problems with quality of care;
- current or future methods to use in assessing quality of care;
- organizations that now engage in various quality assurance activities;
- possible strategies for assuring the quality of health care;
- leadership and coordination of quality assurance programs; and
- needs for further research.

We are seeking the views of a wide range of patient groups, consumer agencies, provider groups and associations, institutional administrators, federal and state governments, and other interested parties on these and other issues related to the quality of health care for the elderly Medicare population. Materials provided by representatives of these groups in written or oral form will be compiled and considered by the Study Committee in its deliberations and preparation of the study's final report.

PART B. KEY QUESTIONS

Please address any or all items listed below that apply to you and your organization. Your written statement may be as long as you choose. Supplementary materials (such as brochures or other publications) are also welcome.

1. What does your organization understand "quality of health care" to mean?

2. What are your views about the level of quality of care now provided to the elderly?

(a) Does your evaluation differ by the type of care, setting of care, or other factors?

(b) Does it differ for different groups within the elderly population?

3. If you believe that quality is a key issue for Medicare today, what do you believe are the major existing or emerging problems? the major strengths?

4. To what extent do you believe that quality of health care is being adequately monitored or assessed today? That is, do you believe quality assessment of the care Medicare beneficiaries receive is too extensive, adequate, or too little to protect the quality of patient care now and in the future?

5. What agencies, institutions, associations, or individuals do you believe should be responsible for assessing and assuring the quality of health care as you have defined it above?

6. In what ways is your organization involved in assessing or assuring the quality of health care? For instance, do you (a) promulgate regulations, (b) license, certify, or accredit individual practitioners or institutions, (c) conduct quality assurance programs within your own institution or for other organizations, (d) conduct training or technical assistance programs, (e) compile information for your members or for public use, (f) participate in research projects or medical technology assessment, or (g) conduct other such activities?

Please describe your activities as fully as possible or include separate explanatory materials.

(a) What kinds of problems do you encounter in conducting quality assessments or in resolving quality-of-care problems?

(b) What would improve the effectiveness of your efforts—for instance, better measurement tools? expanded financing? greater support from management, providers, or patients? greater integration of quality assurance into the organization's other activities? or other factors?

(c) What do you estimate is the cost of your assessment and assurance activities—for instance, dollars spent per case reviewed, or percentage of your total annual budget spent on quality-related activities?

7. How should quality assurance programs be coordinated among the following groups:

(a) among local, state, and federal agencies?

(b) among private accrediting and review organizations? and

(c) between the public and private sectors?

8. If you are subject to quality assessment and assurance activities:

(a) what kinds of problems do you experience with those efforts?

(b) what do you believe would improve the effectiveness of those efforts?

9. What kinds of activities are the most effective and what are the least effective in improving quality of health care?

10. What do you believe are the primary gaps in our knowledge of how to implement cost-effective quality assessment and assurance strategies?

11. What would your recommendations be for the highest priority areas for research and development in this area?

12. If the above items have not included issues of special interest to you, please tell us what additional topics related to quality of health care for the elderly you believe the Study Committee should pursue.

PART C. FORMAT

Your submission should include information about your organization or agency. Materials already developed, such as a flyer or brochure, would be adequate. All submissions should have a one-page Executive Summary for direct use by the Study Committee. A cover letter should include the name, position or title, and telephone number of a contact person, should IOM staff need to follow up.

Written testimony should be submitted in duplicate. IOM would appreciate receiving testimony no later than July 29, 1988. If you are among those who have been requested to submit written documents to the IOM office by a specific date, you should follow the specific instructions you received.

Address for mailing testimony: Telephone contact
Quality Assurance in Medicare Study   for assistance:
Institute of Medicine   Jo Harris-Wehling
National Academy of Sciences   Molla S. Donaldson
2101 Constitution Avenue, NW   202/334-2165
Washington, DC 20418

APPENDIX B
ORGANIZATIONS SUBMITTING TESTIMONY

Name of Organization	Presented Testimony at Public Hearing[a]
ARA Living Centers	
Academy for Health Services Marketing	
Administration on Aging, Department of Health and Human Services	
Aetna Life Insurance Corporation	DC
American Academy of Facial Plastic and Reconstructive Surgery	
American Academy of Family Physicians	
American Academy of Home Care Physicians	
American Academy of Orthopaedic Surgeons	
American Academy of Otolaryngology-Head and Neck Surgery	
American Academy of Physical Medicine and Rehabilitation	

Name of Organization	Presented Testimony at Public Hearing[a]
American Association of Critical Care Nurses	
American Association of Homes for Aging	
American Association of Retired Persons (AARP)	SF
American Board of Medical Specialties	
American Board of Nutrition	
American Board of Otolaryngology	
American Board of Pathology	
American College of Emergency Physicians	
American College of Physicians	DC
American College of Radiology	
American College of Surgeons	DC
American Congress of Rehabilitation Medicine	
American Diabetes Association	
American Dietetic Association	
American Federation of State, County and Municipal Employees	DC
American Foundation for the Blind	
American Gastroenterological Association	
American Geriatrics Society	DC
American Health Care Association	
American Health Care Institute	
American Hospital Association	DC
American Medical Association	DC
American Medical Peer Review Association	DC
American Nurses Association Council on Computer Application in Nursing	
American Nurses Association, Inc.	DC
American Occupational Therapy Association	
American Pharmaceutical Association	
American Physical Therapy Association	
American Podiatric Medical Associates, Inc.	
American Psychiatric Association	
American Psychological Association	
American Red Cross	
American Society for Gastrointestinal Endoscopy	
American Society for Parenteral & Enteral Nutrition	

Name of Organization	Presented Testimony at Public Hearing[a]
American Society of Anesthesiologists	
American Society of Plastic and Reconstructive Surgeons	
American Society on Aging	SF
American Urological Association	
Arkansas Foundation for Medical Care	
Asociacion Nacional Pro Personas Mayores	
Association for Advancement of Higher Education	
Bay Area Health Resources Center	SF
Blue Choice (Rochester, N.Y.)	
Blue Cross and Blue Shield Association	
Blue Cross and Blue Shield of Arizona	SF
Blue Cross and Blue Shield of Kansas	
Blue Shield of California	DC
Bureau of Health Professions, Health Resources Services Administration, Public Health Service	DC
California Medical Association	SF
California Medical Review, Inc.	SF
Center for Study of Drug Development, Tufts University	
Colorado Foundation for Medical Care	
Commission on Legal Problems of the Elderly, American Bar Association	DC
Community Health Care Plan (New Haven, Conn.)	DC
Community Home Health, Inc. (Boise, Idaho)	
Department of Defense, Office of Assistant Secretary	
Empire State Medical, Scientific and Educational Foundation (New York PRO)	
Federation of American Health Systems	
Georgetown University School of Nursing	
Gray Panthers of San Francisco	SF
Group Health Association of America, Inc.	DC
Health Care Purchasers Association	SF
Health Data Institute, Baxter	
Hewlett Packard	SF
Home Health Review - Erie County (New York)	
Hospital Association of New York State (HANYS)	

Name of Organization	Presented Testimony at Public Hearing[a]
Illinois Council of Home Health Services	
Independent Health Association (Buffalo, N.Y.)	
Institute for Health and Aging, University of California - San Francisco	SF
InterStudy	DC
International Association for Enterostomal Therapy, Inc.	
International Union, United Auto Workers	
Joint Commission on Accreditation of Healthcare Organizations	DC
Kaiser Foundation Health Plan, Inc.	DC
Kansans for Improvement of Nursing Homes	
Keystone Peer Review Organization (KePRO)	DC
Kentucky Association of Health Care Facilities	
Kentucky Medical Association	
Levindale Hebrew Geriatric Center and American Medical Directors Association	DC
Massachusetts Peer Review Organization (MassPRO)	
Mathematica Policy Research	
Mt. Zion Medical Center, Institute on Aging	SF
National Association of Healthcare Providers, Inc.	
National Association of Board of Examiners For Nursing Home Administrators	
National Alliance of Senior Citizens	
National Association for Home Care	DC
National Association of Private Psychiatric Hospitals	
National Association of Quality Assurance Professionals	
National Association of Retired Federal Employees	
National Association of Social Workers	
National Center for Nursing Research, National Institutes of Health	
National Council on the Aging, Inc. (NCOA)	DC
National Hospice Organization	
National Institute on Adult Day Care, NCOA	
National Institute on Aging, National Institutes of Health	DC
National League for Nursing	
National Medical Association	DC

Name of Organization	Presented Testimony at Public Hearing[a]
National Medical Audit	SF
National Multiple Sclerosis Society	
National Rural Health Association	SF
National Senior Citizens Law Center	
Nursing Home Advisory and Research Council	
Office of Technology Assessment, Congress of the United States	
Older Women's League (OWL)	DC
Omaha Visiting Nurse Association	
OnLok Senior Health Services	SF
Over 60 Health Clinic	SF
PEERVIEW (PRO for Indiana)	
Professional Review Organization for Washington	
Professional Review Organization for Washington, Alaska Division	
Pacific Telesis	
Paralyzed Veterans of America	
Pharmaceutical Manufacturers Association	
Prospective Payment Assessment Commission	
Providence Hospital (Anchorage, Alaska)	
Public Citizens Health Research Group	
Sanford Feldman, M.D. (Consultant)	
Service Employees International Union	DC
Sisters of Mercy Health System	
Society of General Internal Medicine	
SysteMetrics	DC
Thompson, Mohr and Associates, Inc.	
University of Washington School of Nursing	
Visiting Nurses Association of Washington, D.C.	DC
Veterans Administration	
W.K. Kellogg Foundation	
Washington State Aging and Adult Services	
Wellspring Gerontological Services (Evergreen Park, Ill.)	
Windermere Senior Health Center (Chicago, Ill.)	

[a]DC, presented testimony at Washington, D.C. Public Hearing; SF, presented testimony at San Francisco Public Hearing.

3

Results of the Medicare Beneficiary and Physician Focus Groups

Allison J. Walker

In order to design a strategy for quality review and assurance in the Medicare program, the Institute of Medicine (IOM) study committee judged it necessary to learn more about definitions, expectations, and concerns regarding quality of care. To this end, two separate studies were conducted using a focus group methodology. Although initially only one series of focus groups was planned—among Medicare beneficiaries—the activity yielded a wealth of information and generated further interest in this approach. Because of the need to reach more physicians in private practice than the original study design and committee structure permitted, it was decided that a second series of focus groups would be held among practicing physicians. This chapter describes the methods and results of the two sets of focus groups.

BENEFITS AND LIMITATIONS OF FOCUS GROUPS[1]

Focus groups are open-ended, but structured, discussions led by a trained moderator. They provide a practical and useful way to identify issues relevant to, and concerns about, a given topic. In contrast to other survey research methods that require the investigators to ask respondents a uniform set of questions, focus groups can be used to collect information in participants' own words about how they view, define, understand, or evaluate the topic under discussion. The focus group methodology was initially developed by sociologists Robert K. Merton and Patricia L. Kendall over 40 years ago (Merton and Kendall, 1946). This technique has been advanced and improved over numerous applications since the original work.

We designed the first set of focus groups to elicit attitudes and concerns of Medicare beneficiaries in five main areas: (1) personal experience and satisfaction with health care; (2) views on the concept of quality of medical care; (3) knowledge of quality assurance activities; (4) desire for information; and (5) ideas about how to improve the quality of health care. Similarly, the focus groups among practicing physicians were designed to elicit attitudes and concerns in six main areas: (1) positive and negative aspects of caring for elderly patients; (2) views on the concept of quality; (3) the Medicare program and its effect on quality of care; (4) identification of quality problems; (5) effectiveness of quality assurance mechanisms; and (6) ways to improve quality of care.

Although focus groups do not involve "rigorous" survey methods that permit results to be generalized to an entire population, they add a very human element that is often absent in more quantitative research. Discussions guided by open-ended questions permit a more in-depth investigation of salient issues than do rigid survey instruments. Issues and insights can surface that otherwise might be missed. Focus group research is widely used and, some have argued, is the most "psychologically valid" form of opinion research in the United States.

Nonetheless, the limitations to the generalizability of information derived from the focus groups should be understood. First, the sample size of participants is usually smaller than that which is required for statistical generalization. Second, regardless of how they are recruited, focus group participants are not representative of the population; willingness to participate in focus groups is not randomly distributed throughout the population. Third, unmeasurable bias can be introduced by differences in question sequence and phrasing in each focus group. An important component of statistical reliability in survey research is the requirement that each respondent will be exposed to the questions in the same order and manner. This cannot be easily achieved in focus groups.

In the present case, the ideas that focus group participants expressed about quality in health care provide an understanding of common attitudes and opinions among Medicare beneficiaries and physicians treating Medicare patients. The findings supplement information available to the committee from the literature and through public hearings and site visits.

STUDY METHODS

Subcontractor Selection

The subcontractor for this activity, Mathew Greenwald and Associates, Inc., was selected on the basis of several criteria: (1) previous experience with focus groups involving elderly people; (2) experience with focus groups on health care issues; (3) experience using focus groups for policy studies; and (4) proposed budget.

Mathew Greenwald and Associates arranged for the use of focus group facilities and audiotaping and transcription for each group. In conjunction with IOM staff, the company drafted the screening criteria by which participants were recruited and also prepared the moderator's guide listing the questions to stimulate the group discussions. Mathew Greenwald and Associates supervised the recruitment of participants, and Dr. Greenwald, president of the company, moderated all focus groups.

Focus Group Site Selection

Four main criteria guided the selection of sites for each set of focus groups:

1. The sites had to contain a high concentration of Medicare beneficiaries within a specific geographic region, for ease in recruiting both beneficiaries and physicians whose Medicare patient population was to be at least 20 percent.
2. Locating facilities and recruiting participants had to be relatively straightforward, essentially restricting the activity to urban areas.
3. At least two sites for each set of focus groups had to have a high concentration of health maintenance organizations (HMOs).
4. For the groups among beneficiaries, the four major census regions had to be represented. For the physician groups, at least two had to be comprised primarily of rural physicians.

For the beneficiary focus groups, study staff selected New York City; Miami, Florida; Minneapolis, Minnesota; and San Francisco, California as the study sites that best met these four criteria. For the focus groups among practicing physicians, study staff selected Philadelphia, Pennsylvania; New Orleans, Louisiana; Chicago, Illinois; Los Angeles, California; and Albuquerque, New Mexico. All the focus groups except two were conducted at facilities with which Mathew Greenwald and Associates had had previous experience. One group in New Orleans was conducted at a hotel in conjunction with the annual conference of the American Academy of Family Physicians (AAFP), and the group in Albuquerque was conducted at the offices of the New Mexico State Medical Society, in conjunction with its annual meeting.[2]

Development of the Moderator's Guide

For both sets of focus groups, the subcontractor and the study staff jointly developed the moderator's guides. Different guides were developed for separate focus groups of fee-for-service beneficiaries, nursing home residents, and HMO enrollees. (Refer to Appendix A for one example of the moderator's guide.) Each guide addressed the same five topics but was modified as appropriate for the group in question. For the focus groups among practicing physicians, one moderator's guide was developed to provide direction on the six topics to be discussed (Appendix B).

The Recruiting Process

Recruiting focus group participants can be done in several ways. Two of the more common approaches are to use files previously developed by the research facilities and to use randomized telephone dialing. Each approach has drawbacks and advantages, including a tradeoff between cost and unbiased selection.

To minimize disadvantages and maximize advantages, we decided to combine the two approaches to ensure some degree of randomness and to decrease the bias that might be associated with using only one of the previously mentioned methods. Thus, in most of the groups, half of the participants were recruited through the use of facility lists, and half were recruited from telephone listings selected randomly from telephone directories. Each research center was responsible for recruiting its own sets of participants according to these methods.

All participants in the New York City beneficiary focus groups were recruited exclusively through the use of facility lists because of the high cost of recruiting through random digit dialing in that city. For the group of nursing home residents, participants were selected on the basis of ability to travel and attend the focus group session at a facility outside of the nursing home. Recruiting for the AAFP physician group was conducted using the conference pre-registration list and random dialing, and the group in New Mexico was selected by the Executive Director of the state medical society.

Focus Group Composition

Although it is not realistic to seek representativeness or to estimate population parameters using focus groups, we went to some lengths to achieve diversity. By design, therefore, we obtained elderly participants who brought with them perspectives that may be affected by age, race, sex, recent health care experience, and HMO membership, and in the case of physicians, practice in the fee-for-service or prepaid group practice sector, rural or urban location, and specialty.

Pre-recruitment Specifications of the Beneficiary Focus Groups

Eight beneficiary focus groups were conducted: two each in New York City, Miami, Minneapolis, and San Francisco (in that order). The composition of the groups was varied by design: two groups comprised participants ages 65 to 74; two groups had participants ages 75 and above; and one group was diverse by age with all participants being at least 65 years old. Most participants in these five groups obtained their health care largely through the fee-for-service system. Two other groups (one in Miami and one in Minneapolis) consisted of only HMO enrollees, both groups being diverse by age. One group (in Minneapolis) had only nursing home residents.

The recruitment criteria required that each focus group should have as even a male-female ratio as possible and some ethnic diversity. The groups in New York City, San Francisco, and Miami were to have at least three nonwhite or Hispanic participants; the groups in Minneapolis were to have at least one nonwhite or Hispanic member. Finally, each group was to have at least four people with recent "acute" or "nonroutine" health care experience; for instance, care in an emergency room, outpatient surgery, a hospitalization, admission to a nursing home, or home health care.

Pre-recruitment Specification of the Physician Focus Groups

Eight physician focus groups were conducted: two in Philadelphia, two in New Orleans, one in Chicago, two in Los Angeles, and one in Albuquerque (in that order). Again, the composition of the groups was varied by design. The variables included specialty, HMO concentration, and urban-rural mix, and the recruitment criteria required that each focus group should have as even a male-female ratio as possible and some ethnic diversity.

Final Composition of the Groups

For the beneficiary focus groups, individuals were invited to participate in each group through recruitment procedures based on a screening instrument fielded by the focus group facility. (Appendix C gives an example of the recruiting "screener.") To ensure that an adequate number of persons would be available, 14 individuals were invited with an aim of having groups of 10 participants. Ultimately, five groups had 10 participants, one group in New York City had 11 participants, one group had 9 participants, and the nursing home group had 6 participants, for a total of 76 participants.

At those facilities where more than 10 recruits appeared on the day of the focus group, selection to reduce the number of participants was made on the basis of previously mentioned criteria to achieve the desired diversity in participants. People who were not asked to stay were thanked and reimbursed for their time and travel expenses by the research facility staff. Those who did stay for the session were also paid a nominal fee by the research facility for their time and travel expenses.

Table 3.1 displays the main characteristics of the beneficiary groups. Overall, we had 39 women (51 percent of the total) and 37 men. The youngest participants were 66 years of age (eight individuals); the oldest were 90 (in the nursing home group) and 87 (in a community-resident group). The participants were overwhelmingly white (79 percent); four groups (both of those in San Francisco, one in Minneapolis, and one in New York City) met the target for ethnic diversity. The groups were less likely to have had recent acute or nonroutine health care experience than we had initially planned; 12 persons in the fee-for-service groups reported such an encounter in the previous 3 months. All the HMO participants (in Miami and Minneapolis) reported that they had had an encounter with their HMO since being covered by Medicare, although most of the encounters were considered to be nonacute. Finally, a considerable number of participants (55 individuals or 71 percent) reported having some form of Medigap insurance to supplement their Medicare coverage.

For the physician focus groups, 12 individuals were invited to participate in each group through recruiting procedures similar to those used for the beneficiary groups. (Appendix D gives an example of the recruiting "screener".) In these groups, the aim was to have 8 to 10 participants. Ultimately, two groups had 10 participants, two groups had 9 participants, three groups had 7 participants, and one group had 6 participants, for a total of 65 participants. Table 3.2 describes the main characteristics of the groups.

Focus Group Process

Before each session, participants were asked to complete a form to verify basic demographic information including age, sex, and primary occupation or medical specialty. In addition, the participants were served lunch, dinner, or light refreshments, depending upon the time of the session.

The moderator then explained the purpose of the focus groups and indicated that the sessions were being tape-recorded and observed through a one-way mirror. Finally, the moderator explained the "three rules" of focus group sessions: (1) that people speak freely and honestly; (2) that discussion be among participants and not directed only to the moderator; and (3) that only one person speak at a time to ensure that everyone is heard.

To open the discussion, the moderator began by posing a question: "What are the most positive aspects of medical care, and what are the most negative aspects of medical care?" Participants then discussed the question in subgroups of two or three people before reporting their views to the rest of the group. This approach helped to make people comfortable with speaking among themselves as well as with the moderator. The moderator then proceeded through the remaining sections of the guide. Each focus group session lasted approximately 2 hours.

FINDINGS OF THE BENEFICIARY FOCUS GROUPS

This section summarizes the main points that emerged across the eight beneficiary focus groups. These main themes are illustrated in the verbatim quotations from the participants. Notations following each quote signify the location, type of group, and sex of the participant.[3]

Personal Experience and Satisfaction with Health Care

Recent Experience

Before being asked any questions about "quality of care," participants were asked about their experiences and satisfaction with medical care. As would be expected, some of these Medicare beneficiaries had had considerable experience with the health care system. Twenty-one participants reported during the screening stage that they had some acute or nonroutine care in the previous 3 months. At the focus group sessions, 16 participants said that they had used emergency rooms, 4 had received home health care, and 3 had had outpatient surgery. Most of the participants believed they were in good health.

Satisfaction with Care

Almost all the focus group participants expressed satisfaction with their own primary physician and the medical care they received. High among the positive aspects of the health care system was the Medicare program itself. Many beneficiaries asserted that adequate health care would be a financial burden without the assistance of Medicare. (As recorded in Table 3.1, however, many also rely on other insurance to supplement their Medicare coverage.)

The general perception among participants was that medical care is very good in the United States—much better than in most other countries. Other positive aspects of medical care frequently mentioned were scientific advances, the high state of medical technology, increased efficacy of drugs, and a higher skill-level among providers of care.

> "As far as I'm concerned, the general medical care you get has been pretty good. I mean, I've come across a lot of competent doctors." (NYC, 65+, M.)

> "The best is the high state of development that has been attained and what it can do for the individual. It's a great process of medical development." (NYC, 65–74, M.)

Participants occasionally experienced "system" problems such as financial and access barriers. A majority of the negative points focused on these

TABLE 3.1 Selected Characteristics of Focus Group Participants

Group	Sex	Age	Race[a]	Recent Health Care Experience[b]	Has Medigap Insurance[c]
Group 1	F	74	H	Y	Y
	F	72	W	N	Y
New York City	F	71	H	Y	Y
Community residents	F	70	W	N	Y
Fee-for-service Medicare	F	68	W	N	Y
Ages 65 to 74	F	67	W	Y	N
	M	72	W	N	Y
	M	69	W	N	Y
	M	69	W	N	Y
	M	69	B	Y	N
	M	66	W	N	Y
Group 2	F	86	W	N	N
	F	79	B	Y	N
New York City	F	78	W	N	Y
Community residents	F	78	W	N	Y
Fee-for-service Medicare	M	87	W	N	N
Ages 75+	M	79	W	Y	N
	M	78	B	Y	N
	M	77	W	Y	N
	M	77	W	N	Y
	M	75	W	N	Y
Group 3	F	73	W	N	N
	F	71	W	N	N
Miami, Florida	F	70	W	N	N
Community residents	F	67	B	N	N
HMO enrollees[d]	F	67	B	N	N
Ages 65+	M	82	W	N	N
	M	76	W	N	Y
	M	76	W	N	N
	M	72	W	Y	Y
	M	68	W	N	N
Group 4	F	78	W	N	Y
	F	70	W	N	Y
Miami, Florida	F	69	W	N	Y
Fee-for-service Medicare	F	66	W	Y	Y
Ages 65+	M	82	W	Y	Y
	M	78	W	Y	Y
	M	72	H	N	Y
	M	70	W	N	Y
	M	68	B	Y	Y

Group	Sex	Age	Race[a]	Recent Health Care Experience[b]	Has Medigap Insurance[c]
Group 5	F	80	W	N	N
	F	79	W	N	Y
Minneapolis, Minnesota	F	69	W	N	Y
Community residents	F	67	W	Y	Y
HMO enrollees[d]	F	66	W	N	Y
Ages 65+	M	82	W	Y	Y
	M	80	W	Y	Y
	M	75	W	Y	Y
	M	69	B	N	Y
	M	68	W	N	Y
Group 6	F	90	W	N	N
	F	81	W	Y	Y
Minneapolis, Minnesota	F	77	W	Y	Y
Nursing home residents	F	74	W	N	N
Fee-for-service Medicare	M	83	W	Y	Y
Ages 65+					
Group 7	F	74	B	N	Y
	F	74	W	Y	Y
San Francisco, California	F	69	H	N	Y
Community residents	F	66	B	N	Y
Fee-for-service Medicare	F	66	W	N	Y
Ages 75+	M	70	W	Y	Y
	M	68	W	N	Y
	M	66	W	N	Y
	M	66	H	N	Y
	M	66	W	N	Y
Group 8	F	83	B	Y	Y
	F	79	W	N	Y
San Francisco, California	F	78	W	N	Y
Community residents	F	76	H	N	Y
Fee-for-service Medicare	F	75	W	N	Y
Ages 65 to 74	M	86	H	N	N
	M	77	W	N	N
	M	77	H	N	Y
	M	76	W	N	Y
	M	76	W	N	Y

[a]B is black; H is Hispanic; W is white.

[b]Y is yes and signifies that the participant reported a "nonroutine" encounter with the health care system (e.g., a hospitalization, a visit to the emergency room, or services from a home health agency) in the previous 3 months; N is no.

[c]Y is yes and signifies that the participant reported having some form of a supplemental health insurance in addition to Medicare; N is no.

[d]Although very few HMO enrollees reported an encounter with the health care system in the form of a hospitalization, a visit to the emergency room, or services from a home health agency, all reported that they had received care from their HMO since being covered by Medicare.

TABLE 3.2 Characteristics of Physician Focus Groups

Sex	Age	HMO Affiliation[a]	Specialty
		Philadelphia 1	
M	<45	N	Orthopedic Surgery
M	<45	Y	Thoracic Surgery
M	<45	Y	Neurosurgery
M	<45	N	Ophthalmology
M	<45	N	Colon & Rectal Surgery
M	<45	Y	Ophthalmology
M	<45	Y	Urology
F	≥45	N	Obstetrics/Gynecology
F	≥45	Y	Obstetrics/Gynecology
		Philadelphia 2	
M	<45	N	Internal Medicine
M	<45	N	Internal Medicine
M	<45	N	Internal Medicine
M	<45	N	Gastroenterology
M	<45	N	Dermatology
M	≥45	Y	Pulmonary Disease
M	≥45	Y	Cardiology
F	≥45	Y	Neurology
F	≥45	Y	Allergy
F	≥45	N	Oncology
		AAFP	
M	≥45	N	Family Practice
M	≥45	N	Family Practice
M	≥45	N	Family Practice
M	≥45	N	Family Practice
M	<45	N	Family Practice
M	<45	N	Family Practice
M	<45	N	Family Practice
		New Orleans	
M	≥45	Y	Urology
M	≥45	Y	Dermatology
M	<45	N	Ophthalmology
M	<45	Y	Internal Medicine
M	<45	Y	Dermatology
F	≥45	N	Obstetrics/Gynecology
F	≥45	N	Obstetrics/Gynecology

Sex	Age	HMO Affiliation[a]	Specialty
		Chicago	
M	≥45	Y	Internal Medicine
M	≥45	N	Ear, Nose, & Throat
M	≥45	N	Obstetrics/Gynecology
M	<45	Y	General Surgery
M	<45	Y	Ophthalmology
M	<45	Y	Thoracic Surgery
M	<45	Y	Internal Medicine
		Los Angeles 1	
M	≥45	N	Family Practice
M	≥45	N	General Surgery
M	≥45	N	General Surgery
M	<45	N	Family Practice
M	<45	N	Ophthalmology
M	<45	N	General and Vascular Surgery
M	<45	N	Ear, Nose, & Throat
F	<45	N	Obstetrics/Gynecology
F	≥45	Y	Ophthalmology
		Los Angeles 2	
M	≥45	Y	Ear, Nose, & Throat
M	≥45	N	General and Vascular Surgery
M	<45	N	Urology
M	<45	N	Urology
M	<45	Y	Internal Medicine
M	<45	Y	Internal Medicine
M	<45	Y	Internal Medicine
F	≥45	N	Family Practice
F	<45	Y	Obstetrics/Gynecology
F	<45	Y	Obstetrics/Gynecology
		New Mexico	
M	≥45	N	Neurology
M	<45	N	Internal Medicine
M	<45	N	General Surgery
M	<45	N	Internal Medicine
F	≥45	N	Anesthesiology
F	<45	N	Oncology

[a]HMO is health maintenance organization, N is no, and Y is yes.

..s, which do not necessarily relate to quality issues. Although the .oderator tried to de-emphasize cost and access issues, these issues surfaced quite frequently as problems faced by beneficiaries. Complaints included excessively high physician and hospital charges as well as balance billing by physicians who do not accept Medicare assignment.

"It's gone way beyond the inflation factor. In other words, general cost of living may be up eight times. But hospital care has gone up about 12 or 15 times." (NYC, 65–74, M.)

"You're talking about cost. But I want to tell you don't forget that doctors are human beings. And basically they are business people today. The monkey only dances when you give him music. And the only thing they understand is money. It's a business like any other business. My doctor charges me $300. The next time I come to see him, I bring him a gift. He's going to treat me right. He's going to give me all the best that he knows." (NYC, 75+, F.)

As previously mentioned, the majority of focus group participants seemed satisfied with their own physicians and rated them above average compared to others. However, some had to change providers at least once to find one with whom they were satisfied. Frequently mentioned as one area of dissatisfaction with physicians was the feeling that fees varied with location, that is, the same services could cost more or less depending upon the part of town in which the physician practices or the patient lives.

Several participants also stated that it was imperative to check every bill because patients were often charged several times for services they received only once or were charged for services never received.

"My dad passed away August 25th. And we got a bill from the doctor, and the bill shows services rendered for August 26th and 27th. I called up the doctor. He couldn't come to the phone. I called again and I said to the girl, I'm refusing to pay. She got very indignant. I said, it's very simple. Since the doctor says he gave services two days after my father died, how do you account for this? And if I get another bill I'm bringing it up to the AMA. Never heard another word from them." (FL, 65+, F.)

"One man in our building got a gynecology bill, something that a woman would have had taken care of. He called, and it was about $1,000." (FL, 65+, F.)

Additionally, some participants expressed concern about Medicare fraud as a reason for excessive charges and cautioned against signing blank reimbursement forms.

"I think Medicare gets ripped off sometimes, because when I got a copy of my bill, it was 11 or 12 pages . . . some things you remember and some things you don't. And I saw a number of items on there that I *know* I did not get service on." (MN-HMO, 65+, F.)

> "I just got a bill from the hospital and it gives me $32,000 worth of charges. And I see that on one day, four times we get charged for the same thing. And Medicare is paying for it. In the ultimate long run, I'm really paying for it; we are. Don't you think you ought to do something about it? Guess what the answer was? We don't care. It's just part of the charge." (FL, 65+, F.)

Although students of health care find it useful to distinguish "cost" problems from "quality" problems, these focus group discussions suggest that these issues are often linked in people's minds. Patients sense that some physicians are so motivated by money—indeed, are willing to commit fraud—that they may not really be interested in their patients' well-being. The loss of confidence that accompanies the suspicion that the provider's primary motivation is financial was an unmistakable undercurrent in some discussions.

Many other comments pertained more directly to quality of care. These included difficulty in scheduling appointments, perceived differences in the treatment for elderly patients compared with that for younger patients, and staffing deficiencies (specifically nurses) resulting in increased waiting times and less personalized attention.

> "The attitude from what I hear and what I see is when you're old, to hell with you. You're too old, so you're going to die anyway." (NYC, 75+, F.)

> "I wonder why they are cutting back on the nursing profession. And the girls are good and they want to spend time with the patients. But there aren't enough to go around." (SF, 75+, F.)

The principal area of dissatisfaction that related to quality of care was the feeling that differences exist between physician practice in the office setting and in the hospital. With respect to hospital care, physicians were described as being less friendly, offering less personalized attention, and often hurrying patients more than those in office practice.

> "It's going to be different. The doctor just runs through your room in the hospital. At the office, they've got you in a room, and you talk." (NYC, 65–74, M.)

> "At the office I get a chance to find out everything I want. In the hospital I didn't find out anything." (NYC, 65–74, M.)

Premature discharge was another concern expressed by participants, although none actually seemed to have experienced this. Financial incentives of the Medicare reimbursement system were cited as the main reason for premature discharge, with insufficient home health care and nursing home beds viewed as serious related problems.

> "I think it's a crime with the hospitals we have and the equipment the way they shove people out when they're still sick. What have we got hospitals for?" (MN-HMO, 65+, F.)

"They push the older people out sooner than they really should go. From what I've read, it's a bonus factor in there to get you out sooner." (NYC, 65–74, M.)

"DRGs. Medicare pays the hospital X number of dollars for a period of days. As a result, many people have been pushed out before they are well. And it has been documented. I know of a particular case where the man died because he was pushed out of the hospital before he was able to be discharged. And that's wrong too . . . and we don't say anything. We don't open our mouths and it goes on and on and on." (NYC, 75+, M.)

View of the Concept of Quality

A general theme that surfaced quite frequently during the focus groups is the perception that those who receive medical care define and judge the quality of that care in ways that are different from those who provide care. Whereas professionals evaluate quality in terms of complex clinical indicators and outcomes, patients use "art-of-care" or interpersonal indicators when describing what they mean by quality of care. They may acknowledge (at least indirectly) a lack of information or capacity for making other types of judgments.

"There are very few of us around who can understand what quality is as far as the medical field [is concerned]." (FL, 65+, M.)

Competency of the physician, along with the outcome of treatment (see below), was mentioned a few times as a factor by which to judge quality, but most responses centered on the physician's personality and interpersonal skills. These included the amount of time doctors spend with a patient, how much interest they show in who the patient is and in his or her well-being, how much information they provide, and whether they are compassionate and understanding.

"I think you can sum it all up in just a couple words, compassion and understanding. This denotes the quality of the doctor." (FL, 65+, M.)

"Well, even before the man gives you medicine he can make you feel good. But if he comes in, [and] his attitude is not good, then the cooperation is lacking. Then you become sure enough just a patient." (NYC, 65–74, M.)

"I feel if a doctor I'm seeing introduces himself to you, sits down and talks to you and doesn't hurry you and even asks you things that do not pertain to what you went in for, and when you do start to tell them what's wrong with you, they start asking questions. When they seem to take an interest in your health, I think that's good care. But if they come in, and out he goes, I think, hey, I don't want that doctor anymore." (SF, 75+, F.)

"The quality care is exactly how good a doctor is as a diagnostician. If he can diagnose your trouble, your problem is 99 percent of the cure. Bedside manner doesn't mean a thing to me or how much time he spends with you. If he can pinpoint your illness, you've got it licked because the cure comes shortly afterwards through medication. That's quality care to me." (FL-HMO, 65+, M.)

Outcomes of care were noted by several participants as an indicator of quality. Most participants used positive or negative outcomes to make broad judgments about quality. They tended not to relate outcomes to the severity of illness or other factors outside the physician's control that may negatively affect the results of treatment.

"This lady and I might be going to the same doctor. He takes the same care of both of us. But she is cured of all her ailments. I'm not. She thinks the doctor is great. I think he's lousy." (NYC, 65-74, M.)

Medicare fraud and honesty were mentioned again in the context of defining and judging the quality of a physician. Patients felt they could not trust a physician who is "ripping off" the Medicare system through professional preoccupation with financial incentives rather than with the patient.

Quality of hospitals and nursing homes was judged on overall cleanliness, friendliness and helpfulness of the staff, and tastiness of the food. Also important was going to a hospital that is "*not* like a factory." The quality of an HMO was judged by how easy or difficult it is to schedule an appointment and the amount of waiting time in a physician's office. Again, very few clinical indicators of quality were mentioned.

"The difference between a good and bad HMO [is] when the doctor doesn't have a million patients and you [don't] have to wait for 5 hours to get to see him for 5 minutes." (FL-HMO, 65+, F.)

Quality of Care and Medicare

When asked to rate "the quality of care received while on Medicare," some participants saw no connection between who pays the bill and the quality of care. (This view was contradicted, however, by others in the context of who *should* be responsible for monitoring the quality of care, as discussed below.)

"Medicare is all I have, so it doesn't make a difference. Whether he's a good doctor or a bad doctor, he's going to send a Medicare form in." (NYC, 65-74, M.)

"Medicare has nothing to do with it. Medicare is nothing but an insurance company set up by the government who pays medical expenses. They pay the bills. That's all they do." (FL-HMO, 65+, M.)

Other participants voiced concern about how Medicare's payment system affects quality of care, perhaps leading to underprovision of services or premature discharge. Yet other participants noted that decreases in services do not necessarily reduce quality of care.

"Well, there's a lot of good and bad points since they've increased the number of seniors. . . . Lower the rates, get the people in, make the money, and then cut down your care. Because the physicians are too overworked. They'll give you 15 minutes, and if you're not through, that's too bad. And that's very unfortunate. I think a lot of people are missing a lot of things they normally wouldn't." (MN-HMO, 65+, F.)

"Medicare restricts the hospitals from doing things for you and the doctors. I feel that I'm not getting the same care I did before I was 65." (MN-HMO, 65+, F.)

"Well, I think getting the necessary tests that you need, not a lot that you don't need. I think maybe physicians are a little more conscious of that now because of DRGs and the way medical costs have risen above the cost of living. So I think that just getting the necessary things is part of quality." (MN-NH, 65+, F.)

Quality of Care Now and in the Past

Most focus group participants contended that the health care available today is better than that available 10 years ago. Reasons cited include improved technology, better trained providers, and increased longevity.

"There have been new discoveries in the field of medicine. Longevity has been prolonged. And many of the hospitals that can afford it have gotten new equipment. On the whole I would say that medical care today is much better than it has been." (NYC, 75+, M.)

"The doctors today, they're better educated. More facilities [are] available to them. And they have staff members just doing the same expertise-type of medical care. And they talk with each other, and you conduct conversations before they make a move on you. Before, a room of doctors looked at you and said, well, let's try it and see if it works." (SF, 75+, M.)

Participants in the two New York City groups felt that health care was better 10 years ago because of recent staffing shortages (specifically nurses), less personalized attention, and increased prices.

"Everything's changing. The help, the hospitals and everything has changed so much that I guess that's true of everything. It's a changing world." (NYC, 65–74, F.)

"Well, in some respects, it was better then. Of course now they have more tests and things. They've made a lot of progress. But as far as the hospital is concerned, they were cleaner, they had more nurses." (NYC, 65–74, F.)

Understanding How Health Care Is Monitored

How Respondents Handle Problems

Most participants agreed that if they had problems with a particular doctor, they would leave that doctor and find a new one. A few people mentioned reporting the problem doctor to other patients; others would call the "medical association." Most, however, would simply look for a new doctor.

> "You can drop one primary doctor and go to another if you feel as though you're not getting the right thing." (FL-HMO, 65+, F.)

> "We all have our good runs and our bad runs with the doctors. If you don't like your doctor, you're not obligated to see him again. When you call to make your next appointment you can say I want Dr. Timbuktu. I just don't want this doctor. And a lot of people do it." (SF, 75+, M.)

> "I had one doctor who never realized I was sitting in his office. He was writing and writing, and I figured I'd be in a book one day. But he wasn't paying any attention to me. So I just stopped him. One day I met his nurse in town. She asked what happened, and I said I don't think he knew I was there most of the time. I feel like I'm the only sick person in the world when I walk into that doctor, and I want him to look after me." (SF, 75+, F.)

When asked what they would do if they experienced problems with a particular hospital, most participants agreed that they would report the problem to their doctor or the head nurse first. If that did not work, then they would proceed to the next level, the administration. Some participants believed that there are times when nothing can be done about problems in the hospital; although they were a minority, their view was stated with some vehemence.

> "Over the years I can only say you're at their mercy and there's not much that can be done. There's always people worse off than you are. And you say, well, [there] but for the grace of God go I. So keep your mouth shut, don't bitch too much about anything. Just get out of there." (SF, 75+, F.)

HMO enrollees evidently would handle perceived problems in much the same manner. They might, however, be more likely to bring up an issue to an administrative person at the HMO rather than to their doctor.

> "If it's a serious matter, the consumer council in the HMO has a committee dealing with complaints about physicians, real or imaginary, which are then referred to the administrator or director of the hospital. Now if it's a serious matter, you sue the doctor. We're talking about relatively adjustable matters. You deal with the administrator, or your own physician and then the administrator." (NYC, 75+, M.)

When asked how problems in a nursing home should be handled, the non-nursing home respondents seemed to view the nursing home situation as presenting a different set of problems and that the patient has fewer options for taking action. Most thought that a family member or friend would have to raise the problem issue for the resident, rather than the resident himself or herself.

"If you're in a nursing home, then generally speaking, you're pretty sick. Secondly, you're going to be a little intimidated by trying to complain yourself. You're going to have to rely on your family or friends, whoever's taking care of you. You're not going to do it yourself." (NYC, 65–74, M.)

Nursing home residents themselves had a different idea of what to do about problems. Some said family members could raise the issue, but many residents do not have family in close proximity to the home. The nursing home residents said they would raise problems themselves, through the nursing home complaint procedure or the ombudsman program.

"They always say the squeaking wheel gets the oil. So I've learned to squeak . . . If you want anything, that's the way to go. It seems to get the results, anyway." (MN-NH, 65+, F.)

"Well, if they speak up and voice their concerns [they get results]. Otherwise, they're going to lay there and just suffer." (MN-NH, 65+, F.)

With very few exceptions, the nursing home residents responded to the moderator's questions in much the same manner as the rest of the focus group participants. The only major difference involved the way they handled problems within the nursing home versus the way they were perceived (by those outside the home) to handle problems. It should be stressed, however, that the nursing home residents who were able to participate in our focus group are probably not typical; for instance, they were sufficiently mobile to be able to come to the focus group center. We had originally intended to conduct this group in the nursing home in order to gain the participation of typical residents, but the practical barriers proved too difficult to overcome in the time available to us.

Awareness of How Medical Care Is Monitored

Many focus group participants did not think health care is monitored very closely. Others clearly assumed it is evaluated to one degree or another through accreditation of hospitals, licensure of physicians and nursing homes, or government monitoring.

"We presume they're monitored. But I don't think anybody can tell. Because how would we know?" (NYC, 65–74, M.)

"It would be the head of the staff in the hospital. They know what's cooking in the hospital. So they observe the doctors. I'm assuming they do. How close they do, I don't know. But I'm assuming they do." (SF, 75+, M.)

"Well, hospitals do get accreditation, whatever you call it. So I assume that there's some monitoring going on for them to be accredited. But I don't know exactly what it is." (FL, 65+, F.)

"There's enough complaints to the state government that somebody would interfere and say, what's going on here? There's got to be regulations from the state in some manner. Otherwise, it would just be running rampant. But I do not know." (MN-HMO, 65+, M.)

In general, participants were not sure who is currently responsible for performing these functions and believed that care is not monitored closely enough. The increase in the rate of malpractice suits was mentioned several times as resulting from a lack of monitoring.

As to what agencies or groups *should* monitor the quality of care provided through Medicare, the participants' responses were quite varied. Some mentioned that it should be done by Medicare, because "they pay the bills"; this view was most forcefully expressed by HMO enrollees. Others were skeptical of this role for Medicare, evidently believing that Medicare may not be in a good position to "be its own watchdog." Some participants presumably extended this skepticism to the professions more generally.

"I think Medicare must have control. Because they're paying hundreds of dollars a month for every patient . . . they must have some strings attached. They don't just give it up willy-nilly." (MN-HMO, 65+, M.)

"They [Medicare] should have qualified personnel to go out and check these different doctors and different offices and see the quality of care. If an office is overcrowded, or if an office is understaffed, and the only reason the doctor is there is for the purpose of making money, but not to take care of the patients. Monitor different doctors." (FL-HMO, 65+ F.)

"The more you have that Medicare monitors them, the less they'll take assignment. You have to have a different organization monitoring them." (FL, 65+, M.)

Across all the groups, participants expressed a number of ideas about other possible ways for the quality of care to be monitored. These included patients themselves, ombudsmen, boards of directors at hospitals, insurance commissioners, and medical associations.

"Nursing homes are monitored by ombudsmen that are appointed by your state legislature. So the nursing homes are monitored more closely than hospitals. And my suggestion is that there should be ombudsmen appointed to monitor hospitals." (FL, 65+, F.)

Desire for Information About Quality of Care

Much of today's health policy rests on notions of competition and the related concepts of information and choice. We touched on these issues indirectly during the focus groups. One question for the participants was whether Medicare beneficiaries want to be able to select their own physicians and other providers (as is presently guaranteed to them in the fee-for-service portion of Medicare). Related questions concerned variation across providers in quality of care and how patients learn about which practitioners or facilities provide what levels of quality.

Patient Choice

Most focus group participants agreed that being able to choose their own physician is very important to them. The ability to do so seemed especially relevant because they evidently perceive that different providers do render different levels of quality of care (see below).

HMO focus group participants acknowledged that although they still choose their own physicians, they have a smaller, predetermined set from which to choose. Several (seven persons in Miami and five in Minneapolis) had had to change their physicians on joining the HMO, but they generally did not view this as a problem.

Most respondents claimed that they generally have enough information available to choose a primary care physician. They received a majority of that information from two sources: friends (through word-of-mouth or their friends' experiences) and physicians (referrals and recommendations). Nevertheless, participants also believed there is a certain amount of luck involved in choosing a physician for the first time.

"There's always an element of chance." (NYC, 65–74, M.)

"You have to go through the experience. You never know." (NYC, 65–74, F.)

With regard to choosing specialists and hospitals, most participants said that their primary care physician refers them to specialists as well as to hospitals. For instance, they would go to the hospital where the physician was on staff and, therefore, would not actually have a great deal of input in choosing a hospital. Participants evidently did not question this pattern very often.

"I would say if you have full confidence in your own physician, you go along with him." (NYC, 65–74, F.)

With respect to selecting a nursing home, three of the participants in the nursing home focus group said they made their own choice as to which home to enter and that they had enough information available to make this choice. Of the remaining participants, two reported that their family members made the decision as to which home to enter, and one was referred to the nursing home by her physician.

Variations in Quality of Care

Participants strongly believed that providers of health care are not uniform with respect to quality of care. They were nearly unanimous in claiming that differences exist in the quality of care available to patients in different hospitals, from different physicians, and from different HMOs. Most people say they avoid those physicians, hospitals, and health plans that they feel offer substandard or inconsistent care. Their comments reveal a great deal about what they think of as quality of care.

> "There are some doctors that are fine, that you can absolutely trust, and others that for some odd reason don't want to work very hard on a patient and are rather short with you or cursory." (MN-HMO, 65+, F.)

> "There is no real consistency. There's no uniformity. Depending upon the doctor you get. . . . In other words, different doctors will give you different treatments. You could go to one hospital and get one kind of treatment. You could go to another hospital and get another kind of treatment. Some hospitals are personal; some are very impersonal." (NYC, 65–74, M.)

A few participants implied that this variation in quality is not necessarily related to the range of services or equipment offered. The general sense was that quality would not be harmed if different hospitals provided different or limited arrays of services instead of all hospitals providing all services.

> "Some of the things about the new equipment—they should have better administration. Because I think one hospital should have all those things. Not all the different hospitals. Every hospital thinks they have to have certain things, and they don't." (MN-HMO, 65+, F.)

Sources of Health Care Information

Apart from information about health care from friends and primary care physicians, Medicare beneficiaries also reported health care associations and the media as sources of information. When asked from which sources they would like to receive additional information, several people mentioned the American Medical Association (AMA). A few mentioned federal and state government and other health care associations.

Types of Information Desired

Although most participants felt that they generally have enough information available to choose a physician or a health plan, many sensed that they do not have enough information to judge adequately the clinical quality of care they receive. As previously mentioned, participants evaluate their health care according to interpersonal or art-of-care indicators, partly because they lack either clinically based information or the ability to use it. Some participants contended that they rely heavily on their physician to supply as well as interpret this type of information.

> "Well, the question is when you make these decisions or you just listen to someone . . . does it really help to have more information? Or do you just have to do what the doctor or specialist says?" (SF, 75+, M.)

> "It's probably my fault. Because I really just don't know what to ask when he suggests these things. I know he has made examinations . . . and things have really helped me. But I don't know. He doesn't sit down really and explain things to me. And I don't know what to ask." (MN-NH, 65+, F.)

Participants were asked about the availability and usefulness of certain types of information relating to health care and, at least by implication, to the quality of that care. Four types of information that are commonly suggested (in health policy circles) as useful in this regard were specifically raised by the moderator: (1) hospital mortality rates; (2) the frequency with which a physician performs a particular operation; (3) the number of malpractice claims against a particular physician; and (4) nursing home inspection reports.

The majority of respondents agreed that these four types of information would be very useful in making decisions about health care, but they did not feel that this information was readily available. Interestingly, several noted that mortality rates need to be looked at in relation to the severity of the cases and the type of hospital (e.g., teaching hospital versus community hospital).

> "We don't know the circumstances. The people who come to one type of hospital that handles emergencies, the rate of deaths will be higher than another hospital that handles less severe situations." (FL-HMO, 65+, M.)

> "That [mortality rate] in itself doesn't mean anything. Because some hospitals take very seriously ill patients. Others won't admit them. You have to know the average age of the person and how sick they were." (NYC, 65+, M.)

> "He [the doctor] can't guarantee a life. He's going to open you up and use a knife on you. He's going to do the best he can. But he has no way of knowing how you look inside." (SF, 75+, F.)

Some participants remarked that the number of malpractice suits must be looked at in relation to the number of successful claims.

> "The information should state how many times the doctor won and how many

times he lost. Just to say he's been sued . . . anybody can bring suit. Anybody with a frivolous cause can bring suit." (NYC, 75+, M.)

Some respondents suggested that nursing home inspections need to be more comprehensive and that perhaps nursing homes should be rated on a scale in the same manner that restaurants are rated. Participants were especially interested in these reports as they realize the possibility of one day having to enter a nursing home.

Finally, some individuals expressed an interest in having more information about specific diseases, such as the cause of disease, treatment alternatives, and outcomes. This interest was volunteered; the moderator had not probed directly on this point.

Knowledge of Medicare Part B

Toward the end of each focus group session, the moderator asked how many participants were covered by Part B of the Medicare program. He then probed their understanding of how the program works (e.g., what Part B covers, how much the premium costs, and who is eligible).

Those participants who were covered by Part B were very well informed. They knew the amount of the monthly premium almost to the penny, that it covered physician services as opposed to inpatient hospitalization, and that it was a voluntary program paid for by a monthly premium.

"My impression is that Part A is for hospitalization, and that's mandatory. You get that automatically. And Part B is for the doctor. And that's what you pay the $24.00 for." (SF, 75+, M.)

The participants who were not covered by Part B, however, seemed not to understand the different aspects of the Medicare program. Although this may not be too surprising, given that they were not covered by Part B, it does suggest that some Medicare beneficiaries lack the information they need to make certain health care decisions.

"Part A is all medicine, and the B would be the hospitalization." (SF, 65+, M.)

"One pays the doctor and the other pays the hospital. I think B pays the hospital and A pays the doctor." (MN-NH, 65+, F.)

Suggestions for Improving the Quality of Medical Care

The last section of each focus group centered on ideas for improving the quality of medical care in the future. In fact, responses from participants went far beyond quality of care per se. We have grouped the specific points that arose during these free-ranging discussions into three main categories: (1) quality issues, (2) cost issues, and (3) generic issues relating to health care.

Recommended actions with regard to quality included increased staffing levels for nurses and allied health professionals, which may help to ensure more personalized attention and more time with the physician (two important criteria that participants use to judge the quality of their health care). More "regulatory" suggestions included raising the level of monitoring of care, increasing the number of investigations, and enforcing stronger punishment for Medicare fraud. These steps were seen as a way to decrease the number of malpractice claims and to reduce questionable billing practices, both of which also have implications for reductions in cost.

The most frequently mentioned ways to address rising Medicare costs involved the adoption of a catastrophic coverage plan (which should include prescription drugs) as well as a long-term-care insurance package. Participants expressed a great deal of concern about rising nursing home costs and the possibility of developing a catastrophic illness. Lowering the cost of hospital care was another suggestion to improve medical care in the future.

Two other suggestions related to patient costs for outpatient care. One was to encourage physicians to accept Medicare assignment. The other was for Medicare to increase its payments to physicians in order to eliminate balance billing for amounts not reimbursed through Medicare.

Finally, two general suggestions relating to Medicare were advanced. The first was to ensure that Medicare will be available for future generations. The second suggestion was to continue speaking with more Medicare beneficiaries. Focus group participants felt that it is extremely important to obtain the views of the population being served by the Medicare program because they know how well the program works (or does not work) through first-hand experience. Interestingly, the suggestion was made several times to conduct more focus groups among Medicare beneficiaries throughout the country (similar to these conducted for the IOM study).

"I think Medicare should be widened, broadened. These people are saying we have enough money for Medicare now, next few years. But maybe for our children's children, will they have Medicare for them? Will they be taken care of?" (SF, 75+, M.)

"I would say that Medicare should question the patient, and ask the patient, was he satisfied with the treatment? Are there any suggestions he would like to make?" (NYC, 75+, M.)

"I think what you're doing right now. In that little tape recorder and the gal back there writing down the notes. It lets somebody smarter than us take care of it." (MN-HMO, 65, M.)

FINDINGS OF THE PHYSICIAN FOCUS GROUPS

Positive and Negative Aspects of Medical Care

This section summarizes the themes from the eight focus groups conducted among practicing physicians, with points illustrated by verbatim quotes. Notations following these quotes signify the location and sex of the respondent.[4]

As a warm-up question, the moderator asked the physician participants to describe either the most positive and negative aspects of medical care in general or the most and least rewarding aspects of caring for elderly patients in particular.

The most frequently mentioned positive aspect of medical care was that health care was readily available to virtually everyone. In addition, it was felt that physicians still have the freedom to practice medicine the way they want (although this is changing) and have access to state-of-the-art equipment and technology to complement their practices. Finally, our respondents frequently mentioned the feeling of being able to do something good for other people as an important positive aspect of practicing medicine.

"I think the positive aspect that I see is that we have quality health care available for everybody in this country in comparison to other countries throughout the world." (PA2, F.)

"One of the up sides of medicine here is that you're allowed to choose what you want to do, go in what specialty, open where you want to, go independent, go with a group, do whatever you want in that regard. So there's some choice." (PA1, M.)

"I guess the best aspect of it is the feeling. And it's a feeling that when I go home 98 percent of the time you've done a good job for the public." (PA2, M.)

The most frequently mentioned negative aspect of medical care was the extent to which the quality and availability of care (mainly the amount and type of care, not initial access to care) depended on the financial status of the patient. The continual threat of a malpractice suit was also mentioned.

One of the more rewarding aspects of caring for elderly patients was the fact that the elderly appreciate the physician's care more than younger patients do. The elderly often question their ability to survive, and the physician's reassurance is very welcome. Also, caring for the elderly population presents many more challenges. Multiple medical conditions and limited financial resources make the physician's job more difficult and a positive outcome more rewarding. Finally, elderly patients have a wealth of experience that they share with the physician.

"I think one of the most rewarding things is that patients of that age have serious doubts as to whether they're going to be able to survive. And when you're able to reassure them or allay some of their fears, I find them very much more appreciative than younger people who perhaps expect to have good health and they're angry if they don't." (CH, M.)

"I think the reward to me is to have the privilege to treat a population of patients who constantly are presenting real challenges to your abilities as a physician. They tax all your ingenuity and ability to treat them with the highest quality of medicine you can provide them." (CH, M.)

The least rewarding aspects of caring for the elderly population include constraints related to the Medicare payment system. Reimbursement policy and medical liability create opposing forces; to be covered against the threat of malpractice, the physician performs extra tests and services (defensive medicine) that may not be reimbursed. In addition, the amount of regulation, paperwork, and monitoring associated with Medicare reimbursement was often cited as a negative aspect of caring for the elderly.

"And the whole thing too is when you brought him in the hospital you have to find a certain diagnosis. Then you have overutilization and underutilization. And your final diagnosis, whether that agreed with your initial diagnosis and whether you did the correct test. All these things go through your head. You're worrying so much about the guidelines that you almost forget about the patient. You're worried about following all the rules in the book." (CH, M.)

"I had dinner with a friend who is still in private practice. And he had a Medicare patient for whom he gave a B-12 injection. That patient was sent a letter from the government saying that this B-12 shot was not indicated, should not have been given, that this was bad medicine. Interestingly enough, this patient has a diagnosis of pernicious anemia. This sort of thing is absolutely unreal and yet it is happening all the time and it is getting worse and worse." (AAFP, M.)

"The stack of regulations are creeping. I mean, one of these days we're going to have certification exams for janitors and maids." (NM, M.)

Our respondents also commented on other negative aspects of caring for this population that are not the result of the reimbursement system. For example, they noted that elderly patients demonstrate less compliance to treatment plans than do younger patients, perhaps because older patients may not understand or remember their treatment plan. In addition, elderly patients require a greater amount of support outside the acute care facility, which may not be available or covered under Medicare. Finally, the physician has no control over a large set of social issues that affect the elderly population.

One final point should be made about caring for the elderly. On the one hand, Medicare has made health care available to people who previously might not have been able to afford care. On the other hand, many people have been accustomed to receiving essentially as much medical care as they want because of generous third-party insurance. When the person becomes eligible for Medicare, he or she may not realize that Medicare coverage and payment policies may be more restrictive. This causes great anxiety among those seeking health care.

"I think Medicare has made medical care available to many people who would not have had it otherwise. But the reverse is true, too. People have been used to having good care with good insurance. So when they get old everything seems to be shrinking on them. And the medical cost is not shrinking. It's a very sudden change in life for them. As long as they're working they have good insurance. Once they retire, it's different. I think they're in a big dilemma." (NO, F.)

Views on the Concept of Quality

One finding from the beneficiary focus groups was that those who receive medical care think they define and judge the quality of that care in ways that are different from those who provide care. For example, the elderly evidently believed that professionals define quality in terms of complex clinical indicators and outcomes whereas patients use interpersonal indicators to describe what they mean by quality of care.

The focus groups among practicing physicians did not substantiate this distinction. Most of the definitions of quality that we heard from physician participants did not center on clinical indicators of care, although competency of the physician and the outcome of treatment were mentioned several times. (For example, one physician stated that quality involves making the correct diagnosis and formulating an effective treatment plan—it is more than being nice to the patient.) Many of the physicians' definitions of quality were similar to those offered by the beneficiaries. These included providing the care you would like your family to receive, giving the patient what they need and not giving them what they do not need, using reasonable judgment in rendering decisions, and recognizing one's (i.e., the physician's) limitations.

"I think quality care is the care you would like for your very best friends and your family to receive. I think it means if you need certain medications you provide them. I think it also means if you don't need a lab and X-ray test you don't do it and you don't do anything to make the situation worse." (AAFP, M.)

"Quality of care is not just medicine. It's taking care of the patient, coddling him, getting through whatever. I think it's not just what you've learned in medical school, but what sort of human being you are. I don't think just knowing how to work a computer or to work an instrument, being able to give the right amount of pills is quality of care." (PA2, M.)

These physicians definitely felt that quality does not depend solely on the physician, but also on the care provided by others and on the patient's physical condition and diagnoses.

"I don't think we should delude ourselves, either, to think that quality of care is directly related to the physician. I can name a hundred instances where nurses and other ancillary health professionals made the difference between life and death." (PA1, M.)

"It's a standard of care for a community. And it's very difficult to be more specific because we all represent different specialties. And what's quality care for someone who has a cold, or what's quality of care for someone who has a brain tumor is very different. But what it means is a competent physician delivering what is currently acceptable treatment as would be found in a current textbook. And of course, that physician should have some personal qualities." (PA1, M.)

Although most of the physicians offered definitions of quality, a few felt that not enough information is available to define and identify quality accurately, other than as a minimum standard of care. This skepticism carried over to their views about quality assurance as well.

"Quality assurance has always been the business of looking at what goes on either from a structure point of view, from a process point of view, and from an outcome point of view. Then you take all that stuff and show it to the people who did this and you say, what do you want to do about this? And then you say, based on the data from so and so, we know we need this and that. So it comes down to providing some sort of feedback. Then at point X later on you look and say gee, did it work? That's what it's supposed to be. The problem is, for me at any rate, I don't think we know enough to do that sort of thing." (AAFP, M.)

"Quality of care is like pornography. I know it when I see it. It's more difficult to define, though." (AAFP, M.)

Does the Medicare Program Affect the
Quality of Care Physicians Provide?

When asked about the Medicare program and its effect on quality of care, most physicians agreed that the Medicare reimbursement system may affect the *way* care is delivered but not the *quality* of care per se. The physicians also stated that they see no difference between the quality of care provided to Medicare beneficiaries and that which is provided to others. (This same point was made in the beneficiary focus groups. They did not feel that quality of care differed by virtue of whether it was received before or after being eligible for Medicare; evidently this was because they viewed Medicare simply as a payment system for health care services and not a delivery system.) Our physician respondents recognized that having Medicare coverage may influence whether or how easily someone is initially accepted into the health care system, but they believed that once a patient was in the system, Medicare would not affect the quality of care that patients obtained.

> "A Medicare patient or any other patient gets exactly the same type of care. There is no difference. I don't pay any attention to what's going on in age or anything else." (CH, M.)

> "It [Medicare] doesn't affect how I treat a patient. It may affect whether or not we initially accept them as a patient. But once we've taken the responsibility for their care, everyone's treated the same." (PA1, F.)

When asked how the Medicare program affects the way care is delivered, the physicians spoke about the reimbursement policies and the restrictions these policies placed on caring for elderly patients with respect to treatment settings, length of stay, and covered services. They also spoke about ways to "get around" these restrictions.

> "You see, what's happening is you're putting the doctor in a vise between what he feels he wants to do for the patient and what the hospital administrator wants to tell the doctor about how he should take care of the patient. There are a lot of MBAs between us and the patient telling us what care we can administer, for how many days, what they will pay for and what they won't pay for." (NO, F.)

One example of the perceived restrictions on treatment settings cited in two different groups is that of same-day, outpatient hernia repair. Although outpatient surgery may be appropriate for a 35-year-old patient, the same setting for a hernia repair on a 70-year-old patient may not be appropriate because of age and physical condition of the patient. The 70-year-old patient typically requires hospitalization, which is not reimbursed by Medicare unless the patient has a specific complication that warrants admission. Therefore, the physician will indicate a complication on the chart so the patient can be hospitalized and the procedure reimbursed by Medicare.

> "Medicare doesn't really recognize the differences in patients. The same rules and regulations we're supposed to follow for outpatient procedures apply to a patient who is 66 years old as well as a patient who is 86 years old." (NO, M.)

> "Getting them in [the hospital] when they ought to be in—you have to be very imaginative sometimes. And keeping them in when they ought to be in—you have to be imaginative. And the hospital says, well, if you just put it in the notes that this patient still had chest pains today, nobody's going to argue

with you. So you sit and you say, but she didn't tell me that. Should I put it in?" (CH, M.)

Restrictions on length of stay [as determined by payment policies directly applied by hospitals in response to the Medicare prospective payment system (PPS)] were cited as having a possible effect on quality in the form of premature discharge. (This had also been mentioned in the beneficiary focus groups; many of the participants had heard about premature discharge, although none had actually experienced it.) The physician participants stated that they would keep a patient in the hospital as long as medically necessary, regardless of the pressure to release the patient, and they were also willing to take responsibility for this action.

> "Having to send patients home prematurely after their recovery. That makes physicians feel guilty. They'd like to keep the hospital fiscally sound and not send it down the tubes. But at the same time, the patient is the primary responsibility. And you're a patient's only and best advocate. You talk about quality of care. But that's quality—fighting for the patient and deciding that you're not going to let the hospital or members inside it intimidate you into discharging a patient prematurely." (CH, M.)

Also perceived by physicians to affect the overall quality of care were denials of payment and letters of noncoverage or "substandard care." The respondents were especially angered by the notices sent to the patient without the physician's knowledge.[5]

> "There's a new situation where the patient now receives a letter from Medicare stating that the quality of care you received was inadequate. I've had one or two friends who have received notification of some of these letters. The letters were initially sent to the patient, which leaves a wide door open for litigation." (NO, M.)

With respect to coverage, our respondents frequently mentioned that Medicare does not adequately cover preventive services, home health care, or prescription drugs. Most physicians in the focus groups believed that prevention is one of the main ingredients for quality care. To ensure that preventive care is reimbursed, the physician will list on the bill false diagnoses and treatments that the patient did not receive. One physician in the group thought that the government is not a very prudent buyer of health care because it does not invest in preventive services that may save money in the long run, nor does it invest in home health care, which may be less expensive than inpatient care.

> "One of the main problems in terms of quality of care is that Medicare doesn't cover preventive screening. The government can recommend that everyone have their cholesterol checked. But if you put down a routine exam as the reason you had the cholesterol, they won't pay for it. The standard of care

includes preventive medicine. That is good medicine. And they're not paying for good medicine." (NO, M.)

"You talk about patients remembering to take their medication. But how about affording the medication? I spend an hour or more a week talking to drug reps [representatives], which I don't care the slightest about, so I can get free medicines from them to give to the people that can't afford them." (NM, M.)

"With respect to Medicare, the ability of these people to get home care supplied to them afterwards is a real drawback. If the interest is in saving money, it's a lot cheaper for them to be taken care of at home. It cuts down on the expense." (NM, M.)

Similarly, the argument was made that reimbursement limitations may cause underutilization of certain services. This affects quality and continuity of care if patients avoid seeking necessary care.

"Older people don't come to the doctor enough because they're worried about cost. Therefore, I find that they're a lot sicker than they ought to be. And they've suffered a lot more than they should have at home, by themselves. And I think that's the system. From a personal point of view that upsets me." (AAFP, M.)

Finally, the amount of paperwork required for Medicare reimbursement, the continual monitoring and oversight of physician activities, and the time it takes to deal with regulations were seen by many to be significant burdens. Our participants speculated that some physicians may leave the medical profession and others may stop accepting Medicare patients because they are beginning to feel overwhelmed and perceive the declining benefits from practicing medicine. Specifically, physicians were becoming impatient with nonmedical personnel in the Medicare reimbursement offices; they were also tired of having to explain their treatment plans to government agents who they claimed know little about the intricacies of medicine, only about "cookbook methods" of care.

"We put people in the hospital and the first thing that often happens to me is that I start getting reviews from the Medicare provider [i.e., the Peer Review Organization (PRO) or Medicare contractor], saying how long is this person going to be in? What drugs am I going to use to treat them? As soon as somebody comes in, the monitoring and the pressure to push [the patient] out comes, and I feel that. And I don't think that at this point in my life I have changed what I would do based on the fact that someone is pushing me, it just adds time to my day because I have to take telephone calls from so-and-so, and I resist the urge to be nasty on the phone saying, what do you think I'm going to treat this case with? I'm going to treat them with whatever I see fit, thank you." (NM, F.)

"We appeal every single thing that's denied [by Medicare] and we always win. But it just takes three or four letters and a lot of time to do it." (NM, M.)

Identification of Quality Problems

After a discussion about quality and the Medicare program, the physician focus group participants were asked to identify, first, some general quality problems and, second, more specific problems with respect to overuse of services, underuse of services, and poor physician skills.

Government restrictions and gaps in benefit coverage were the most frequently cited general quality problems. In several sessions the physicians stated that the amount of regulation and monitoring imposed by government is excessive. They also believed that government policies are changing the physician-patient relationship, in part by removing decision making from the hands of practitioners and patients and in part by making doctors responsible for societal choices, not single patient-provider choices. Woven throughout this was the subtheme of concern about malpractice liability.

"The problem is the government doesn't know how to practice medicine. And it's trying to tell us how to treat people, patients. They are now in the business of practicing medicine. And they don't belong there." (LA1, F.)

"We as doctors are being asked to be much more cost effective and by various councils to be assuring people of quality of care. Frankly, I could take some of these issues and turn them back on the bureaucracy. Is the bureaucracy cost effective? Is the bureaucracy assuring quality?" (CH, M.)

"The government has done everything it can to break up the physician-patient trust—everything to make the physician and patient adversaries rather than trust. They've changed our ability to keep confidentiality because we have to report certain things. To a certain extent they've changed our ability to practice in the way we want because they're regulating certain things we can do. And the threat of malpractice always tells you that no matter how much you like this patient, this patient is a potential adversary." (PA1, M.)

With respect to more specific quality problems, almost all the physician participants stated that overuse of services was common and more pervasive than underuse of services. They offered several reasons for this view.

First, many physicians feel compelled to provide a full range of tests and services to protect themselves against the threat of malpractice, even though all these tests and services may not be clinically indicated.

"It's a legal defensive type thing in some cases. In some cases it's pure ignorance. In some cases it's financial gain—ordering a study that maybe you are interpreting or you own your own machine. And then there's this nebulous category where a patient is complaining bitterly about something. And you want to show the patient and the family how much you care by ordering a whole myriad of tests." (PA2, M.)

"There is a certain amount of overuse in defensive medicine. That may be overuse to you. But it's not overuse to me who pays tens of thousands of dollars a year in malpractice insurance and doesn't want to pay anymore. To me that's a necessary realization." (PA2, F.)

Second, some physicians may overuse certain services for financial gain, especially those with high reimbursement rates. This was cited, however, as more of an institutional than an individual problem.

"I think that services are provided where reimbursement is also provided. So the pressure to overutilize, I suppose, would be where reimbursement is high. The pressure to underutilize would be where reimbursement is low." (AAFP, M.)

Third, overuse may occur from the desire to do everything clinically possible for the individual patient, perhaps in response to patient or family wishes or complaints.

"Because I (as a neurologist) see so many elderly patients, I wonder virtually every day if what I'm doing aggressively to treat a very elderly patient, and I'm talking about a population 85 and older, is really appropriate. Specifically, when a 90-year-old patient ends up in the ICU [Intensive Care Unit] on a respirator and is in the hospital for 5 weeks before they die. And it is very unclear to a lot of us what is appropriate in that kind of situation." (PA2, F.)

Finally, limitations in physician skills and knowledge may be a factor in overuse of services; for example, when a physician is uncertain about the appropriate course to take and orders every possible test.

Almost all of the focus group physicians found it very difficult to estimate the amount of overuse of services. Some groups felt that approximately 10 percent of all services provided could be categorized as overuse, but another group estimated it to be between 20 and 30 percent. However, all groups cautioned that overuse varies by individual provider, institution, and geographic area.

"I think overutilization is very difficult to define because not everybody arrives at a diagnosis or uses the same type of treatment. All doctors are individuals, do different things. And what may be overutilization for one person is a standard way of operating for another person. And we have run into a lot of difficulties when the government or some outside person tries to define what overutilization or inappropriate utilization is." (LA1, M.)

As previously stated, underuse of services was not seen to be as pervasive a problem as overuse, although one group estimated the amount of underutilized services to be approximately 10 to 20 percent. Reasons for this include lack of coverage for services (financial barriers to access), lack of knowledge about what is covered and to what extent, and geographic barriers to access.

"I think underprovision of services is somewhat encouraged by Medicare rules and regulations. For example, in nursing homes, visits are allowed only once a month. So if a nurse calls you up and says your 76-year-old male patient has a little fever and cough, well that may be pneumonia. But you already saw him last week. So if you go and see him again, you probably won't get reimbursed. If you lie and write down that there's a diagnosis, then they'll pay you another $14.40 for that diagnosis. That didn't help me the last time I went to a nursing home. I got a parking ticket, which cost me $22.00." (AAFP, M.)

"It's a task to keep up with the latest things that are happening in medicine. But above and beyond that, to keep up with what Medicare is or is not paying for currently. And a lot of time, you're the physician, and you have to express, well, this is not really in my hands to determine. And you have to get involved with the counselors in the hospitals about what they are and are not paying for." (CH, M.)

The physician with poor skills was the final problem area specifically probed by the moderator. Most participants believed that there are and will always be physicians with poor skills. The number, however, is fairly small because the health care market is competitive enough to eventually "weed out" these physicians through word-of-mouth or legal action. Again, the participants found it difficult to estimate the number of physicians with poor skills, but they believed the range to be from less than 5 percent to approximately 10 percent. When asked whether the physician with poor skills could improve his or her competency, the participants felt that 90 to 95 percent could theoretically improve with education and monitoring but that probably only about 65 percent actually do improve.

"There are certain physicians you see that lie on the fringe. And there will always be problems. We're human beings just like everyone else." (NO, M.)

"The marketplace is competitive enough that a physician who does not meet the standards is weeded out very quickly. If not by his colleagues, by the hospital. And God forbid, if not by the hospital, by the legal system that will hit everybody." (CH, M.)

"I think the way to address the outdated or poor skills is education, because I think the average person who's got poor skills has either been undertrained or has just lost contact for a while." (PA1, M.)

"There's probably a lower percentage of bad docs than bad insurance salesmen. But nobody really cares about that." (NM, M.)

Almost all the focus group participants believed that it is very difficult to deny privileges or revoke licenses of physicians with poor skills. The legal system was cited as a big roadblock.

"Attempts have been made to deny privileges, to pull out medical society membership or to call this person on it and say, listen, you can't keep doing strange things. And the reaction that was obtained was, you try to yank my privileges and I'll sue you." (NM, F.)

Effectiveness of Quality Assurance Mechanisms

The effectiveness of specific mechanisms for maintaining or improving quality was explored by the moderator in several categories. Participants were asked to evaluate individually focused mechanisms, hospital-based mechanisms, and external quality assurance mechanisms.

The individually focused mechanisms for quality assurance included state licensure, board certification, and continuing medical education. Across the eight physician groups, we heard no real consensus about the effectiveness of these mechanisms. Some participants felt they were very instrumental in assuring quality whereas others felt that they played no part. Although most participants felt that state licensure was necessary, they said that it was a very low hurdle to jump and, therefore, not very effective.

"It's [licensing] a very basic minimum. I think that's about it." (PA1, M.)

"I think the licensing helps, but I don't think you weed out many people that way." (NM, M.)

Initial board certification was viewed as a positive step in assuring quality of care, but the idea of recertification met with mixed views. Some participants believed that recertification is necessary to assure that practicing physicians keep up with changes in their fields. Others, however, said that recertification is expensive, takes a great deal of time to prepare for, and tests the ability of the physician to take an examination, not the clinical competency of the physician.

"A lot of the questions they ask are of no clinical application. It would have to be something that would be related to what the clinician practices in medicine, what he is seeing. The academicians do have a slightly different view of what's going on than the people in the trenches." (NO, F.)

"I see these things every day, 30, 40 times a day, day in and day out . . . if it was a clinical test it wouldn't be any problem for me. Is it going to be to anyone's advantage for me to take this test every 6 years? I'm not so sure. Would it prove my level of medical care? I'm not sure. Because with practice every day, I just get better and better every time." (NO, M.)

"I think there are good test takers who are terrible clinicians." (NO, M.)

Finally, with respect to individually focused mechanisms for quality assurance, our participants broadly debated the effectiveness of continuing medical education (CME). Some physicians felt that CME is worthwhile for those who are truly interested in keeping up with advances in medicine. Others believed that CME is a waste of time and money. Opinions differed about the value and cost-effectiveness of courses versus reading the published literature in medical journals.

"Education is one answer. The government can require us to fill out all kinds of paper and crap like that. It's irrelevant. But to require us to have education in our own subspecialty once we've finished our training is reasonable." (CH, M.)

"It depends on what value you place on your time. To me it's better to go to meetings and spend a couple of days to learn the most important things than it is to spend time trying to separate wheat from chaff in all these journals. You could literally spend hours reading, whereas you can get most of the important stuff from CME. And I think it's probably the most important thing a physician can do." (NO, M.)

"It's very hard to justify these courses on a cost-effective basis. They're $450 to $600 for 2 to 3 days. You can learn just about as much by subscribing to $80 worth of journals." (NO, M.)

One type of education that was valued by most physicians was hospital-based clinical conferences, where problems are discussed among peers and proper diagnosis and treatment plans are formulated using "real-life" examples. In essence, physicians can learn from other physicians in a nonthreatening manner.

"And you talk about CME. A point comes across very strongly. When an error is made and you say to yourself, gee, I could have made that same error. And a specialist gets up and tells you what the proper approach to the problem should have been, then that's a form of CME. That is more educational than listening to some guy ramble on about the new methods of treating whatever." (PA2, M.)

"I do think that certainly having your peers review your work or criticize your work in the form of mortality and morbidity conferences is good. I think this is a strong conference in every hospital or it should be. I think that's the conference that either makes you or breaks you as a doctor." (CH, M.)

In general, hospital-based or internal peer review was thought to be more effective in quality assurance than any other mechanism, especially more effective than the external review of the Peer Review Organizations (PROs).

"Review should be done. But it doesn't have to be done through the government, through some outside agency. It can be done through individual hospitals that set up policies for quality assurance and review. It doesn't have to be some outside guy coming into a strange hospital and reviewing charts. It should be a colleague reviewing the chart who works with the physician and knows him and what kind of patient he has and what kind of care he gives." (PA2, M.)

These physicians were, however, concerned about confidentiality and legal liability in an internal peer review system. Many physicians stated that although they were willing to serve on peer review committees, they were worried about the possible ramifications of having to implement corrective action against another physician.

> "You have to assure confidentiality in any kind of peer review mechanism that the physician who works in that peer review, utilization review, and quality assurance will not be threatened himself with the actions he wants to take, say legal action or something like that." (NO, M.)

Immediately following the discussion about the internal peer review, the moderator probed the effectiveness of external review by PROs. Again, most of the physicians felt that internal review was much more effective for assuring quality than the external review of PROs. Many of the physicians equated PRO review with harassment, saying that PROs are capricious and that they should publish their review criteria so that the physicians would know what they are being judged against. Our participants also felt that PROs may be able to weed out "gross abuse" but that they mainly do fiscal, not quality, reviews. Finally, there was some criticism as to who was actually doing the PRO reviews.

> "They're very capricious. You never know what they want. They review only charts, they never look at the patients. So you don't know what is expected, what they're looking for. They should publish their screens that they're going by so you know what their criteria is." (NO, M.)

> "The PROs—they're nothing. It's a fiscal review. I don't think it's quality of care." (NO, M.)

> "I find that more and more what's happening is that the government is trying to create a system, using a cookbook and rather cheap labor by paying LPNs [licensed practical nurses] and RNs [registered nurses] to sit and review charts, to see if for every diagnosis certain things were done. The point is that it's very difficult to quantify quality of care. And that's what the government would like to do. And I don't think it's going to work. I think a much better way is to have doctors at their own hospitals reviewing the charts within their hospital, reviewing their colleagues. I think that's a much more effective way of dealing with the problems internally rather than the government doing it. Coming in and hiring cheap labor and labor that's ill-informed to go over these charts. I don't think a nurse can adequately do that, even the best." (PA2, F.)

Ways to Improve Quality of Care

The last topic discussed during the physician focus groups was ideas for improving the quality of medical care in the future. Although many of the suggestions from the beneficiary groups were related to cost, most of the ideas for improving quality from the physician groups centered on education (both physician and patient education) and on decreasing the amount of government regulation.

Some focus group participants believed that nationwide CME is one way to improve the quality of medical care. Currently, fewer than one-half the states require CME.

> "The skills of the physicians will always be represented by a bell-shaped curve. What we ought to try to do is move the whole bell upward or forward. Just try to make everybody better. And the way to do that is education."
> (CH, M.)

These respondents also advocated stronger patient education efforts. They believed such activities will improve quality as people learn what to expect from their medical care, how to judge quality, and how to use the health care system to get the most from their health care dollars.

In addition, participants suggested that caps on malpractice insurance premiums and on amounts of malpractice settlements would ultimately affect quality in a positive manner by reducing the threat of litigation and its negative consequences. Also, allocating more money for preventive care or adding a preventive care benefit to the Medicare package would benefit quality. Ultimately, less money would be spent on expensive, inpatient hospital care as problems were detected earlier and treated in less expensive, outpatient settings.

The last category of ideas to improve quality of care involved decreasing the amount of government regulation and allowing physicians to practice medicine the way they were trained instead of constantly worrying about meeting regulatory requirements. In addition, the physicians felt that internal or hospital-based review, which allows actual peers to review cases, will improve quality more than relying on external PRO review.

> "You give them full autonomy to decide when it's proper to send a patient home or bring one into the hospital without imposing all the constraints that basically challenges the physician's independence as a professional. And I think it weakens the soul to know that you've spent all these years in medical training and your professional decision is being challenged by nonmedical people or people who don't have a clear idea of what you're trying to achieve. It really taxes all of your cunning, your style, your ability to withstand a lot of the pressure that has been imposed by government." (CH, M.)

> "The quality was there long before Medicare. The best thing that could be done for improving the quality of care would be allow us to deliver. Medicare does not allow us to deliver. It creates roadblocks." (NM, M.)

Finally, many participants felt that quality of care is as good as it is going to be and that nothing can be done to improve it further except the natural course of progress in medicine.

"You talk like it's poor quality care and we're trying to tell you that the quality of care is good. It's the quality of the bureaucracy that's bad." (NM, F.)

"The quality of care in this country has become too good. We are keeping people alive for a longer period of years. The technology has been advanced. People live into their 80s and live useful and productive lives. It would have been unthinkable two or three generations ago. But now all of a sudden nobody wants to pay for this care. We've done our job too well." (NO, M.)

CONCLUDING REMARKS

The primary objective of the focus group projects was to elicit opinions and attitudes of both Medicare beneficiaries and physicians who treat Medicare beneficiaries about the quality of the health care received and provided under the auspices of the Medicare program. This information was intended to aid the IOM study committee in identifying key issues of concern that should be addressed in designing a more coherent strategy for reviewing or assuring quality of care in the program.

Findings from the Beneficiary Focus Groups

Overall, as would be expected from the large literature on people's general satisfaction with care, our beneficiary participants were basically satisfied with the medical care they received. The major areas of concern related to the costs of care and basic access to services, especially services that are presently not covered or covered only very minimally in the Medicare program.

The concepts and dimensions to quality of care of greatest importance to patients and beneficiaries were not markedly dissimilar to those of practitioners and professionals. By and large, the participants' definitions of quality center on the "art of care" and interpersonal aspects of the medical encounter, rather than on more technical or clinical areas. Although the beneficiaries emphasized interpersonal aspects in making judgments about care from physicians and hospitals, they recognized that it is a limited basis for evaluating quality. Very little information is available to them, however, about technical aspects of care.

In emphasizing interpersonal dimensions of care as the basis on which they evaluate physicians and the care they render, our elderly participants seemed to be seeking more than a friendly relationship with someone they like. Rather, they saw or sensed important links between the way a physician relates to the patient and the likelihood that the patient will benefit from the encounter. That physicians spend time with their patients, get to know them, and are patient and considerate were also very important. These behaviors help physicians uncover problems that patients might not otherwise mention and will generally reinforce the considerable reservoir of confidence and trust that patients have in their physicians.

The complaints about physicians' behaviors were neither about technical aspects of care nor about disappointing outcomes but were about disinterest in patients and excessive interest in financial matters. Some comments related to unfair or fraudulent billing practices, which raised the possibility to respondents that their own health interests were not of primary importance.

Beneficiaries attached great importance to being able to select their own physicians, at least in the area of primary care. They reported that they rely heavily on suggestions from family and friends about physicians. If initial choices prove disappointing, they tend generally just to seek a new physician rather than to try to remedy the situation or to voice complaints anywhere. Our respondents were relatively comfortable with letting their primary physicians recommend specialists, consultants, and hospitals. This behavior is consistent with the points made earlier about the extent to which patients trust and rely on their primary physicians (or want to be able to do so).

The average age of our participants was almost 78 years, which means that most have been covered by the Medicare program for many years. That they did not see the program per se as having much effect on quality of care is of interest, even recognizing that their views are not necessarily generalizable. The one exception concerned the perceived effect of "DRGs" on hospital care (i.e., diagnosis-related groups as the basis for PPS hospital reimbursement)—specifically, on the likelihood of being discharged so early that one's health might be put in jeopardy. Nonetheless, most apparently believed that the care available to them now is better than it was a decade ago, owing mainly to technologic and scientific advances and not to changes or improvements in the program.

Elderly participants knew little about whether and how the quality of health care is monitored, although they assumed that something was being done by someone. They were largely unaware that professional organizations or governmental agencies (i.e., PROs) might be involved in systematic programs, or that quality-related information might be available to them. Not surprisingly, these individuals *also* believed that quality needed to be monitored more thoroughly than they believe it is today.

Finally, we were intrigued by the interest in these topics expressed by the members of these focus groups. Even allowing for the substantial self-selection bias inherent in this process, these participants were willing to engage the issues forcefully. Their general satisfaction with the health care available through the Medicare program was leavened by the expressed desire to be asked about how well the program is working and how satisfied they are and to have a way to make suggestions for improvement. In this, they are certainly in line with the emerging recognition of "patient satisfaction" as an important dimension of the quality of care—that is, the domain most directly related to measuring the interpersonal aspects of care.

Findings from the Physician Focus Groups

Three main themes can be drawn from the physician focus groups. First, they believed that the Medicare program does not affect quality of care per se, but it does greatly influence the setting for care and the way in which care is delivered. Second, quality of care is often defined in terms of the "art of care" as well as technical and clinical terms. Third, hospital-based peer review programs are viewed as the most effective means for monitoring quality of care.

Overall, as we anticipated from the results of the focus groups among Medicare beneficiaries, most of the physicians did not feel that Medicare patients were different from those patients under age 65 or that the quality of health care differed between the two groups. However, they felt that reimbursement policies place far more constraints on the delivery of care to Medicare patients than to patients under age 65 and that government intervention and paperwork imposed a huge burden on physicians. As a result, some physicians thought that they may in the future serve fewer Medicare patients and may eventually stop accepting them altogether. Some of these points appear to correlate with issues raised by the Medicare beneficiaries themselves.

Many dimensions to quality of care of importance to physicians matched those of greatest salience to patients. That is, art-of-care and interpersonal aspects of the medical encounter were important to physicians in addition to the technical or clinical aspects of quality, which one might assume would be of greatest importance to clinicians. The Medicare beneficiaries in our focus groups saw a link between the way a patient is treated by a physician and the likelihood that the patient will benefit from the encounter. The physicians echoed some of the same feelings and described quality to be the care you would want your family or friends to receive. Even though physicians can and do judge quality on the basis of technical and clinical indicators, they recognize the importance of interpersonal skills in effectively treating the whole patient. Technical and clinical indicators were viewed as important aspects of quality, and good interpersonal skills would not substitute for poor technical skills.

The feeling that hospital-based peer review programs are probably the most effective and well-received quality monitoring systems among physicians has implications for the future of quality assurance. The punitive, confrontational aspects of public and external quality assurance programs were decried, and PROs were not seen as effective quality assurance mechanisms. There did not seem to be consensus about the value and effectiveness of CME, although some positive views were expressed about consumer-patient and physician education. Other professional issues raised involved the general loss of autonomy ("others" making decisions and taking control out of the hands of the physician and patient) and conflicting pressures of malpractice, cost-containment, and professional judgment.

NOTES

1. The assistance of Mathew Greenwald, of Mathew Greenwald and Associates, Inc. (a Washington, D.C.-based company specializing in focus group activities around the nation), in preparing this background description and in conducting the focus groups is gratefully acknowledged.

2. We would like to acknowledge the help of Randy Marshall, Executive Director of the New Mexico State Medical Society; Robert Graham, M.D., Executive Vice-President, AAFP; and Daniel Ostergaard, M.D., Vice-President, Education and Scientific Affairs, AAFP. We greatly appreciate the time they devoted to our focus group project and their interest in our study.

3. The codes are as follows: NYC, New York City; FL, Miami; MN, Minneapolis; SF, San Francisco; HMO, the Health Maintenance Organization groups; NH, the nursing home groups; 65+, the groups diverse by age; 65–74 and 75+, the groups with restricted age ranges; F, female; M, male.

4. Codes for the notations are as follows: PA1 and PA2 are the two groups in Philadelphia; CH is the Chicago group; AAFP is the group conducted among family practitioners at their annual meeting in New Orleans; NO is the other group in New Orleans; NM is the group conducted in Albuquerque at the state medical society meeting; LA1 and LA2 are the two groups in Los Angeles; F, female; M, male.

5. Chapter 8 on the Medicare Peer Review Organization program describes this issue in more detail. Close to a year after these focus groups took place, this policy was changed so that physicians are notified and given an opportunity for the case to be reconsidered before a payment denial or "substandard care" letter is sent to the beneficiary.

REFERENCE

Merton, R.K., and Kendall, P.L. The Focused Interview. *American Journal of Sociology* 6:541–547, May 1946.

APPENDIX A
MODERATOR'S GUIDE FOR THE BENEFICIARY FOCUS GROUPS
Fee-For-Service, Non-Institutionalized Groups

I.   INTRODUCTION AND WARM-UP (15 MINUTES)

A. Purpose of focus group

B. Use of tape recorder and one-way mirror

C. Objectivity of respondents and moderator

D. Collect basic demographic/categorical questionnaire

E. Warm-up Question: Ask half the group, "What are the most positive things about health care today," other half of group, "What are the most negative things about health care today."

II. PERSONAL EXPERIENCE WITH HEALTH CARE (10 minutes)

A. What sorts of health care experiences are represented around the table here? (Get a show of hands)

In the past year or so,

1. How many have been in the hospital?
2. How many have had home health care?
3. How many have had outpatient surgery?
4. How many have had to go to the emergency room?
5. Other?

B. For those of you who have had a recent experience with health care, what would you say you learned about health care as a result?

PROBE POINTS: FACTORS OF QUALITY OF CARE, AVOID COST OR PERSONAL ASPECTS OF THEIR HEALTH CONDITION

C. Based on your experiences, how satisfied are you with the health care available to you today?

1. What things were good?
2. What things were not so good?

PROBE POINTS: FINANCING, ACCESS, AVAILABILITY, TECH-NOLOGY, QUALITY, PERSONAL CARE ISSUES

3. How does your doctor and hospital compare with what you think the average is?

D. How would you rate the quality of care you've received while on Medicare?

1. Why do you say/think that?

III. PERSONAL VIEWS ON THE CONCEPT OF QUALITY MEDICAL CARE (45 min)

"I'd like to get a feeling for what the group thinks about the quality of health care, in general, and the quality of the care available to them . . ."

A. How would you define quality health care?

GO AROUND THE TABLE, ASKING PEOPLE TO EACH ADD A
DIMENSION TO THE DEFINITION OF QUALITY HEALTH CARE

    1. What differentiates good health care from poor health care?

B. You people are all on Medicare; is there anything different about
the care you get through Medicare than in other types of health care?

    1. Why do you say/think that?

C. How would you rate the quality of care you've received while on
Medicare?

    1. Why do you say or think that?

D. Costs are always a problem, but what do you feel are other problems people face in getting quality health care?

    1. Is good health care readily available?

E. Do you have any major concerns about:

    1. doctors?
    2. hospitals?
    3. emergency rooms?
    4. home care?
    5. nursing home care?
    6. care you might get through a health maintenance organization?
    7. any other health care provider?

F. How does the health care available today compare to the care available 10 years ago? 20 years ago?

(avoid cost issues, probe for definition of improving or deteriorating
quality. PROBE POINTS: CLINICAL, PERSONAL, OUTCOME)

G. Do you believe there are any differences in the quality of care
available to patients in different hospitals or from different emergency
rooms?

    1. How large are those differences?
    2. Are they big enough to make you avoid some hospital facilities
and choose others?

H. Do you believe there are any differences in the quality of care
available from different doctors or other types of practitioners such as
home health care agencies?

    1. How large are those differences?
    2. Are they big enough to make you avoid some physicians or
practitioners or to choose others?

IV. UNDERSTANDING OF HOW HEALTH CARE IS MONITORED, REVIEWED (15 min)

DO QUESTIONS A, B, C, D FOR HOSPITALS, HOME CARE AND (if time) NURSING HOMES

A. If you were unhappy or had a problem with the quality of your DOCTOR'S/HOSPITAL'S/HOME CARE PRACTITIONER'S/ NURSING HOME CARE, what would you probably do?

B. Where would you turn for advice if you felt the need to know more about the quality of your health care?

C. In your opinion, how closely is the quality of your DOCTOR'S/ HOSPITAL'S/ HOME CARE PRACTITIONER'S/NURSING HOME'S care monitored?

    1. Who is doing it?

D. Who should be responsible for making sure DOCTORS/HOSPITALS/HOME CARE PRACTITIONERS/NURSING HOMES provide good quality care?

V. DESIRE FOR INFORMATION ON QUALITY OF CARE (30 min)

A. How important is it that you be able to choose your *own* doctors, hospitals, home care nurses, or other health care providers?

B. Do you generally have the information you need when choosing a doctor?

    1. Do you feel you need more information?

        a. If so, where could you get it?

SAME QUESTION FOR HOSPITALS, HOME CARE, EMERGENCY ROOMS, NURSING HOMES, HEALTH MAINTENANCE ORGANIZATIONS

C. Do you think patients need help in identifying or choosing who would be the best hospital, doctor, or other health care providers for them?

    1. If so, what sort of help would they need?
    2. Should the Medicare program play a role in helping you select a hospital or doctor?

D. If you needed the care of a specialist, who do you think should pick your specialist—that is, should it be you, or your doctor, or somebody else?

    1. Should Medicare play any role here in picking a specialist?

"Now I'd like to explore a little more the question of where you get information on the quality of health care services."

For instance:

E. Where do you usually get most of your information on the quality of health care?

F. What do you hear about heath care quality on TV or the radio?

    1. What do you read about it in the newspapers or magazines?

G. What other kinds of information do you think is available to you about the quality of health care services?

    USE AS EXAMPLES

    1. Hospital mortality rates
    2. How often a type of operation is performed by a doctor or in a particular hospital
    3. Information on malpractice claims or physicians inspector's reports on nursing homes

H. From what sources would you like to receive additional information on the quality of health care?

I. Would you be likely to make use of such information services if they were available?

    For instance:

    1. If you or someone close to you were going into the hospital for surgery, would you like to know beforehand the mortality rate of that hospital or of particular physicians for that kind of operation?
    2. Would you like to know the mortality rate of hospitals in your area, in case you ever had to go to one in an emergency?

VI. SUGGESTIONS FOR IMPROVING THE QUALITY OF MEDICAL CARE (15 min)

    (At this point, the moderator will leave the room to confer with the observers to see if they have any points they would like the group to address in greater depth)

"What is the one thing that most needs to be done to improve quality of care?"

        ASK EACH PERSON IN GROUP

APPENDIX B
MODERATOR'S GUIDE FOR THE PHYSICIAN FOCUS GROUPS

I. INTRODUCTION AND WARM-UP (10 minutes)

A. Introduction of the moderator

B. Introduction of sponsor and purpose of the focus group

"The Institute of Medicine is part of the National Academy of Sciences. It is a private research institution established in 1970 to conduct studies for and provide advice to a wide range of government agencies and private concerns and foundations.

Congress has asked the Institute of Medicine to develop strategies to review and assure quality within the Medicare program.

As part of this process, last spring the Institute conducted a series of focus groups around the country with elderly Medicare beneficiaries to understand their views about quality of care.

The expert committee overseeing this study is also holding public hearings with testimony from physician groups, hospital groups, consumer groups, and other health care organizations. A series of site visits are under way to cities around the country to talk with people in hospitals and other health facilities.

The focus group you are participating in today is one of eight to be held in different areas of the country in which we are specifically seeking the views of office-based physicians who care for the elderly. I will be asking for your opinions and advice about assuring quality of care for Medicare patients."

C. Stress focus on quality, not cost. Not intended as criticism, but opportunity to give physicians a chance to provide input on important issues pertaining to health care.

D. Description of focus group process and ground rules

Mention tapes, observers, confidentiality, one-at-a-time, and refreshments.

E. Introduction of participants

Introduce and identify specialty and type of practice. Rotate asking most rewarding aspect of providing care for Medicare patients and most difficult part of providing care for Medicare patients.

II. DEFINITION OF QUALITY HEALTH CARE (15 minutes)

A. "Before we talk about the Medicare program, can we talk in general about defining "quality" in medical care? How would you define quality in medical care—what are the dimensions of quality?"

B. What differentiates good health care from poor health care?

III. QUALITY OF CARE IN THE MEDICARE PROGRAM (10 minutes)

A. General Quality Issues

"Now let me turn the discussion to the Medicare program. From your perspective as a practicing physician . . ."

1. "Does the Medicare program and the way it is run affect the quality of care you and other doctors provide to your patients?" (focus on any limitations caused by the Medicare payment system, review system, or other factors)

B. Location of Quality Problems

"We've been talking about a lot of different issues so far. If you could generalize about problems in care affecting Medicare patients, what would you say that the main problems in quality are?"

PROBE IF NOT MENTIONED SPECIFICALLY:

1. overuse of services
2. underuse of services
3. poor physician skills
4. outdated physician skills
5. physician training/retraining
6. poor lab services or other support services
7. personal problems of physicians (substance abuse, etc.)
8. something else?

PROBE: HOW SERIOUS OR PERVASIVE ARE THESE PROBLEMS?

C. Other issues to probe (OPTIONAL)

"I'd like to ask about some specific quality of care issues we have been hearing about from the elderly and in our public hearings."

SKIP ANY ISSUES THAT HAVE ALREADY BEEN RAISED

1. lack of information for decision-making
2. not enough time with physicians

    3. continuity of care—who is responsible
    4. conflict of interest
    5. differences among physicians and hospitals in the same area

PROBE POINTS: HOW SERIOUS OR PERVASIVE ARE THE PROBLEMS AND WHAT ARE THE REASONS FOR THEM?

IV. AREAS TO TARGET FOR QUALITY ASSURANCE (30 minutes)

A. Focus of Quality Assurance Efforts

"In terms of all the quality-of-care issues that the Medicare program might be concerned with, what (in your view) is the relative importance of dealing with *poor practitioners* as contrasted with trying to improve the *general or "average"* quality of health care provided?"

B. Analysis Using Schematic Aid

"I'm handing out to you a schematic table with two dimensions along which problems in health care quality exist that are under the control of the physician."

DESCRIBE HANDOUT

    1. Where would you say most of the problems in quality lie?
    2. For each category, what proportion of care by all physicians could be put under each category?
    3. What proportion of doctors can be defined as outliers?

HANDOUT

Type of Quality Problem	Average Physician	Outlier Physician
Over Provision of Services		
Under Provision of Services		
Poor Physician Skills or Knowledge		
Outdated Physician Skills		

4. For each problem, what would be the most effective quality assurance mechanism?

V. ASSESSMENT OF MAJOR QUALITY ASSURANCE MECHANISMS (40 minutes)

  A. Knowledge of Quality Assurance Mechanisms

  "Now I'd like to turn our attention to something different—the mechanisms for maintaining or improving quality."

  1. What procedures or systems are most important for assuring the quality of medical care?

  PROBE UNDERSTANDING OF PEER REVIEW SYSTEM

  2. For each of the problem areas we have been talking about:

     a. What ideas do you have for addressing the problem?
     b. How difficult/costly would it be to address the problem?
     c. What role should Medicare play in addressing the problem?
     d. How much progress do you think can be expected?
     e. Is it worth it?

  B. Are there any other mechanisms of quality assurance?

IF ANY OF THE FOLLOWING HAS NOT BEEN MENTIONED, ASK ABOUT IT.

  1. Individually focused mechanisms

     a. state licensing and state board of medical examiners
     b. specialty board certification/periodic recertification
     c. continuing medical education

  2. Hospital-based mechanisms

     a. hospital privileging process
        1. admitting privileges
        2. privileges to perform certain kinds of procedures
     b. master physicians who serve as proctors (as corrective actions for doctors identified as providing poor quality)
     c. hospital peer review activities
     d. private review such as Joint Commission accreditation

  3. Externally based mechanisms

     a. PRO program for Medicare
     b. exclusion from the Medicare program
     c. the legal system - malpractice

4. Information-based mechanisms

a. analysis and feedback of physician or provider-specific information
   1. making public certain kinds of information about the quality of care of hospitals or doctors
   2. public disclosure of hospital-specific mortality rates
b. review of office-based records against physician-developed criteria
c. surveying patients about practitioners

C. How do physicians acquire new skills or upgrade existing skills once out in practice?

D. To what extent can a physician keep up with the knowledge explosion in medicine? How do they do so?

RELATE TO QUALITY ASSURANCE MECHANISMS OF LICENSING, CERTIFICATION, RECERTIFICATION, PRIVILEGING, CONTINUING EDUCATION, MASTER PHYSICIANS, AND PEER REVIEW.

E. How effective are these quality assurance systems?

1. generally
2. for dealing with the outlier physician

F. Addressing Specific Problems

"The study committee has been asked to consider some specific kinds of problems. So, how adequately do you think existing quality assurance methods address each of the following problems?"

1. the impaired physician (psychological or substance abuse)
2. a physician whose skills and knowledge are out of date
3. a provider in a rural or otherwise isolated setting who gives substandard care
4. a physician or hospital that has a pattern of poor performance or patient outcomes

G. What can Medicare do to address each of these problems?

MODERATOR LEAVES THE ROOM
TO CONFER WITH THE OBSERVER

H. Suggestions for Change (15 minutes)

1. "What one change do you think practicing physicians would most readily support that would most improve the quality of care Medicare patients receive?"

APPENDIX C
RECRUITING SCREENER: MEDICARE BENEFICIARY
FOCUS GROUPS

Fee-For-Service Groups
New York City, NY
San Francisco, CA

Hello, I am _____ from _____ . We are conducting a study of health care for the Institute of Medicine of the National Academy of Sciences. For this study, we are seeking the opinions of people ages 65 and over.

1. Do any men age 65 and over live in this household?

    a. YES—May I speak with him please?
    b. No—Do any women age 65 and over live in this household?

        1. YES—May I speak with her please?
        2. NO—terminate.

QUOTA: AT LEAST 6 MALES IN FINAL GROUPS, AND NO MORE THAN 8

(When speaking to the appropriate person) Hello, I am _____ from _____ . The Institute of Medicine of the National Academy of Sciences is doing a study of health care today. We will be inviting a small number of older Americans to take part in a research discussion of their experiences and views about health care. We would like a diverse group for this discussion, and would, therefore, like to ask you a few questions. All of your responses will be kept confidential.

First, I need to ask you a few questions.

2. Are you covered by Medicare?

    a. YES
    b. NO—terminate

3. May I ask your age?

    a. YES _____

    b. NO—May I ask if you are: GROUP A: 65 - 74
        a. 65 - 74   GROUP B: 75 AND OVER
        b. 75 and over

If respondent will not give age, terminate conversation.

QUOTA: AT LEAST 5 PEOPLE IN EACH GROUP NEED TO ANSWER "YES" TO QUESTION 4

4. In the past 3 months, have you (or your spouse) been a patient in a hospital, had surgery when you did not have to be hospitalized, had to go to a hospital emergency room, or had nursing home or home health care?

   a. YES
   b. NO—IF QUOTA NOT MET, TERMINATE CONVERSATION

5. Has your primary occupation been in the health field; that is, have you been a doctor, nurse, hospital administrator, or other health care professional?

   a. YES—terminate
   b. NO

6. As I mentioned before, we would like to learn the views on health care of a diverse group of people. As such, may I ask your racial or ethnic background?

   _____ QUOTA: AT LEAST THREE NON-WHITE OR HISPANIC IN EACH GROUP

   We would like to invite you to join us for a discussion group on health care issues. The sponsor of the group is the Institute of Medicine of the National Academy of Sciences. Our purpose is to learn about people's views toward health care. No one will try to sell you anything. The discussion group will be held on _____ at _____ . Refreshments will be served. We are located at _____ . The discussion will take approximately two hours. The discussion leader will be an expert in this area, whose name is Mathew Greenwald. About 10 other people like yourself will participate. You will receive $30 for your time and participation, and your transportation expenses will be paid.

7. Will you be able to attend?

   a. YES
   b. NO —is there anyone else in your household above age 65 who might be able to attend?

      1. YES—May I speak with him/her?
         — repeat screener
      2. NO—terminate conversation

NAME: _____

ADDRESS: _____

_____

TELEPHONE: _____

Let me repeat your name and address to make sure we have it correct.

REPEAT NAME AND ADDRESS

Would you like me to repeat the discussion group date, time, and location to make sure you have it written down correctly?

IF YES, REPEAT DATE, TIME, AND LOCATION

Thank you. You will be receiving a reminder post card and we will call again to make sure you will be able to attend.

APPENDIX D
RECRUITING SCREENER: PHYSICIAN FOCUS GROUPS

High HMO Concentration Groups
　　Los Angeles, CA

Hello, I am _____ from _____ . We are conducting a study of the quality of health care for the Institute of Medicine of the National Academy of Sciences. For this study, we have been asked to contact a group of doctors in your area. Dr_____ 's name was selected at random, and we would like to ask him/her a few questions for this study.

1. Is doctor ——— available to speak with us?

　　a. YES—May I speak with him/her for just a few minutes?
　　b. NO—ARRANGE FOR A RETURN CALL OR CALL BACK TIME

(When speaking to the appropriate person) Hello, I am _____ from _____ . The Institute of Medicine of the National Academy of Sciences is conducting a study of physician's opinions about quality of health care. We will be inviting a small number of doctors from your area to take part in a research discussion of their views about health care quality. We would like a diverse group for this discussion, and therefore, need to ask you a few questions. All of your responses will be kept confidential.

2. First of all, do you maintain an office-based medical practice?

　　a. YES—Are you affiliated with an HMO or IPA? (NOTE: HEALTH MAINTENANCE ORGANIZATION OR INDEPENDENT PRACTICE ASSOCIATION)

　　　　1. YES—With which HMO are you affiliated?

　　　　　　_____

　　　　2. NO

  b. NO—Are you a staff physician for an HMO (Health Maintenance Organization)?

     1. YES—With which HMO are you affiliated?
     2. NO—terminate conversation.

QUOTA: AT LEAST 4 HMO PHYSICIANS, AND NO MORE THAN THREE FROM ANY ONE HMO

3. Would you say that at least 20% of the patients you have treated over the past year were over age 65?

  a. YES
  b. NO—terminate conversation.

4. What is your medical specialty?

TERMINATE CONVERSATION IF DOCTOR IS A PSYCHOLOGIST, AN ALLERGIST, A PEDIATRICIAN, OR AN EMERGENCY ROOM PHYSICIAN.

QUOTAS: RECRUIT NO MORE THAN *TWO* FROM EACH OF THE FOLLOWING SPECIALTIES:

INTERNAL MEDICINE
  Cardiovascular Disease
  Gastroenterology
  Pulmonary Disease
  Neurology
  Dermatology

FAMILY MEDICINE
GENERAL PRACTICE

SURGERY
  General Surgery
  Neurology
  Otolaryngology (ENT)
  Colon and Rectal Surgery
  Thoracic Surgery
  Urology
  Obstetrics and Gynecology

5. Are you under age 45 or older?

  a. under 45
  b. over 45

6. DON'T ASK, BUT RECORD SEX

  a. Male
  b. Female   QUOTA: AT LEAST TWO FEMALES

7. Have you been a participant in a focus group within the past three months?

  a. YES—terminate conversation
  b. NO

We would like to invite you to join us for a discussion group on health care issues. The sponsor of this group is the Institute of Medicine of the National Academy of Sciences, a private research institution not associated with any government agency. Our purpose is to learn about physicians' views towards the quality of health care. No one will try to sell you anything. The discussion group will be held on_____ at _____ . Refreshments and a buffet will be served. The discussion will take approximately two hours and you will be paid_____ for your time and participation. About 10 other doctors will participate. The discussion leader will be Mathew Greenwald, who has a great deal of experience with research in this area.

8. Will you be able to attend?

   a. YES—get name/address information
   b. NO—Is there another physician in your office who might be able to attend?

      1. YES—May I speak with that doctor please?

      REPEAT SCREENER

      2. NO—thank and terminate conversation.

NAME: _____

ADDRESS: _____

_____

TELEPHONE: _____

Let me repeat your name and address to make sure we have it correct.

   REPEAT NAME AND ADDRESS

Would you like me to repeat the discussion group date, time, and location?

   IF YES, REPEAT DATE, TIME, AND LOCATION

Thank you. You will be receiving a reminder post card and we will call again to make sure you will be able to attend. Should your schedule change, making it impossible for you to attend, please let us know as soon as possible so that we may find a replacement. Our number is _____ .

4

Site Visits

Molla S. Donaldson and Kathleen N. Lohr

The site visits occupied a central place in fact-finding for this study. The Institute of Medicine (IOM) study committee comprised individuals whose diverse backgrounds and experience provided breadth to the committee's deliberations. Because of this diversity and the range of settings and issues included in the legislative charges, the committee chose to devote a substantial amount of time to site visits; the committee members believed such activities would provide a collective understanding of the variety of methods, concerns, and viewpoints of groups with roles in quality assurance. Site visits of this kind are often carried out in IOM projects precisely to bring committee members to some common understanding of the issues under study.

The committee members emphasized the educational objectives of the site visits. The principal goals were as follows: (1) to increase their understanding of the strengths and limitations of methods of quality assessment and assurance from the point of view of those involved in them; (2) to come to appreciate the kinds of problems that are (or are not) identified by such techniques; (3) to learn more about the types of quality assurance interventions that are implemented by various quality assurance programs around the country; and (4) to use this information in generating recommendations for the Medicare program. The committee did not, therefore, try to evaluate the soundness or effectiveness of any organization's quality assurance program.

The remainder of this chapter describes the site visit process and documents the main groups, organizations, and facilities visited. It also discusses major issues raised during the visits and gives examples of the types of quality-of-care problems that health care providers identify through their quality assessment systems or that they consider basic health care systems issues.

METHODS

Site Visit Schedule and Planning

IOM staff began site visit planning in mid-1988. They selected locations that included different regions of the country as well as organizations that conduct quality assurance activities and those that are the object of external quality assurance. For instance, a Medicare Peer Review Organization (PRO) and providers such as hospitals, risk-contract health maintenance organizations (HMOs), and practicing physicians were all included.

In addition, the staff and committee believed it important to visit large urban, small community, and rural settings and to see a range of facilities, for instance large and small institutions and academic and nonacademic settings. They also believed it important to visit groups with "exemplary" quality assurance programs and those struggling to implement programs. To tap community perceptions, staff planned site visits to include representatives of consumer and local community groups. Finally, special meetings were also arranged with experts in quality assurance, ethics, geriatrics, and related issues.

Early in the study, members of the study committee and this study's technical advisory panel were asked to recommend organizations and contacts. The staff first contacted possible site visit locations and visitees by telephone and then sent a confirming letter that outlined the objectives of the site visit (see Appendix A). Staff also determined potential dates for all major site visits and the dates on which committee members could be available and then assigned individuals to specific site visits. Some effort was made to have committee members visit cities and states outside their own location. When committee members could not remain for an entire site visit, they were asked to participate at least partially in more than one visit.

The nine major site visits took place between October, 1988, and March, 1989. Each lasted about 3 days and included two or more committee members and two IOM staff members. During April and May, 1989, several 1-day site visits were made. Tables 4.1 and 4.2 identify the states and cities visited and list the major organizations visited and main meetings conducted.

Visits to Organizations

During the site visits to organizations such as hospitals, hospital associations, HMOs, home health agencies (HHAs), and Medicare PROs, the committee generally used the "Guide for Site Visitors" (Appendix B). Individual committee members and staff were, however, also guided by their own interests and those of the group being visited.

Each site visit included an introduction of participants and an overview of the study objectives presented by a committee member. Generally, the formal site visits then included an overview of quality assurance concerns and activities from the site visitees and a broad discussion of issues in defining and measuring quality. When appropriate, the work of Medicare PROs and concerns directly related to care of the elderly were discussed. Organizations were asked to identify important quality problems faced by the elderly, the kinds of quality problems identified by their quality assessment programs, and the strategies used to correct those problems. During some visits, the participants broke into smaller groups for more informal discussions.

Meetings

All site visits included meetings organized around specific themes or groups representing various views of health care delivery. A highly selective listing includes:

- physicians in office practice (Minnesota, Virginia, and Texas);
- HMO representatives (Minnesota, Texas, California, and Massachusetts);
- hospital administrators and medical directors (Washington, including representatives from Idaho);
- HHAs (Washington);
- geriatric experts (Pennsylvania and Washington);
- rural health care (Washington and Texas);
- data base development and retirement benefits (Illinois);
- community and minority health concerns (New York and Georgia);
- ethical aspects of quality assurance (Virginia).

In several instances, committee members and IOM staff met with experts in a particular area of quality assurance, health services research, nursing quality assurance, or geriatrics. Although all of the meetings concentrated on quality assurance for Medicare, each brought forward somewhat different views.

Documentation

After the site visits, each IOM staff member and some committee members prepared lengthy trip reports based on written and tape-recorded observations. Materials gathered at the site visit or forwarded to the study committee later were logged and filed. A study consultant cataloged this material for later reference and use (particularly for Chapter 6 of this volume). At the committee meetings following the site visits, time was allotted for

TABLE 4.1 States and Cities Visited on Major (Multi-day, Multi-city) Site Visits to Major Organizations, and Meetings with Participants from Several Organizations

---

Illinois (October 12-14, 1988): Chicago and Naperville

Organizations
Crescent Counties Foundation for Medical Care (PRO) (Naperville)[a]
Edward Hospital (Naperville)
Illinois Health Care Cost Containment Commission (Chicago)
Joint Commission on Accreditation of Healthcare Organizations (Chicago)
Michael Reese Health Plan (Chicago)
Rush–St. Luke's Presbyterian Medical Center (Chicago)

Meetings
Experts in data base development and employee retiree benefits (Chicago)
Metropolitan Chicago Hospital Council and member hospitals (Chicago)

New York No. 1 (November 2–4, 1988): New York City, Albany, and Troy

Organizations
Beth Israel Medical Center (New York City)
Hospital Association of New York State (Albany)
Health Insurance Plan (HIP) of Greater New York (New York City)
Health and Hospital Corporation (New York City)
New York State Department of Health (Albany)
St. Mary's Hospital (Troy)

Meetings
New York Community Trust, Center for Policy on Aging (New York City)
Practicing physicians in Albany area (Albany)

New York No. 2. (November 2–4, 1988): New York City, Rochester, and Buffalo

Organizations
Buffalo General Hospital (Buffalo)
Columbia Presbyterian Medical Center (New York)
Health Care Plan (Buffalo)
Island Peer Review Organization (PRO) (Rego Park)
Physician's Network (Rochester)
Rochester Area Hospitals Corporation (RAHC) (Rochester)
Sisters of Charity Hospital (Buffalo)
Strong Memorial Hospital (Rochester)
Visiting Nurse Service of Rochester (Rochester)

Meetings
New York Community Trust, Center for Policy on Aging (New York City)
Rural-urban hospitals in Rochester area (Rochester)

Pennsylvania (November 30–December 2, 1988): Lemoyne, Harrisburg, Blue Bell, and Philadelphia

Organizations
Hospital Association of Pennsylvania (Harrisburg)
KePRO (PRO) (Lemoyne)
Pennsylvania Health Care Cost Containment Council, Data Commission (Harrisburg)
Thomas Jefferson University Hospital (Philadelphia)
U.S. Healthcare (Blue Bell)

Meetings
American Board of Internal Medicine (Philadelphia)
Experts in gerontology and functional assessment (Philadelphia)
Hospital quality assurance representatives—quality assurance and use of Medis-Groups in teaching, community, and rural hospitals (Philadelphia)
Joseph Gonnella, M.D., Dean and Vice President, Jefferson Medical College (Philadelphia)

Minnesota and Iowa (December 13–15, 1988): Minneapolis, St. Paul, Golden Valley, Excelsior, Minn.; Des Moines and West Des Moines, Iowa

Organizations
Becklund Home Health Care (Golden Valley)
Blue Plus (St. Paul)
Fairview Hospital System, Southdale Hospital (Minneapolis)
Healthcare Education and Research Foundation (St. Paul)
Honeywell (Minneapolis)
Iowa Foundation for Medical Care (PRO) (West Des Moines)
Iowa Methodist Medical Center (Des Moines)
Minnesota Coalition on Health (St. Paul)
Minnesota Hospital Association (Minneapolis)
Quality Quest (the Medicare peer review organization for HMOs) (Excelsior)
United Hospital (St. Paul)

Meetings
Health Policy Corporation of Iowa and Iowa Health Data Commission (Des Moines)
Hennepin County Medical Society and Minnesota Medical Association (Minneapolis)
Medicare risk-contract HMOs in Minneapolis (Minneapolis)

TABLE 4.1 continues

TABLE 4.1 Continued

Washington (January 9–11, 1989): Seattle, Davenport, and Spokane

Organizations
Group Health Cooperative of Puget Sound (Seattle)
Lincoln County Hospital (rural hospital) (Davenport)
Peer Review Organization of Washington (PRO) (Seattle)
Providence Medical Center (Seattle)
Visiting Nurse Service (Seattle)
School of Nursing, University of Washington (Seattle)

Meetings
Health Care Purchasers Association (Seattle)
Home Care Association of Washington and representatives of several home health care agencies
Medical directors and hospital administrators of hospitals in eastern Washington State and western Idaho (Spokane)
Medical directors of major Seattle hospitals (Seattle)
Physician staff of the Pike Market Community Clinic (Seattle)
Representatives of Area Agency on Aging, home health care agencies, and local geriatric programs in Spokane and eastern Washington State (Spokane)
James LoGerfo, M.D., University of Washington (Seattle)

Texas (January 30–February 1, 1989): Austin, San Antonio, Houston, and Pasedena

Organizations
Bexar County Health District (hospital and outpatient clinic) (San Antonio)
Pasadena–Bay Shore Hospital (Pasadena)
PruCare (Southwest Region headquarters) (Houston)
St. Luke's Episcopal Hospital (Houston)
Texas Medical Foundation (PRO) (Austin)
Wilford Hall Air Force Medical Center (San Antonio)

Meetings
Practicing physicians from southwest Texas (San Antonio)
Carmault B. Jackson, Jr., M.D., Medical Advisory Services (San Antonio)

California (February 13–15, 1989): Los Angeles, Santa Monica, and San Francisco

Organizations
California Medical Review, Inc. (PRO) headquarters (San Francisco) and regional offices (Los Angeles)
Kaiser Foundation Health Plans–Northern California Region (San Francisco)
The RAND Corporation (Santa Monica)
University of Southern California Medical Center (Los Angeles County)
Value Health Sciences (Santa Monica)

Meetings
HMO Medical Directors and experts in HMO quality assurance and California
    Department of Corporations (Los Angeles)
Hospital Council of Southern California and member hospitals (Santa Monica)
Professional Risk Management Group, Institute for Medical Risk Studies (Los
    Angeles)
Michael McCoy, M.D., University of California, Los Angeles (Los Angeles)

*Virginia and Georgia (March 13–15, 1989): Annandale and Richmond, Va.; Atlanta
    and LaGrange, Ga.*

Organizations
Instructional Visiting Nurse Association Home Health Care (Richmond)
Medical Society of Virginia Review Association (PRO) (Richmond)
Richmond Community Hospital (Richmond)
Richmond Memorial Hospital (Richmond)
West Georgia Medical Center (LaGrange)
West Paces Ferry Hospital (Atlanta)
Woodburn Internal Medicine Medical Associates (private office-based internal
    medicine practice) (Annandale)

Meetings
Representatives of HCFA Regional Office and State Office of Regulatory Ser-
    vices (Atlanta)
Representatives of the Virginia Society of Internal Medicine (Richmond)
Community, minority, and geriatric issues (Atlanta)
Robert Centor, M.D., Medical College of Virginia (Richmond)
Edward Hook, M.D., University of Virginia, Charlottesville (meeting in Richmond)

NOTE: PRO is Peer Review Organization, HMO is Health Maintenance Organization, and HCFA is Health Care Financing Administration.

[a]Location of meeting shown in parentheses.

committee members and staff to report on their observations at the site
visits and to compare their findings.

ISSUES

Topics discussed during the site visits can be divided into two major
classes: issues of concern to study committee members and staff or to site
visitees (some of which were couched as "recommendations" or "messages"
to the Health Care Financing Administration); and quality-of-care problems

TABLE 4.2 Single City Site Visits

Bolling Air Force Base (January 31, 1988)
   Col. Michael Torma, Surgeon General's Office
Cleveland, Ohio (April 4, 1989)
   Meeting of multispecialty group practices (Lahey, Mayo, Oschner, and Cleveland
      Clinics)
Washington, D.C. (April 17, 1989)
   Kaiser Permanente Foundation Health Plan (Mid Atlantic)
Boston and Brookline, Massachusetts (April 25, 1989)
   Massachusetts Board of Registration in Medicine (Boston)
   Harvard Community Health Plan (Brookline)
   New England Medical Center (Staff of Institute for the Improvement of Medical
      Care and Health) (Boston)
Madison, Wisconsin (May 19, 1989)
   Wisconsin Peer Review Organization (PRO)

---

identified by the quality assurance programs of those organizations and facilities that had such programs. These issues are briefly summarized here.

Among the subjects raised fairly consistently across the site visits were the following:

• general health care issues including special health care needs of the elderly;

• benefits and reimbursement issues in the Medicare program;

• environmental issues such as shortages of nurses and other health care professionals and of community-based long-term-care beds;

• consumer education and participation in health care decisions;

• setting-related topics of health care delivery and quality assessment and assurance that focused on particular difficulties or circumstances of ambulatory care settings, home health care, teaching hospitals, and small and rural hospitals;

• internal health care organization issues such as leadership, systems of health care delivery, and accountability for quality;

• quality assessment methods, including data issues, guidelines, and outcomes assessment;

• quality assurance methods, including concerns about duplication of efforts, the value of education and feedback of quality-of-care information, disclosure, dealing with very poor practitioners, legal issues in peer review, and improving average practice;

• the Medicare PRO program.

Because of the salience of the PRO program to the core issues of this study, the site visits allotted considerable time to hear the views of PROs and of the health care institutions subject to PRO review. Among the more contentious topics were the overall focus of the PRO program, case-finding techniques (e.g., usefulness of generic screens), the need for flexibility in responding to local or special problems, the strengths and weaknesses of "peer review," problems with sanctions and other corrective actions and the need for more innovative interventions, the "paper burden" of providing medical records, and rules regarding review. Many site visitees noted both beneficial effects (which some believed is a "sentinel" effect for their own organization-based programs) and the perverse effects of PRO review on health care providers. These issues are also discussed in Chapter 8 of this volume.

PROBLEMS OF QUALITY AND QUALITY ASSURANCE

The organizations and facilities we visited identified many different types of problems. Some problems were classified as the most important problem for Medicare, some as the most important problem at the institution, and some simply as examples of problems found by the quality assurance program of the facility. Although some problems are narrowly clinical, the majority can and should be seen as problems of "systems," rather than of individual providers. The emphasis on systems problems, rather than on problems attributed to individual practitioners, was an important finding from the site visits.

Problems Reported by PROs and Other External Regulatory Bodies

Generic Screens

The first set of problems were those identified by the inpatient generic screens[1] that PROs use in their retrospective review of hospital charts.[2] PROs reported that the screens frequently flagged the following problems:

• abnormal results of diagnostic services that are not addressed and resolved or where the record does not explain why they are unresolved;
• care resulting in serious or life-threatening complications that were not related to admitting signs and symptoms, generally involving the neurological, endocrine, cardiovascular, renal, and respiratory systems;
• medical instability at discharge;
• nosocomial infections (specifically, temperature elevation greater than 2 degrees more than 72 hours after admission and indications of infection following an invasive procedure);
• trauma suffered in the hospital (specifically, hospital-acquired decubitus ulcer).

One PRO downplayed the value of generic screens in identifying quality problems. Instead it noted that the best yield of quality problems came from review of cost outliers, readmissions, some beneficiary complaints, and some calls and reports from physicians and fiscal intermediaries.

Other Problems

PROs also reported a broad range of more general problems. These included poor access to care and inappropriate or inadequate resources (transitional, extended care, home care) in the community that led to use of acute care hospitals for convalescence. They also mentioned lack of knowledge and understanding of the Medicare program or of how to obtain care through an HMO as problems.

Various PROs noted the following: lack of thorough diagnosis and appropriate follow-up;[3] poor monitoring of patient status; premature discharge; poor technical knowledge of physicians; specialists who practice beyond their competence in performing some procedures; surgical specialists not calling in medicine consultants soon enough; nurses not calling in physicians appropriately (as a function of inexperience and work overload); lack of supervision of house staff (particularly in large public hospitals); and general problems of quality of care in rural areas.

Among the specific clinical problems mentioned by PROs were appropriate use of pacemakers (a particular problem earlier in the PRO program) and improper respiratory therapy. Poor medical management of critical care patients included diagnosis, treatment, and monitoring of cardiopulmonary pathophysiology (often among rural physicians and nurses) and, especially, difficulties with fluid and electrolyte management, recognition of arrhythmias, and advanced cardiac life support. Among the diagnoses noted as posing particular patient management problems were diabetes and "infectious disease"; especially troublesome in the latter case was the use of cultures and sensitivities in identifying the infectious organism and prescribing appropriate antibiotics. Pharmacology, especially cardiac[4] and pulmonary drugs and antibiotics, poses its own significant problems. Problems relating to surgery included appropriate use of procedures, surgery in geriatric patients, and post-procedure management.

The New York State Department of Health (NYSDOH) has considerable experience with a form of generic screening and incident reporting. With respect to incident reports (relating mainly to generic screens) from all their hospitals (8,000 to 9,000 reports for all ages), one-third concerned patient falls resulting in fracture, and most of the rest involved administration of medications. The NYSDOH incident reporting system also highlighted two particular problems for the elderly; pneumothorax following placement of central lines, and adverse reactions to contrast media (including anaphylactic reactions).

Problems Reported by Hospitals

The comments from one hospital illustrate a widely held belief about the types of quality problems found in hospitals: "Eighty percent of problems are system problems, not medical diagnosis and management problems." These system problems include timely receipt of laboratory test reports, X-ray films and interpretations, and reports of consults; delayed or missing medical records as patients are transferred from site to site or even cared for within a site was also a significant issue. One hospital noted that their procedures for "intake and admissions" and for "communication and information transfer" all needed improving. One unusual issue was timeliness of autopsies. Hospital staff could not find the charts necessary to do the daily mortality review of the deceased patients because records were being held in the pathology department pending autopsy.

Several hospitals raised poor documentation as a particular problem. Among the specific examples were lack of documentation of reasons for sinus surgery and lack of documentation of preoperative status. More generally, poor documentation in medical records and information flow were mentioned by site visit participants.

Other system-oriented clinical problems reported by hospitals were the following: infiltrates of intravenous lines; problems with central line catheters; aspiration pneumonia; unplanned transfers to the intensive care unit (ICU); nosocomial infections and patient falls (both of which are PRO generic screens); and lack of informed consent. Long waiting times to go from the emergency room to the ICU or hospital bed were cited at one facility.

Diagnosis-specific problems included phlebitis in stroke patients and dementia-related problems (e.g., excessive use of medications, poor use of occupational therapy). Problems linked to surgery were complications of coronary artery bypass graft (which was traced to length of intubation), hematomas after cardiac catheterization, and post-anesthesia headaches. One institution mentioned that generic screens had helped them discover that a particular type of spinal anesthesia was resulting in slower patient recovery.

Inappropriate use of drugs and medications always figures high in quality problems. Cases in point included inappropriate use of coumadin, misuse of antibiotics, and prolonged use of prophylactic antibiotics both before and after surgery. Falls related to medications were reported by at least one hospital.

Blood transfusions and general overuse of blood products are other traditional quality problems that were noted by more than one hospital. In some cases, the blood usage problem was confined to a single department (e.g., orthopedic surgery) rather than present across the facility.

Infection is a common problem. Among the examples cited were penicillin-resistant organisms and an increase in postoperative pneumonia rates (which, in the reporting institution, was attributable to lack of training of inhalation therapists). One hospital's ambulatory review program found readmissions for hospital-acquired wound infection to be a problem, which was traced to inadequate discharge planning and instruction about wound care. Another hospital reported a high incidence of wound infections after open-heart surgery; the source of the problem was eventually tracked to the blood-clotting tanks, which were filled by ice buckets that had a small amount of old water left in the bottom of them.

Only rarely were technical skills mentioned as an important problem. One hospital mentioned skills needed for gastrointestinal procedures. Another mentioned poor placement of feeding tubes, for which a new policy prohibiting blind passage of feeding tubes was developed. A third cited an emergency room physician who missed some fractures on x-ray. One hospital noted an unacceptably high complication rate for retrograde cannulated sphincterotomies, which prompted them to discontinue the procedure.

Overutilization of procedures was mentioned more than once. Sometimes this issue was couched as "indications for" admission to the hospital (instead of a more appropriate setting) or for a certain procedure such as cataract surgery. At one facility, site visit participants stated that providers for the elderly (1) prescribed too many medications, (2) initiated more aggressive therapy than appropriate, and (3) failed to recognize that quality of life may be more important than length of life. Finally, one respondent cited "overuse" generally and claimed that the "PROs don't see it."

Site visit participants occasionally mentioned problems that can affect patient satisfaction. These included excessive waiting times (e.g., in hospital outpatient facilities) and problems of access (e.g., reaching the institution by telephone).

External "environmental" problems were also raised. In one hospital, use of the APACHE database helped it to identify increased morbidity that was linked to a decreasing nurse to patient ratio in its ICU, presumably a reflection of a broader problem with a shortage of nurses. The nursing shortage was cited by other hospitals as a significant limitation on quality of care. Another facility noted morale problems from a low ratio of support personnel. Aging physical plants and lack of funds to undertake the needed capital improvements came up more than once, as did access to and the quality of care in nursing homes.

Finally, some institutions noted limitations of quality assurance itself. For example, programs often do not know how to address problems of overutilization. Further, institutions find it difficult to convince physicians of the value of, and need for, quality assurance and to obtain their willing participation in quality assurance activities.

Problems Reported by HMOs

Prepaid group practices were as likely to report problems with ambulatory care as with inpatient care. With respect to ambulatory care, underuse of preventive services (vaccination, cancer screening) was often noted. A low rate of vaccination for pneumococcal pneumonia among elderly patients (17 percent) was aggressively tackled by one HMO visited. Poor compliance with Pap smear screening guidelines was an issue at another site; poor follow-up for Pap smears and positive fecal occult blood tests was noted at another. Issues related to both diagnosis and ongoing care of common conditions were prominent; for instance, the timeliness of cancer diagnosis and management of hypertension. Failure to follow up abnormal tests was also cited as a problem. Finally, underuse of mental health services was noted by one large system, as illustrated by the appearance in the emergency room of patients in need of psychiatric admission who had not had prior outpatient mental health care.

Other potential quality problems cited were unscheduled return visits to the emergency room (within 48 to 72 hours) and unexpected or problematic admissions to the hospital. As with hospitals, overuse and misuse of drugs and medications were cited as significant quality problems. One example was overcoagulation of patients with transient ischemic attacks. Other issues were polypharmacy (the use of many medications that have potentially conflicting effects, or the use of multiple medications in the same class), use of outdated medications, and psychotropic drug use.

Patient dissatisfaction arose from problems with telephone contacts, waiting times, and, perhaps most importantly, the patient-physician relationship. Lack of coordination of care was also raised (one example being polypharmacy); little or no case management, appropriate post-hospital care, and follow-up are all seen as manifestations of this problem. Patient complaints noted by the HMOs visited included those relating to benefits, access, and referrals to specialists.

Failure of system integration and documentation surfaced as issues for several HMOs. Examples included accuracy of demographic data, presence and accuracy of discharge summaries, and general problems of record-keeping. One provider mentioned lack of documentation of earlier breast examinations as a an obstacle to appropriate breast cancer screening, diagnosis, and care.

Problems Reported by Physicians for Office-Based Practice

Inadequate patient follow-up, particularly of abnormal diagnostic findings, was an issue in fee-for-service outpatient care as it was for prepaid group practice. Poor compliance with preventive care guidelines (in one case, influenza immunizations; in another, breast cancer screening) was also noted as a problem in office-based practice.

As in every other setting, record-keeping and documentation is a concern. One respondent noted that medical records are not built around a standardized database. Another noted that formal hospital discharge summaries are not in the office chart; that is, the office medical record has no formal place to identify dates of, reasons for, and other clinical information about hospitalizations, especially hospitalizations generated by different physicians.

Office-based physicians face some patient-generated problems that they believe are a cause of poor quality. Among the examples cited were patient requests for abusable, addictive drugs and, more generally, difficulty in getting families to agree to "less technology."

Problems Reported by HHAs

HHAs face some problems that differ in degree or kind from those encountered in more traditional settings. One is lack of coordination of services and continuity of care. The many caregivers involved may give conflicting advice to patients (or their families) and yet overlook some aspects of care altogether. Another problem is the discharge of patients from teaching hospitals, when no physician assumes responsibility as liaison to the HHA staff. This is a significant problem when care plans have to be changed, because there is no responsible physician to approve the changes. Conversely, some HHAs evidently find that with case management, their patients are not always sure if "my doctor" is in charge or knows what is happening to the patient.

As with hospitals, staffing can be a problem, especially in regard to registered nurses and therapists, and the availability of full-time staff may be severely limited. One HHA claimed that aides have basic problems reading and writing, which makes documentation problematic.

Some HHAs noted general "gaps in treatment" as a quality issue. The only diagnosis-specific problem mentioned concerned the teaching of cardio-pulmonary rehabilitation to patients.

CONCLUDING REMARKS

The site visits were central to the information-gathering portion of this study. They gave committee members an unparalleled opportunity to learn about a wide range of quality problems and to hear opinions about quality assurance and similar topics directly from health care providers and practitioners; from community, business, and elderly interest groups; and from quality assurance experts across the entire country. This staying-in-touch with the real world was considered imperative for a study that could easily have become quite academic.

The locales and institutions visited represented a very broad set of viewpoints and expertise in health care delivery and in quality assurance. The documents and reports provided during and after the site visits demonstrated forcefully the breadth of quality problems that can be identified by good quality assessment and surveillance programs and the many different, often idiosyncratic, approaches that are taken to solve these problems. The variety of issues and problems mentioned in this chapter underscores this immense diversity, adding to the perception that inflexible and centrally directed quality assurance will not be able to identify, let alone properly address, these deficiencies in quality of care.

This chapter has not documented the different ways that our site visit participants dealt with the quality-of-care problems they identify or encounter. These quality assurance methods, which are discussed more fully in Chapter 6 of this volume, are as diverse as the problems they are intended to overcome. It became quite clear that there is much ferment about, experimentation with, and lingering hostility to quality assessment and assurance. Notwithstanding the latter, the interest in this study and the responsiveness of those visited are hard to overstate. The contributions of the site visit participants to our understanding of the many difficulties and opportunities facing a quality assurance effort were very great indeed.

NOTES

1. The six major categories of PRO generic screens are as follows: (1) adequacy of discharge planning; (2) medical stability of the patient at discharge—for instance, signs such as blood pressure, temperature, pulse, or purulent drainage of postoperative wounds at the time of discharge that would indicate that the patient was not stable—as well as abnormal results of diagnostic tests that were evidently not addressed during the hospital stay; (3) certain unexpected deaths; (4) nosocomial (hospital-acquired) infections; (5) unscheduled return to surgery; and (6) trauma suffered in the hospital, for example, falls, certain life-threatening events, and hospital-acquired decubitus ulcer. See Chapter 8 for more details.

2. At the time of the site visits, very few PROs were involved in "intervening care" review of home health agencies or skilled nursing facilities. One that was reported that an important failed quality screen for skilled nursing home care was "signs and symptoms not reported to physician within four hours from the time detected."

3. One PRO offered the following example. A 92-year-old woman was admitted to the hospital in septic shock, but the facility was unable to find a responsible physician for almost 3 hours, as her usual physician was on vacation. She subsequently died. The PRO took the case through to possible sanctioning.

4. One PRO, for instance, reported that a rural hospital stocked tissue plasminogen activator (tPA) but had no protocol available for its use. The PRO gave them one.

APPENDIX A
CONFIRMATION LETTER REGARDING SITE VISIT

INSTITUTE OF MEDICINE
NATIONAL ACADEMY OF SCIENCES

2101 CONSTITUTEION AVENUE   WASHINGTON, D.C. 20418

Dear _____ :

I am writing to follow-up our conversation about the Institute of Medicine Study to Design a Strategy for Quality Review and Assurance in Medicare and to confirm the date and time of our visit to _____ on Tuesday, January 31, 1989 at 3:00 - 5:30 p.m. Each site visit team includes Committee and IOM staff members. I am enclosing a brief description of each member of the site visit team to _____ .

The study is being conducted in response to a request from the United States Congress and will result in a report to Congress early in 1990; it is funded by the Health Care Financing Administration. I enclose a description and an update of study activities for your further information. You will also find enclosed a brochure on the Institute of Medicine.

The study is under the direction of an IOM committee of experts that is chaired by Steven A. Schroeder, MD, who is Chief of the Division of General Internal Medicine and a member of the Institute for Health Policy Studies at the University of California, San Francisco. A list of the other members of the Committee is included on the back of the blue descriptive sheet.

One of the study activities is a series of ten site visits to a number of cities throughout the country; included in the site visits will be provider institutions and associations, PROs, public sector agencies, and the like. The purpose of the visits is to provide Committee and staff members with a more thorough first-hand understanding in the following areas:

(a) the varieties of approaches that exist today for measuring and assuring the quality of health care to the elderly;

(b) the barriers experienced by health care facilities in developing effective quality assurance (QA) programs, and the solutions they may have devised to overcome those obstacles;

(c) the experience of groups responsible for QA activities (e.g., regulatory agencies, Medicare PROs) and of providers and practitioners who are the targets of such activities (e.g., hospitals, health maintenance organizations, ambulatory care centers, home health agencies, private practice physicians) in terms of (1) the effectiveness of these QA or regulatory programs and (2) the direct and indirect monetary or other costs of such programs;

(d) promising initiatives related to quality assurance that are planned or under way (whether or not they are specifically related to the Medicare program); and finally,

(e) the nature and extent of possible problems in the quality of health care delivered to the elderly today.

In short, the intention expressed by the Committee in undertaking these site visits is to gain a "real-world" understanding of what challenges exist in the quality-of-care area, what is being done to meet those challenges, and how well they are being met — beyond what can be learned from published reports. The Committee is also especially interested in hearing your recommendations for increasing the effectiveness of quality assurance strategies for the Medicare program and for health care delivery more broadly.

To achieve our goals for these site visits means that we need to have a frank and open exchange between your group and our site visit team; we need also to hear from people in your organization who have "front line experience" in the quality assurance area. The purpose of the site visits is educational, not evaluative, and the final report will not identify information by individual sites. Please be assured that all information shared will be treated with strict confidentiality.

We believe that it would be helpful to us if the site visitors could meet with a group of no more than 6-8 individuals, including, for instance, a Member of the Board of Trustees or Directors, the Medical Director, the Chairman of the QA Committee, the QA Coordinator, and perhaps the director of your Medical Records or Data Processing Department; it might also be very informative for us to meet with some clinicians on your staff (physicians, nurses, discharge planners and the like) who may have a special perspective on quality review and assurance activities within the institution. We would be particularly interested in learning more about your risk management program and how it may function to improve quality of care.

In discussing their objectives for the site visit Committee members have expressed their strong preference for the site visit to include the following components;

1. A brief introduction to the IOM study by one of the Committee members.

2. A relatively brief (20 - 30 minutes) overview of your quality assurance program (in this regard, we would be pleased to receive ahead of time any background materials).

3. An open discussion of the functioning of your quality assurance program, that will enable us to understand:

- How you know when you might have a clinical quality problem,
- How you analyze the cause(s) of a problem and determine if it is an occasional error or a pattern,
- What kinds of interventions you use to resolve the problem,
- How you know whether what you are doing has an impact,
- The burdens and costs of the program,
- The overall impact of the program in the organization, and
- Your views about what would enable the internal quality assessment/ quality assurance process to be more effective.

4. A discussion of the external (state and federal) environment.

- The overall impact of external programs in terms of both intended and unintended effects, and
- The burdens and costs of responding to external review and regulatory requirements, and your views about how the process could be made more effective.

5. A discussion among those present concerning your thoughts as to the crucial elements of a successful quality review and assurance system that might be applicable to the Medicare program and special quality of care issues related to the elderly. We hope the discussion will include:

- The nature and extent of current and emerging problems in the quality of health care delivered to the elderly today,
- Whether any problems you identify tend to be concentrated in a relatively small fraction of providers, practitioners, or special groups of elderly or are more diffusely spread among the provider community or elderly population,
- Whether quality problems you see are primarily those of overuse, underuse, or misuse of services,
- Promising quality assurance initiatives.

6. During the remaining time the Committee may want to divide into two groups to meet with no more than 1-3 people in each group who are very familiar with the operations of the quality assurance program and could discuss the QA program from a "front-lines" perspective. Perhaps you could help identify for us (at the time of the visit) those individuals you think would be most appropriate for the two groups to meet with.

Again, we would very much appreciate receiving ahead of time any available background materials describing your organization and QA program so that we may be better prepared for the visit. It would be particularly useful if you could provide us at the time of the visit with an estimate of the annual cost of your QA activities (direct costs for personnel, data processing, etc., for both internal review and in response to external requests). Also, might we have copies of any quality indicators, screens, guidelines, and clinical protocols that are currently in use? These would be of great interest to the Committee and staff for use as background materials in preparing the final report. No materials will be quoted or duplicated outside the Committee.

On behalf of the Study Committee and the Institute of Medicine, I would like to thank you for sharing your time and allowing us to visit. We are certainly looking forward to our visit. I or someone from our staff will call your office before the visit for any specific location directions. If you should have any questions I can be reached at 202/334-2165.

Sincerely,

Molla S. Donaldson, M.S.
Associate Study Director

Enclosures:
Study description
IOM Brochure
Description of site visitors

APPENDIX B
GUIDE FOR SITE VISITORS
STRATEGIES FOR QUALITY REVIEW AND
ASSURANCE IN MEDICARE

PLANNING

Site visitors should meet for at least a half hour every morning to plan strategy.

DEBRIEFING

• The site visit team should try to meet for an hour at the end of each day and definitely before the departure of team members for a general debriefing.

• Consider taping these debriefings. Try to cover at least the following major points: problem identification and verification, interventions, restudy, costs and burdens, and three important three quality problems identified by sites with an internal QA program and members' general observations.

TEAM CAPTAIN RESPONSIBILITIES

The Team Captain (assigned in rotation) should plan to introduce the study, its purposes, and the team members. Suggested points to cover:

1. Introduction
   What the IOM is (part of NAS - independent, nonfederal, private, non-profit, research)
   Who commissioned the study (US Congress)
   Composition of Committee (about 1/2 physicians, health experts, chosen for their own expertise not special interests)
   Due date (Jan. 1990)
   Assumptions or lack thereof (not starting with assumption about HCFA, PROs, etc.)
   Medicare (not Medicaid) study
   Educational purpose
   Focus is truly on quality not cost containment
   Settings
      hospitals, free-standing clinics, MD offices, and HMOs, HHAs
   Other activities of study
      public hearings, written testimony, focus groups, commissioned papers, site visits
   Confidentiality of quality information
   Invite them to speak not only for organization, also as individuals
   Desire for materials now or later - follow-up
   Introduction of those present
   How you would like visit to be organized (large/small groups)

2. Keep questioning on track.
3. Keep track of time for splitting into smaller groups and for departure.

RECOMMENDATIONS TO ALL SITE VISITORS:

Seek specific examples, and ask if we can follow-up, be provided with materials, etc.

GENERAL TOPICS OF INTEREST

Mandate from Congress:

   A. Definitions of quality of care;
   B. The role of structure, process and outcome;

C. Prototype criteria and standards;

D. Adequacy and focus of current methods for assessment and assurance;

E. Evaluate current research on methodologies, needed research;

F. Adequacy and range of methods for assurance;

G. Review mechanisms for promoting, coordinating supervising at the national level;

H. Criteria for establishing priorities in allocation of funds and personnel

also:

Conditions of participation (hospitals)

Topics of interest:

Definition of "quality of health care"

Level of quality of care now provided to the elderly?
- differ by the type of care, setting of care, or other factors?
- differ for different groups within the elderly population?

Major existing or emerging problems? the major strengths?

Is quality of health care adequately monitored or assessed today? (too extensive, adequate, or too little)

Responsible agencies, institutions, associations, or individuals?

Coordination
- among local, state, and federal agencies?
- among private accrediting and review organizations? and
- between the public and private sectors?

What kinds of activities are the most effective and what are the least effective in improving quality of health care?

Research
- conducting
- priorities for needed research

Medicare benefits and access

Effect of gaps in Medicare coverage (benefits) on quality

Effect of Medicare reimbursement on quality

Special characteristics of the Medicare population
- effect on quality

Access barriers
- that exist
- that they have overcome

HEALTH CARE FACILITIES WITH INTERNAL QUALITY ASSURANCE PROGRAMS:

The following is the pool of questions suggested by the Committee. ** (asterisks) mark those questions emphasized at the Committee meeting.

ASSESSMENT

Problem Identification

** How do you identify a potential problem?

** What kinds of problems can your QA system identify, and what kinds can it not identify? For instance; overuse, underuse, a single practitioner or service with a pattern of poor care, bad outcomes, misdiagnosis, missed diagnosis, rates of occurrences, case finding, fragmentation in care by setting, service, or dept.

What data do you use to monitor quality? How do you adjust for confounders such as severity? How do you assure the quality of the data itself?

What data (if any) do you collect that is unique for the Medicare patients? Are there data elements you collect beyond what is required for HCFA?

Does your data system allow you to respond to current HCFA requests for data? For HMOs: Can you provide, for instance, no-pay bills?

Problem Verification

** How do you verify a problem found in retrospective review as a real quality problem? Do you use peer groups, expert opinion, other methods? How do you select a given problem (among a number) for review—set priorities among "competing" problems?

** To what extent do you focus on the occasional error as compared to a pattern of bad care?

** What is the yield of real quality problems compared to potential problems that fail "screens" or other methods of first level problem identification?

** What are three important quality problems you have found recently? (frequency, potential harm to patient) If answer does not include clinical problems, guide questioning to this.

** Are problems concentrated in a relatively small fraction of practitioners or are they more diffuse?

** Are the quality problems, in general, related to overuse, underuse or misuse of services?

INTERVENTIONS/ASSURANCE

What do you do if a practitioner or facility is identified as providing sub-standard care?
 - education, feedback, privileging, jawboning by Chairman
 - anything different if identified internally or externally?

How useful and effective are these interventions?

How many (and what kind of) different methods for assurance have you tried?

What changes have occurred in response to the Patrick case - has peer review been "chilled?" What are the disincentives? Have doctors backed off from making hard decisions?

IMPACT OF INTERVENTIONS/ RESTUDY

** How do you know that your interventions have had an impact?
 - What has been changed as a result of this process?

** Please take one quality problem you have identified in the last year and walk us through the steps in identifying it, verifying it, identifying and implementing changes, and reevaluating the problem or impact? Press for specific answers.
 - Who has been told about the information - Board of Trustees, medical staff, nursing, etc.?
 - What methods of information sharing are used?

** What would improve the effectiveness of your efforts?
 - for instance, better measurement tools? expanded financing? greater support from management, providers, or patients? greater integration of quality assurance into the organization's other activities? or other factors?

COSTS AND BURDENS (for internal and external review)

** What is the effect of your internal QA program on the institution, medical staff? What is the effect of the external QA review on the institution, medical staff?

How much burden does the quality assessment system place on providers? Have you identified ways to reduce the burden? Have you identified ways to reduce the burden but haven't been able to implement them because of regulatory restrictions?

For HMOs: What has been your experience with PRO (or QRO) review of care (e.g., the "13 conditions?") and with hospitals and PROs for review of acute hospital care?

How much of your time is spent on quality assessment in comparison to utilization review? Has this changed recently? What is your opinion of the distribution?

What do you estimate is the cost of your assessment and assurance activities—for instance, dollars spent per case reviewed, or percentage of your total annual budget spent on quality-related activities?

What is the local environment for health care quality issues? For instance, does the press or a business coalition affect your internal activities?

How does your QA system affect other actors within the health care system (e.g., physicians)?

As a subject of external quality assessment and assurance activities (PRO review, licensure, accreditation, etc.)

   • What kinds of problems and benefits do you experience with those efforts?

   • What do you believe would improve the effectiveness of those efforts?

How many (and what kind of) different methods for quality assessment have you tried? How do they compare for yield, cost, validity, and ability to identify true quality problems?

ADVOCACY/ SHARED DECISION MAKING

Is there a well-defined role for "patient advocates" in your organization? If so, what are their responsibilities? To whom do they report? What are institutional/organizational objectives of the patient advocacy process? What methods do you use for grievance resolution?

What are the established mechanisms for promoting and targeting provider education - both clinical education and education about the review process?

What are the established mechanisms for promoting, targeting, and monitoring the effectiveness of patient education and participation in decision making?

Is outcome information routinely collected following major medical or surgical procedures or following diagnostic studies? If so, what kinds of outcomes are ascertained? At what point in time?

Is patient satisfaction specifically addressed? Is this information regularly made available to providers? To patients?

Describe any requirements and review mechanisms regarding informed consent.

How does the organization influence providers' decisions about indications for procedures, special care, or hospital admission and length of stay?

How do you (your institution) make decisions about patient care when a particular service is scarce (e.g., ICU beds)?

Are there any mechanisms designed specifically to blunt volume-driven, fee-for-service incentives, or capitation-based disincentives, to perform procedures or render care?

Are decisions to perform or forego major therapeutic interventions reviewed? If so, how are procedures and specific cases selected for such review?

5

Defining Quality of Care

Jo Harris-Wehling

One of the major decisions of the Institute of Medicine (IOM) committee was to adopt a definition of quality of care. Discussions about quality assurance strategies have been shaped (and sometimes complicated) by definitions of quality of care. In the early stages of the committee's work, frequent reference was made to the meaning of quality of care and how a definition might guide the committee's later work. To facilitate the committee's debate about the definition it might ultimately adopt, study staff compiled and analyzed many available definitions of quality of care. This chapter documents that analysis and presents the committee's final definition, which became a focal point for the committee's report.

METHODS

During the study a large number of definitions of quality of care and sets of parameters that should be considered in defining quality were assembled. Definitions in this context are statements that assert what quality of care is according to the organization or individual proposing the definition. By contrast, the sets of parameters are collections of concepts that the organization or individual believed should be included in any definition. For ease of exposition in this chapter, however, we will refer hereafter to both types of statements simply as definitions.

Most of these definitions were submitted to the study through the public hearing testimony; other sources include site visits, focus groups, publications, and a commissioned paper (Palmer and Adams, 1988). Staff reviewed about 100 definitions (more precisely, 50 definitions and another 50 sets of parameters). The Appendix gives excerpts from 52 of these definitions that are used as examples in this chapter. Numerical citations to the list are given as superscripts immediately following the examples.

A preliminary analysis of the definitions yielded 24 dimensions or concepts that could be used to classify elements of these 100 definitions. This first-round analysis gave a sense of (1) the key terms used by others (such as use of the term "patient"), (2) the variations in terms applicable to a given dimension (such as patient versus consumer or client), and (3) the specific combinations of dimensions that tended to appear in this material.

For the main analysis, staff retained 18 dimensions (Table 5.1); the decision about which dimensions to keep was made more on the basis of qualitative judgment than on quantitative findings, such as frequency of mention. First, we combined cost-effectiveness and resource constraints, which were initially considered as separate dimensions. Second, we combined two aspects of accessibility to care. Finally, four preliminary dimensions (reference to a particular setting such as inpatient or home health care; generic reference to outcome; generic reference to process and outcome; and ge-

TABLE 5.1 Quality Dimensions and Frequency of Occurrence in 100 Definitions of Quality

Dimensions[a]	Frequency of Occurrence
Scale of quality	22
Nature of entity being evaluated	21
Type of recipient identified	24
Goal-oriented	15
Risk versus benefit tradeoffs	10
Aspects of outcomes specified	12
Role and responsibility of recipient asserted	16
Constrained by technology and state of scientific knowledge	16
Technical competency of providers	34
Interpersonal skills of practitioners	30
Accessibility	30
Acceptability	27
Constrained by resources	21
Standards of care	13
Constrained by consumer and patient circumstances	13
Documentation required	8
Continuity, management, coordination	6
Statements about use	3

[a]The first 8 dimensions were explicitly incorporated in the committee's definition. They are given in the order of their appearance in that definition. The remaining 10 dimensions are listed in descending order of the frequency with which they occurred in the 100 definitions analyzed.

neric reference to structure, process, and outcome) were dropped because the analysis yielded little evidence of their importance as independent concepts in this context.

In the following discussion we use specific examples from the Appendix. The final section of this chapter discusses the definition of quality of care adopted by the study committee and identifies the dimensions explicitly incorporated in its definition.

KEY DIMENSIONS USED BY SEVERAL GROUPS IN DEFINING QUALITY

The first 8 dimensions discussed in this section are those ultimately included in the committee's definition. They are discussed in the order in which they appear in that definition. The remaining 10 dimensions are discussed in descending order of the frequency with which they occurred in the 100 definitions analyzed.

A Scale of Quality

The dimension of scale can be used in multiple ways. It can indicate a commitment toward excellence and toward continuous improvement. Scale can indicate a belief that assessment methodologies can, or should be able to, distinguish gradations of quality. Scalar terminology can be used in a definition to distinguish superior quality care from minimal levels of acceptable care, a distinction relevant to the different objectives of internal quality assurance systems and external regulatory efforts. A definition without a scale dimension could imply that quality is a level of care only above the unacceptable (disquality) and that no distinction can (or should) be made between high, middle, or low quality.

Examples of language used in definitions that include the scale dimension include the following:

"The degree of adherence to . . . "[2]

"Level of excellence produced . . . "[5]

"The highest quality . . . is that care that best achieves . . . "[8]

"Quality of care is understood to be the highest scientific care . . . "[37]

"Achieving quality means the continuous improvement of services . . . "[52]

The Nature of the Entity Evaluated, or the Quality of What?

Terms such as health care, medical care, and patient care are frequently used interchangeably. Some individuals and groups, however, perceive significant differences among these terms. For instance, the term "health care" may imply a greater breadth of services (and outcomes) than does the term "medical care."

Donabedian (1988) stated that a relationship exists between the specific elements used to define quality and the specific subject being assessed. The subject could be (1) the performance of the practitioners, (2) the care received by patients, or (3) the care received by communities. The definition of quality (and the subsequent assessment of that quality) thus becomes narrower or more expansive, depending on how narrowly or broadly one has defined the concepts of health and care.

Examples of the terms used for this dimension include the following:

"Criteria for quality of medical care: . . . "[12]

" . . . health care services . . . "[18, 20]

"Quality health care . . . "[23, 24, 25, 30, 31, 33, 39, 46]

"Quality is a variety and intensity of humane treatment modalities . . . "[26]

"Quality patient care is . . . "[28]

"Care that is medically appropriate . . . "[32]

Type of Recipient

Who is the recipient of the care for whom a definition of quality is developed? Is it an individual or a population, or both? And what shall be the precise term used?

Individual-specific terms used in quality definitions are patient, customer, consumer, elderly individual, and Medicare beneficiary or enrollee. Population-specific terms treat these individuals as groups or subgroups but could also be expanded to include terms such as society, societal well-being, and public health. Quality definitions that focus on process and structure dimensions rather than outcome dimensions frequently do not refer to a recipient of care.

"Patient" is by far the most frequent term used to describe the recipient in the definitions we reviewed. The term "population" is used by Palmer and Adams (1988)[10] and in the 1974 IOM definition.[14] The American Nurses Association[43] uses the term "consumer" as do the Pharmaceutical Manufacturers Association[49] and the American Diabetes Association (ADA).[22] The ADA also uses the term "patient" in its definition.

The Office of Technology Assessment (OTA)[36] uses the term "patient" in their quality definition, although they frequently use the term "consumer" in their recent report on quality (OTA, 1988). In that report, OTA explicitly notes that it does not evaluate the quality of the entire U.S. health care system and that it excludes cost and efficiency considerations. The report

611

on the quality of medical care provided by hospitals and
individual patients.

"consumer" connotes very different things depending on one's
﹐. Compared to the term "patient," it can imply more active
.ion in and responsibility for one's health care. It is in this active
that OTA uses the term "consumer." Others may find the term
"con﹒ ﹒mer" distasteful, associating it with perceived negative aspects of the
commercialization of health care and the marketing of quality.

Goal-Oriented Care

According to Steffen (1988), quality is the capacity of the elements of
care, such as structure and process, to achieve a goal, such as to improve
outcomes. The explicit or implicit goals of a health care encounter (or a
long-standing provider-patient relationship) determine to a great extent the
dimensions or properties that will be used to assess the quality of that
encounter or relationship. Health care goals differ depending on whether
they emanate from government, patients, administrators of hospitals or other
facilities or agencies, health care practitioners, or other participants in the
health care system such as third-party payers. In many situations, health
care goals are jointly developed among several parties. Not surprisingly,
therefore, goals that may be embedded in a definition of quality will differ
depending on what parties are involved in developing the definition.

Not all goals of patient care are technical or scientific in nature. Nonmedical goals such as patient satisfaction and consistency with patient preferences are considered by many to be of great importance and a critical
dimension of quality care for the elderly.

Several definitions consulted in this analysis are fairly specific regarding
the goal dimension, which in essence describes an action with a specific
aim such as "helping a patient to maintain independent living." Among
them:

" . . . High quality care deals with the physical, emotional, mental and spiritual or meaningfulness dimensions of life, and tries to help the patient integrate all of these areas."[1]

" . . . helping the elderly individual maintain an independent existence for as
long as he or she can."[4]

" . . . either increases or at least prevents the deterioration in health status . . ."[6]

" . . . achieve the health care goals that are determined by the preferences and
values of those patients and populations who receive it."[9]

" . . . make health care more effective in bettering the health status and
satisfaction of a population, . . . "[14]

" . . . selection of the best therapeutic option, be it medical, surgical, psychosocial or environmental for an individual patient . . . "[25]

" . . . produce the optimal possible improvement in the patient's physiologic status, physical function, emotional and intellectual performance and comfort . . . "[42]

"All attempts to define and evaluate quality will fail until all care and services are provided and based on the patient's values and goals."[50]

Risk Versus Benefit Tradeoffs

This dimension acknowledges that regardless of the benefit expected from health care, all health care carries some risks: risks of side effects of treatment; risks of poorer-than-expected outcomes; and risks of unexpectedly poor outcomes. The probabilities of risks and benefits can be forecast more accurately for some health care services than for others. For any given health care service, the ease of predicting probabilities will be greater for some risks and benefits than for others. Predicting the degree of risk or harm in relation to benefit—or net benefit—is also easier for some patients and services than for others.

This dimension implies that a net good or net benefit probability standard has been adopted. Thus, if this dimension were included in a quality definition, quality assurance might allow for some differences in outcome if the appropriate parties were informed of options and the respective risk implications before making health care decisions. This dimension may be stated in various ways.

"The degree to which patient care services increase the probability of desired patient outcomes and reduce the probability of undesired patient outcomes, . . . "[7]

" . . . Contraindicated treatments avoided (medical) and/or lowest feasible incidence of preventable complications."[15]

"Quality of health care is that kind of care which is expected to maximize an inclusive measure of patient welfare after one has taken account of the balance of expected gains and losses that attend the process of care in all its parts."[16]

" . . . and with minimal risk of making the patient worse; . . . "[46]

Aspects of Outcomes Specified or Not

Some definitions refer quite generically to outcomes, sometimes called benefits. Other definitions refer to specific dimensions of health, presumably to underscore the multi-faceted nature of good health or to emphasize a particular domain of health status. Still others strike a middle ground, using terms such as functioning or health status.

Generic terms include the following: anticipated outcome,[2] independent existence,[4] desired patient outcomes,[7, 36] improved health,[10] inclusive measure of patient welfare,[16] level of well-being,[30] and clinical outcomes.[38,44] Examples of terms for somewhat more specific outcomes are as follows: least morbidity and mortality in the population,[5] highest level of functioning,[18] social and psychological well-being,[34] and outcomes that are optimal in arresting disease or restoring function.[24, 42] Finally, one of the more detailed phrases about outcomes refers to the physiological status, physical function, emotional and intellectual performance, and comfort.[21]

Role and Responsibility of Recipient Asserted

This dimension, if present in a definition, implies that the recipient is more than a passive party. The types of responsibilities differ depending on whether the recipient is an individual or a population. In both cases, however, the dimension asserts active participation in the health care process. Many of these participatory elements relate to patient information, informed consent, and active decision making.

This dimension appears in definitions in several ways:

" . . . and tries to help the patient integrate all of these areas."[1]

" . . . with the responsibility of achieving quality dependent on the provider's skills and the time taken to deliver fully the tools (both cognitive and motivational) by which the consumer affects the necessary actions."[22]

"Quality health care should be . . . informed patient consent."[25]

"Quality is . . . with acceptable risk to the patient . . . "[26]

"High quality care is first, care that is desired by an informed patient; . . . "[35]

" . . . It should be reflective of the patient's value system, . . . "[37]

" . . . seek to achieve the informed cooperation and participation of the patient in the care process and in decisions concerning that process . . . "[42]

Constrained by Technology and the Existing State of Scientific Knowledge

This dimension, if incorporated into a quality definition, accepts the limits on the achievable level of quality care imposed by inadequate knowledge of the effectiveness of many technologies and the vast domains of health care science yet unexplored. These constraints affect the quality of care achievable by even the most technically competent practitioner (a dimension discussed next). This dimension implies that quality care will also be delivered in a manner consistent with the best wisdom available and that the state of that wisdom is dynamic.

Examples that include this dimension are as follows:

" . . . based on the best knowledge derived from science and the humanities, . . . "[5]

"Quality health care . . . within the current limitations of medical science."[24]

" . . . based on accepted principles of medical science and the proficient use of appropriate technological and professional resources . . . "[42]

Technical Competency of Practitioners and Providers

This is a traditional dimension of quality. It includes scientific knowledge and cognitive, manual, and perceptual elements. Corporate management skills might be enfolded in it to recognize—in a sense—the formal organized health care delivery system as a provider. The concept of a practitioner having fidelity to a community of patients might also be included.

Examples of this dimension (and in some cases the next dimension on interpersonal skills) are as follows:

"A well-trained, competent, and experienced physician plus a patient who has confidence in his or her physician."[3]

" . . . quality of care consists of two components: 1) the selection of the right activity or task or combination of activities, and 2) the performance of those activities in a manner that produces the best outcome."[6]

" . . . the degree to which adequate therapy is based on an accurate diagnosis and not symptomatology."[12]

"Quality of care = f (technical care + art of care + technical and art interaction)."[17]

"Quality is the best technical rendition of the best options selected for a specific patient with the patient's consent, delivered with the utmost compassion and respect."[29]

" . . . care that is based on the application of the sound judgment of the appropriate professionals involved, applied to the specific individual concerns and needs of the patient; and . . . that is agreed upon and carried out in a relationship of mutual trust and respect."[35]

Interpersonal Skills of Practitioners

This dimension of quality acknowledges a humanistic element of health care in addition to the science of medicine. The trusting relationship between the patient and the health care provider (perceived by many to be the touchstone of high-quality care) evolves through the application of this dimension.

In addition to those examples provided earlier, this dimension might be worded in the following manner:

" . . . Good medical care maintains a close and continuing personal relationship between physician and patient . . . "[11]

" . . . be provided with sensitivity to the stress and anxiety that illness can generate, and with concern for the patient's overall welfare; . . . "[42]

Accessibility

From both the community and the individual perspectives, ease of access and equality of access are important dimensions. Accessibility does not have the same meaning for everyone, however. It can mean care that is needed, wanted, sought, obtained, covered by a third-party reimbursement system, or approved by a managed care plan. The particular meaning of access may be clarified in the definition.

"Encompass adequate means for providing access of the sick to medical care . . ."[27]

" . . . concerns regarding quality of care go beyond only whether those individuals actually receiving care are receiving 'good care'. Quality of care also encompasses whether the level and scope of benefits involved adequately take care of the entire health care needs of the individual . . . "[45]

" . . . these services should be easily accessible to all patients without barriers of any type."[46]

Acceptability

This dimension usually refers to consumer or patient satisfaction with the health care provider, but it can also apply to the satisfaction of a decision-making entity with providers. For instance, an employer-purchaser might use selective contracting as a mechanism to denote its satisfaction with providers. From a similar perspective, the Medicare program "accepts" a hospital as a satisfactory provider of quality care if the hospital meets the conditions for participating in the Medicare program.

Some experts draw a close parallel between the goal-oriented dimension of quality and the acceptability dimension. A patient (or payer) enters into a health encounter with a set of expectations or a goal, which may or may not be realistic from the perspective of the health practitioner; that goal (implicitly) becomes the measurement tool to determine the acceptability of or satisfaction with the encounter. The acceptability dimension in quality definitions is applicable usually to outcomes of the health encounter, although most assessment tools for measuring patient satisfaction also include process and structure variables.

Examples in the definitions that indicate acceptability as a dimension of quality are as follows:

" . . . improved health and satisfaction of a population . . . "[10]

" . . . management designed to satisfy the overall needs of the patient . . . "[13]

" . . . satisfy the reasonable expectations of both provider(s) and patient(s) . . . "[19]

" . . . which is perceived by patient and his/her personal community to be caring, competent, and effective . . . "[28]

"A definition of quality . . . must address . . . whether patients are satisfied."[41]

"Quality of care . . . includes patient's satisfaction which is a function of degree to which their service expectations are met."[47]

" . . . to meet the needs and expectations of the patients, the physicians, the payers, the employees, and the communities we serve."[52]

Constrained by Resources

One major controversy that often arises during efforts to define quality of care focuses on resource availability (usually monetary) and whether the gradations or scales of quality can fluctuate depending on the resources available. If a dimension of resource constraints is used, optimum care, rather than ideal care, can be an acceptable standard of quality. The "social optimum" approach identifies the most efficient means for providing whatever level of care society determines is to be available. This stands in contrast to "ideal care," which accepts no restrictions on the availability of care—even very expensive health services—as long as some marginal net benefit to the patient is likely.

The social optimum standard is usually determined by society; is defined in operational terms rather than explicit budgetary limitations; and, in most cases, is consistent with a principle of distributive justice. This standard may conflict with professional standards of care, which are rarely defined in terms of economics; professional standards of care honor the principles of beneficence and autonomy more so than the principle of distributive justice.

When quality is defined with a resource constraint dimension, at what point on an ordinal or a nominal scale of quality is inadequate care due to resource constraints not acceptable? The acceptable standard is constantly challenged from opposing directions. "Quality" becomes something of a moving target, presenting a unique set of challenges to quality assurance programs. In particular, assessment methods and quality assurance approaches should be able to (1) identify which, and to what degree, structure, process, and outcome elements of health care are affected by the resource constraints, (2) identify the agent or agents that are responsible for the existence of the constraints and that have the authority to address the problems attributed to the constraints, and (3) carry through in some cases with corrective actions and monitoring for improvement in the quality of care.

Examples of the resource constraint dimension are as follows:

"The production of improved health . . . within the constraints of existing technology, resources and consumer circumstances."[10]

"The primary goal . . . within the resources which society and individuals have chosen to spend for that care."[14]

"Quality of health care . . . achieves a cost effective level in terms of both monetary and personal considerations from the patient's point of view."[23]

"Quality of care is a health care system that provides good care at an affordable price to all Americans . . . with particular importance given to quality of life."[33]

Some definitions may deliberately exclude a specific dimension or assert its irrelevance or inappropriateness for quality of care:

"Quality of care is understood to be the highest scientific care available balanced by the quality of life the patient desires and needs. It should be reflective of the patient's value system, and independent of utilization review and resource allocation."[37]

Standards of Care

Palmer and Adams (1988, p. 42) stated that "quality of health care is measured by comparing data describing care received by patients to standards." According to Donabedian (1988), in measuring quality our concepts of quality must be translated to concrete representations (i.e., criteria and standards of structure, process, and outcome) that are capable of some degree of quantification. The standards are generally based on the judgment or the practice of health care professionals.

Examples supporting this dimension as a component of defining quality are as follows:

"Quality patient care is that practice in any given situation which is thought by knowledgeable clinicians to be in consonance with those practices of the pertinent professional community . . . "[28]

"Quality care should be consistent with . . . generally accepted professional standards."[48]

Constrained by Consumer and Patient Circumstances

Many factors beyond a provider's control may affect patient outcomes, including patient characteristics and circumstances. Thus, a comprehensive quality definition, while focusing on the positive role patients may have in assuring good quality (through, for instance, being informed participants in health care decision making), may also acknowledge that consumer and patient circumstances, such as severity of illness or family circumstances constrain what the health care process can achieve.

Examples found in the definitions are as follows:

" . . . the delivery of health care services in such a fashion as to most efficiently, effectively, and humanely return the patient to—or maintain the patient at—his highest level of functioning."[18]

" . . . psycho-social, functional and economic realities; . . . "[51]

Documentation Required

The Medicare Utilization and Quality Control Peer Review Organization (PRO) program and aggressive internal quality assurance efforts tend to increase the overall amount of information documented in patients' records. This emphasis on documentation may or may not directly affect the quality of care, but accurate and thorough documentation is needed to assess care along other key dimensions such as technical competence, constraints of patient circumstances, and continuity.

Examples of definitions that value documentation include the following:

"Level of excellence produced and documented . . . "[5]

"The extent to which it is available, . . . and documented; . . . "[12]

" . . . It should be readily available, . . . and properly documented . . . "[13]

" . . . be sufficiently documented in the patient's medical record to enable continuity of care and peer evaluation."[42]

" . . . such services should be documented and provided with continuity . . . "[46]

Continuity, Management, and Coordination

This dimension of quality relates to the manner in which health care services are delivered, not the range of services available. The management of multiple people, activities, and institutions involved in providing health care to an individual (or population) affects the continuity of the care and thus the overall quality of the care. The complexity and fragmentation of the current structure of the U.S. health care system presents obstacles to the coordinated delivery of health care. This dimension looks beyond the singular units of health care services to a more comprehensive perspective of health care.

Concern with this dimension is frequently expressed through reference to the wholeness of the individual.

> " . . . Good medical care treats the individual as a whole. . . . Good medical care coordinates all types of medical services . . . "[11]

> "Quality of health care . . . considers the health and care of the whole individual . . . "[40]

> " . . . be provided in a timely manner, without either undue delay in initiation of care, inappropriate curtailment or discontinuity . . . and be sufficiently documented in the patient's medical record to enable continuity of care and peer evaluation."[42]

> " . . . such services should be documented and provided with continuity . . ."[46]

Specific Statements About Use

Quality problems can be categorized into one of three broad areas; that is, poor provider skills or performance, overuse, and underuse. Provider competency was discussed above. This dimension goes further to incorporate concerns about overuse and underuse of health services into the definition of quality. Many of the definitions reviewed included generic adjectives such as appropriate and necessary (terms frequently used in utilization review), but their appearance in a definition would not, in itself, be aggressive enough to meet the intent of this key dimension. Two definitions follow that were more explicit in their statements about use of services and resources:

> " . . . extent to which the health services delivered satisfy the reasonable expectations of both provider(s) and patient(s) without either over- or under-utilization of resources."[19]

> "Quality healthcare is the provision of exactly the right measure of service to restore the patient to the level of well-being he/she is capable of achieving."[30]

THE COMMITTEE'S DEFINITION

As defined by the IOM study committee, **quality of care is the degree to which health services for individuals and populations increase the likelihood of desired health outcomes and are consistent with current**

professional knowledge.   As discussed in Chapter 1 of Volume I of this report, this definition has the following properties:

- it includes a measure of scale (. . . degree to which . . .);
- it encompasses a wide range of elements of care (. . .health services . . .);
- it identifies both individuals and populations as proper targets for quality assurance efforts;
- it is goal-oriented (. . . increase . . . desired health outcomes . . .);
- it recognizes a stochastic (random or probability) attribute of outcome but values the expected net benefit (. . . increase the likelihood of . . .);
- it underscores the importance of outcomes and links the process of health care with outcomes (health services . . . increase . . . outcomes);
- it highlights the importance of individual patients' and society's preferences and values and implies that those have been elicited (or acknowledged) and taken into account in health care decision making and policymaking (. . . desired health outcomes . . .); and
- it underscores the constraints placed on professional performance by the state of technical, medical, and scientific knowledge, implies that that state is dynamic, and implies that the health care provider is responsible for using the best knowledge base available (. . . consistent with current professional knowledge).

In this definition, the care provided is expected to have a net benefit (to do more good than harm, given the known risk when compared to the next best alternative care). In turn, that benefit is expected to reflect considerations of patient satisfaction and well-being, broad health status or quality-of-life measures, and the processes of patient-provider interaction and decision making. The values of both individuals and society are explicitly to be considered in the goal-setting process. How care is provided should reflect appropriate use of the most current knowledge about scientific, clinical, technical, interpersonal, manual, cognitive, organizational, and management elements of health care.

CONCLUDING REMARKS

One purpose of a quality assurance system is to achieve the proper balance among the dimensions reflected in a given definition of quality, because, as this analysis has demonstrated, dimensions of quality may well contradict each other. For example, dimensions of financial constraints and accessibility within a single definition may create opposing pressures on health care providers or policymakers.

The committee's definition does not explicitly incorporate all the dimensions reflected in the quality definitions offered by other parties (Table

5.1). However, as discussed in Volume I, operationalizing the committee's definition (i.e., turning it into practical measurement and intervention approaches) and implementing a quality assurance program based on it will require attention to many of these other dimensions. For example, process of care is reflected in dimensions such as technical competence, interpersonal skills, and coordination; these dimensions cannot be neglected in quality review and assurance because they are aspects of health care that can affect the likelihood of desired outcomes.

This compilation and analysis documents the richness and variety of existing definitions of quality of care, and the study committee found this analysis helpful in clarifying the bases for its own definition. This "empirical evidence" significantly contradicts the often-stated view that quality cannot be defined and, thus, cannot be assessed. The committee's definition (and its respective dimensions) provided guidance to the committee in designing the strategy for quality assurance as set forth in Volume I.

REFERENCES

Donabedian, A, The Quality of Care. How Can It Be Assessed? *Journal of the American Medical Association* 260:1743–1748, 1988.

OTA (Office of Technology Assessment). *The Quality of Medical Care: Information for Consumers.* OTA-H-386. Washington, D.C.: U.S. Government Printing Office, 1988.

Palmer, R.H., and Adams, M.E. Considerations in Defining Quality in Health Care. Paper prepared for the Institute of Medicine Study to Design a Strategy for Quality Review and Assurance in Medicare, 1988.

Steffen, G.E. Quality Medical Care. A Definition. *Journal of the American Medical Association* 260:56–61, 1988.

APPENDIX
EXAMPLES AND SOURCES OF DEFINITIONS OF QUALITY*

1. High quality care means caring for and about the quality of life of each of the persons we treat. This includes attending to their physical disease, physiological events, and the medical events they experience, but also transcends these and ultimately may be independent of the physical events or outcomes. High quality care deals with the physical, emotional, mental and

---

*In many examples herein, the author has excerpted the phrases from material submitted to the study. An attempt has been made to retain the actual words used for defining quality but to eliminate extraneous words from the submitted texts. This approach resulted in a number of illustrative phrases rather than complete sentences.

spiritual or meaningfulness dimensions of life, and tries to help the patient integrate all of these areas.

Hattwick, M.M., Woodburn Internal Medicine Associates, Annandale, Va. Provided to study at site visit.

2. The degree of adherence to generally recognized contemporary standards of clinical practice and achievement of anticipated outcome for a particular service, procedure, diagnosis, or clinical problem.

St. Luke's Episcopal Hospital, Houston, Tex. Provided to study at site visit.

3. A well-trained, competent, and experienced physician plus a patient who has confidence in his or her physician.

Provided to study at site visit.

4. Quality health care for the elderly is primarily that of helping the elderly individual maintain an independent existence for as long as he or she can.

West Georgia Medical Center (Liz Watson), LaGrange, Ga. Provided to study at site visit.

5. Level of excellence produced and documented in the process of diagnosis and therapy, based on the best knowledge derived from science and the humanities, and which eventuates in the least morbidity and mortality in the population.

Ochsner Foundation Hospital, New Orleans, La. with acknowledgement to B.C. Payne, M.D., formerly with the Joint Commission on Accreditation of Healthcare Organizations. Provided to study at site visit.

6. The performance of specific activities in a manner that either increases or at least prevents the deterioration in health status that would have occurred as a function of a disease or condition. Employing this definition, quality of care consists of two components: (1) the selection of the right activity or task or combination of activities, and (2) the performance of those activities in a manner that produces the best outcome.

Brook, R.H. and Kosecoff, J.B. Commentary. Competition and Quality. *Health Affairs* 7:150–161, Summer 1988.

7. The degree to which patient care services increase the probability of desired patient outcomes and reduce the probability of undesired outcomes, given the current state of knowledge.

Joint Commission on Accreditation of Healthcare Organizations, *1990 Accreditation Manual for Hospitals,* 1989.

8. The highest quality medical care is that care that best achieves legitimate medical and nonmedical goals.

Steffen, G.E. Quality Medical Care. A Definition. *Journal of the American Medical Association* 260:56–61, 1988.

9. Quality of medical care is the capacity of that care to achieve the health care goals that are determined by the preferences and values of those patients and populations who receive it. Quality therefore depends on processes necessary to establish personal and societal goals as well as the proficiency with which medical knowledge and technology are applied.

Mulley, A.G., Jr. Correspondence to study, 1989.

10. The perspective of the three parties . . . , providers, governments and patients, can be combined to define quality of care as the production of improved health and satisfaction of a population within the constraints of existing technology, resources and consumer circumstances.

Palmer, R.H. and Adams, M.E. Considerations in Defining Quality in Health Care. Paper prepared for the Institute of Medicine Study to Design a Strategy for Quality Review and Assurance in Medicare, 1988.

11.   1. Good medical care is limited to the practice of rational medicine based on the medical sciences.
      2. Good medical care emphasizes prevention.
      3. Good medical care requires intelligent cooperation between the lay public and the practitioner of scientific medicine.
      4. Good medical care treats the individual as a whole.
      5. Good medical care maintains a close and continuing personal relationship between physician and patient.
      6. Good medical care is coordinated with social welfare work.
      7. Good medical care coordinates all types of medical services.
      8. Good medical care implies the application of all the necessary services of modern, scientific medicine to the needs of all the people.

Lee, R.I. and Jones, W.L. *The Fundamentals of Good Medical Care.* Pp. 6–10. Chicago, Ill.: University of Chicago Press, 1933.

12. Criteria for quality of medical care: (1) the extent to which it is available, acceptable, comprehensive and documented; and (2) the degree to which adequate therapy is based on an accurate diagnosis and not symptomatology.

Esselstyn, C.B. Principles of Physician Remuneration. Paper presented at American Labor Health Association National Conference on Labor Health Services, Washington, D.C., June 16–17, 1958.

13. Quality pediatric medical care embodies a scientific approach to health supervision; the establishment of a diagnosis of deviation from optimum health; institution of appropriate therapy; and management designed to satisfy the overall needs of the patient. It should be readily available, efficiently rendered and properly documented. Preventive care should be utilized to assure optimal physical, intellectual and emotional growth and development.

Osborne, C.E. and Thompson, H.C. Criteria for Evaluation of Ambulatory Child Health Care by Chart Audit: Development and Testing of a Methodology. Final report of the Joint Committee on Quality Assurance of Ambulatory Health Care for Children and Youth. *Pediatrics* Supplement 56:625–692, 1975.

14. The primary goal of a quality assurance system should be to make health care more effective in bettering the health status and satisfaction of a population, within the resources which society and individuals have chosen to spend for that care.

Institute of Medicine. *Advancing the Quality of Health Care.* A Policy Statement. Washington, D.C.: National Academy of Sciences, 1974.

15. Essential Criteria for Hospital Care:

1. Objective substantiation of diagnosis or documentation of co-morbidity.
2. Scientifically validated therapy provided (medical) and/or indications for operative intervention met (surgical).
3. Contraindicated treatments avoided (medical) and/or lowest feasible incidence of preventable complications.

Sanazaro, P.J. and Worth, R.M. Concurrent Quality Assurance in Hospital Care. *New England Journal of Medicine* 298:1171–1177, 1978.

16. Quality of care is that kind of care which is expected to maximize an inclusive measure of patient welfare after one has taken account of the balance of expected gains and losses that attend the process of care in all its parts.

Donabedian, A. *Explorations in Quality Assessment and Monitoring. Vol. I. The Definition of Quality and Approaches to its Assessment.* Ann Arbor, Mich.: Health Administration Press, 1980.

17. Quality of care = f (technical care + art of care + technical and art interaction)

Lohr, K.N. and Brook, R.H. *Quality Assurance in Medicine: Experience in the Public Sector.* R-3193-HHS. Santa Monica, Calif.: The RAND Corporation, 1984.

18. Quality of care is the delivery of health care services in such a fashion as to most efficiently, effectively, and humanely return the patient to—or maintain the patient at—his highest level of functioning.

American Health Care Association. Testimony submitted to study.

19. Extent to which the health services delivered satisfy the reasonable expectations of both provider(s) and patient(s) without either over- or under-utilization of resources.

American Academy of Otolaryngology. Testimony submitted to study.

20. Quality of health care generally refers to the value of health care services available, selected, delivered and the resultant patient outcome that ensues.

American Academy of Physical Medicine and Rehabilitation. Testimony submitted to study.

21. Quality care should produce optimal improvement in physiological status, physical function, emotional and intellectual performance and comfort at the earliest time possible.

American Board of Medical Specialties. Testimony submitted to study.

22. For the diabetic patient quality care might be defined as a compassionate and reasonable balance between the resources available and the need of the patient, with the responsibility of achieving quality dependent on the provider's skills and the time taken to deliver fully the tools (both cognitive and motivational) by which the consumer affects the necessary actions.

American Diabetes Association. Testimony submitted to study.

23. Quality of health care encompasses the concept of appropriateness with a satisfactory outcome and achieves a cost effective level in terms of both monetary and personal consideration from the patient's point of view.

American Gastroenterological Association. Testimony submitted to study.

24. Quality health care (in a hospital) is care provided in the appropriate setting, which results in patient outcomes that are optimal in arresting disease or restoring function within the current limitations of medical science.

American Health Care Institute. Testimony submitted to study.

25. Quality health care should be defined as the selection of the best therapeutic option, be it medical, surgical, psychosocial or environmental for an individual patient based on assessment of clinical history and physi-

cal examination, laboratory and imaging results, the technological resources available, the natural history of the disease process itself, and informed patient consent.

Arkansas Foundation for Medical Care. Testimony submitted to study.

26. Quality is a variety and intensity of humane treatment modalities likely to cure, ameliorate or arrest an adverse medical condition with acceptable risk to the patient and at an acceptable cost.

California Medical Association. Testimony submitted to study.

27. Encompass adequate means for providing access of the sick to medical care and then a high level of skill in providing up-to-date diagnostic and therapeutic measures.

Center for Study of Drug Development, Tufts University. Testimony submitted to study.

28. Quality patient care is that practice in any given situation which is thought by knowledgeable clinicians to be in consonance with those practices of the pertinent professional community (a standard defined by the pertinent professional community); which is associated with high probability for good clinical results or outcome (standard supported by professional literature); which is consistent with policies, guidance or general requirements of authorized accrediting bodies (a standard in consonance with legal authority); which is perceived by patient and his/her personal community to be caring, competent and effective (a standard supportive of patient dignity, understanding and outcome).

Department of Defense, Office of Assistant Secretary for Health Affairs. Testimony submitted to study.

29. Quality is the best technical rendition of the best options selected for a specific patient with the patient's consent, delivered with the utmost compassion and respect.

Federation of American Health Systems. Testimony submitted to study.

30. Quality healthcare is the provision of exactly the right measure of service to restore the patient to the level of well-being he/she is capable of achieving.

Health Data Institute, Baxter. Testimony submitted to study.

31. Quality of health care means the degree to which medical services are rendered in a manner that is timely, appropriate to the medical condition

and social needs of the patient, compassionate, and with consideration of the patient's finances and daily living needs.

Kentucky Medical Association. Testimony submitted to study.

32. Care that is medically appropriate—that fulfills the needs of the patient.

MassPRO (Massachusetts Peer Review Organization, Inc.). Testimony submitted to study.

33. Quality of care is a health care system that provides good care at an affordable price to all Americans (with particular importance given to quality of life).

National Association of Retired Federal Employees. Testimony submitted to study.

34. Maintaining or enhancing the social and psychological well-being of patients and families and promoting conditions in the environment which are conducive to this. Quality health care meets psychosocial needs.

National Association of Social Workers. Testimony submitted to study.

35. High quality care is first, care that is desired by an informed patient; second, care that is based on the application of the sound judgment of the appropriate professionals involved, applied to the specific individual concerns and needs of the patient; and third, care that is agreed upon and carried out in a relationship of mutual trust and respect.

National Institute on Aging, National Institutes of Health. Testimony submitted to study.

36. As provided by hospitals and physicians only - The quality of medical care is the degree to which the process of care increases the probability of outcomes desired by patients and reduces the probability of undesired outcomes, given the state of medical knowledge.

Office of Technology Assessment, Congress of the United States. Testimony submitted to study.

37. Quality of care is understood to be the highest scientific care available balanced by the quality of life the patient desires and needs. It should be reflective of patient's value system, and independent of utilization review and resource allocation.

Providence Hospital, Anchorage, Alaska. Testimony submitted to study.

38. Quality management consists of the pursuit of a standard of excellence in care by effective management of the process of care directed toward the highest level of clinical outcomes that are both desirable and feasible within the constraints of available resources.

Sisters of Mercy Health System. Testimony submitted to study.

39. Quality of health care reflects judgments about the degree of excellence inherent in a specified unit of health service delivered to an individual or group of individuals.

University of Washington School of Nursing. Testimony submitted to study.

40. Parameters: Quality of health care includes appropriate biomedical interventions, considers the health and care of the whole individual and emphasizes the importance of the social context of health care delivery.

American Academy of Home Care Physicians. Testimony submitted to study.

41. Parameters: A definition of quality . . . must address . . . whether care is available; whether care is needed; whether outcomes are acceptable; and whether patients are satisfied. A potential fifth dimension of quality is the cost-effectiveness of care.

American Hospital Association. Testimony submitted to study.

42. Parameters: The AMA has identified eight essential elements that characterize care of high quality. The care should: 1) produce the optimal possible improvement in the patient's physiologic status, physical function, emotional and intellectual performance and comfort at the earliest time possible consistent with the best interests of the patient; 2) emphasize the promotion of health and the prevention of disease or disability and the early detection and treatment of such conditions; 3) be provided in a timely manner, without either undue delay in initiation of care, inappropriate curtailment or discontinuity, or unnecessary prolongation of such care; 4) seek to achieve the informed cooperation and participation of the patient in the care process and in decisions concerning that process; 5) be based on accepted principles of medical science and the proficient use of appropriate technological and professional resources; 6) be provided with sensitivity to the stress and anxiety that illness can generate, and with concern for the patient's overall welfare; 7) make efficient use of the technology and other health system resources needed to achieve the desired treatment goal; and 8) be sufficiently documented in the patient's medical record to enable continuity of care and peer evaluation.

American Medical Association. Testimony submitted to study.

43. Parameters: Benefits derived and outcomes attained for the consumer; perceptions of quality of consumers, practitioner, and accrediting organizations; observable and measurable indicators.

American Nurses Association, Inc. Testimony submitted to study.

44. Parameters: Quality is a function of clinical outcome plus appropriate process plus patient satisfaction plus credentialing plus utilization management plus service plus risk management plus . . .

Health Care Purchasers Association. Testimony submitted to study.

45. Parameters: Level of scope of available benefits; human "caring" aspects.

International Union, United Auto Workers. Testimony submitted to study.

46. Parameters: Quality health care should consist of comprehensive, appropriate, medical, diagnostic, therapeutic, and preventive services delivered by and/or under the supervision of a concerned physician and support staff in a timely manner; such services should be documented and provided with continuity, follow-up, outreach and with minimal risk of making the patient worse; these services should be easily accessible to all patients without barriers of any type.

National Medical Association. Testimony submitted to study.

47. Parameters: Quality of care is partly a function of the need for care. Includes patient's satisfaction which is a function of degree to which their service expectations are met.

National Multiple Sclerosis Society. Testimony submitted to study.

48. Parameters: Quality care should be consistent with scientific knowledge and generally accepted professional standards. Need to pay attention to satisfaction and quality of life in addition to morbidity and mortality.

National Rural Health Association. Testimony submitted to study.

49. Parameters: Concept of quality must take into account the perspectives of the following: 1) providers - concerned whether care conforms to standards; 2) consumers - concerned with interpersonal skills of provider, symptom relief and functional improvement; 3) buyers - concerned with cost effectiveness.

Pharmaceutical Manufacturers Association. Testimony submitted to study.

50. Parameters: All attempts to define and evaluate quality will fail until all care and services are provided and based on the patient's values and

goals. Must also incorporate essential role of informal care givers and family. Do not care for the elderly; care about them as individuals.

Wellspring Gerontological Services, Evergreen Park, Ill. Testimony submitted to study.

51. Parameters: a) process; b) outcome; c) physician-patient interaction; d) psycho-social, functional and economic realities; and e) involvement of patient in decision-making.

Windermere Senior Health Center, Chicago, Ill. Testimony submitted to study.

52. Achieving quality means the continuous improvement of services to meet the needs and expectations of the patients, the physicians, the payers, the employees, and the communities we serve.

Hospital Corporation of America. Provided to study at site visit.

6

A Quality Assurance Sampler: Methods, Data, and Resources

Molla S. Donaldson and Kathleen N. Lohr

INTRODUCTION

Purpose of Chapter

Two of the charges to the Institute of Medicine (IOM) study committee in the Omnibus Budget Reconciliation Act of 1986 were to "evaluate the adequacy and focus of the current methods for measuring, reviewing, and assuring quality of care" (Sec. 9313 [G]) and to "evaluate the adequacy and range of methods available to correct or prevent identified problems with quality of care (Sec. 9313 [F]). Because no comprehensive evaluations of quality assurance have been published, responding literally to these charges would have required a series of new empirical investigations that were well beyond the scope of the study. The committee concluded that it could best address its charges by an overview of strengths and limitations of methods of quality assessment and assurance, as provided in Volume I, Chapter 9 of this report, and by a description of the rich mix of methods in use in hospitals, ambulatory care groups, and home health care, as given here.

This chapter describes a wide variety of techniques of quality assessment, drawing on information from several different study sources. It documents the many approaches to quality measurement (and sometimes quality assurance) being pursued by practitioners, facilities, government and private sector agencies, and other interested parties. It provides a large number of exhibits and citations to the pertinent literature.

Sources of Information

Site Visits

We conducted nine major site visits to all regions of the country from September 1988 to April 1989. During them, we visited a range of institutions: public, teaching, community, and rural hospitals; staff and group model health maintenance organizations (HMOs); large multi-specialty clinics; free-standing and hospital-based home health agencies; small group practices; Medicare Peer Review Organizations (PROs); state boards of medical examiners; hospital associations; and accrediting groups. We did not limit our inquiry to methods of quality review used by the Medicare program or by regulatory or external bodies. Rather, the site visits were an attempt to learn about the range of activities in use inside and outside institutions.

It was evident from these site visits that organizations try, modify, and combine numerous approaches to quality assessment and assurance. This apparently happens because no single, dominant theory of quality assessment techniques exists and because information about the relative effectiveness of various techniques to identify serious quality problems is scarce or nonexistent. Some organizations we visited were struggling to implement recent changes imposed by external groups; some had put in place innovative programs that went beyond minimal external requirements. All were very generous with their time and experience. At most health care facilities we were given materials describing plans for and the current approaches used in quality review. Some facilities provided examples of their criteria and data collection forms. A few described examples of the types of problems they found and the corrective actions they had taken. In planning the site visits the IOM staff made a special attempt to identify facilities that would include a range of efforts and levels of commitment.

Other Sources

The "sampler" derived from the site visits is supplemented by examples of methods described in research studies; of reports of model programs in journals such as *Quality Review Bulletin;* and of approaches described in legislation, manuals of accreditation, and guidebooks published by health care associations. Some techniques of quality assessment and assurance, such as credentials review, have become time-honored; some approaches, such as the use of tracer conditions, have been more theoretical than widely implemented; and some, such as generic outcome screening, have been developed so recently that the technology is still rapidly changing and difficult to assess.

We know very little about the frequency with which various methods are used. Data provided to this study from a survey by 13 multi-hospital systems provide an estimate of the allocation of quality review resources in 58 hospitals located in 21 states. Our site visits indicated that resources devoted to quality assessment vary greatly from a small hospital with one staff member responsible for coordination of quality assurance, utilization review, risk management, discharge planning, and infection control to major urban hospitals with numerous staff and considerable computer support devoted to these functions.

We also relied on several papers commissioned for this study, which include the following: Hawes and Kane (1989), for issues in quality assurance in home health care; Reerink (1989), for international experience in quality assurance; Roos et al. (1990), for an examination of the use of administrative databases to detect quality problems; and Smith and Mehlman (1989), for a review of legal issues and regulatory mechanisms related to quality assurance.

Published reports of research studies that validate methods of assessment do not encompass the range of programs and approaches that are under way in organizations such as hospitals, HMOs, and home health agencies. Occasional reports of model programs by institutions only rarely include data on the frequency or type of problems found, the sensitivity and specificity of the methods of assessment, or most importantly, their effect on quality. The more usual publication describes how quality assessment *should* be conducted, but not necessarily how it is conducted. We know even less about the value of various methods of correcting problems.

Organization of Chapter

Quality assessment and assurance activities are not guided by any currently recognized topology (Donabedian, 1988). To provide some structure to this very complex topic, therefore, we have organized the sampler according to three levels: setting of care, purpose of the activity, and focus of the activity. The outline and order that this chapter will follow is shown in Table 6.1.

Setting of Care

First, the *setting of care*—acute hospital, office-based ambulatory, and home health—reflects the three settings of care that the committee emphasized during this study. Some methods apply to more than one setting; for instance, accreditation applies to hospitals, ambulatory care facilities, and home health care agencies. Similarly, physician licensure and board certification apply to physicians as hospital attending staff and as office-based practitioners. Some methods could be applied in several settings but are

TABLE 6.1 Organization of Volume II, Chapter 6

Hospital Setting
- Preventing Problems
  - —External Methods
  - —Internal Methods
- Detecting Problems
  - —External Methods
  - —Internal Methods
- Correcting Problems
  - —External Methods
  - —Internal Methods

Ambulatory Office-Based Setting
- Preventing Problems
  - —External Methods[a]
  - —Internal Methods
- Detecting Problems
  - —External Methods
  - —Internal Methods
- Correcting Problems
  - —External Methods
  - —Internal Methods

Home Health Care Setting
- Preventing Problems
  - —External Methods
  - —Internal Methods
- Detecting Problems
  - —External Methods
  - —Internal Methods
- Correcting Problems
  - —External Methods
  - —Internal Methods

---

[a]Individuals (physicians), institutions, and prepaid or managed health care plans.

more commonly used in one setting; for example, patient care algorithms are most developed in ambulatory care settings. For brevity we discuss these methods in detail only once.

Purpose of Quality Activity

Second, we categorize quality assurance activities according to their purpose—namely, to *prevent, detect, or correct* problems in quality. "Preventing" problems corresponds to those structures that are intended to ensure that care is provided as intended. Methods may be directed at individuals, subsystems within the health care organizations, or the entire organization. For external bodies these approaches consist primarily of licensure of both practitioners and organizations, physician specialty certification, and organizational accreditation by private accrediting groups. For health care organizations, methods include credentialing systems, policies, and patient care systems to structure or guide patient management at both administrative and clinical levels.

"Detecting" problems is the quality *assessment* or *monitoring* function. This includes systematic attempts to monitor the process of care and mechanisms to capture adverse events such as complications. There are three broad categories of assessment methods: case finding, provider profiling that identifies "outlier" patterns of practice, and population-based methods that compare information on preventive care, health status, and outcomes of care for those who use services and those who do not (Steinwachs et al., 1989). Of the three methods, case finding is, by far, the most commonly reported. Case-finding methods use criteria to identify patients who may have received inadequate care. Examples include generic screening, clinical indicators, and surgical and mortality review.

"Correcting" problems refers to the *assurance* function—targeted and specific action taken in response to a recognized problem. Correcting problems that have been identified through quality review implies that the problem is of a known magnitude and that identification was based on measurement using explicit standards, professional judgment, or a verified patient complaint. Correcting problems is also that portion of the quality assurance cycle most often left dangling—left to intuitive approaches or common wisdom after careful and extensive efforts of problem detection have been made.

Two classes of corrective action can be distinguished: corrective action addressed to an individual, based on an individual event or pattern of events, and corrective action addressed to a group or system within an institution. Both may be externally or internally imposed. Corrective actions include feedback of information to the practitioner, educational efforts, incentives, and penalties.

Distinctions among the activities (i.e., preventing, detecting, and correcting) are, in practice, not always clear because activities may have joint purposes and effects. "Correcting" a problem is related to "preventing" further problems (in the sense of secondary prevention), but it is differentiated in practice because it has a specific focus—a setting, a clinical behavior, and sometimes specific individuals as targets. Similarly, malpractice action might have the effect of preventing problems (e.g., practitioners taking extra care to document their actions or to inform patients), detecting problems (when a claim is filed), or correcting problems (e.g., resulting in withdrawal of hospital privileges).

Locus of Activity

Third, we emphasized in Chapter 2 of Volume I that our overall quality assurance model should distinguish *external* and *internal* programs, even though these distinctions are not always clear cut. Many internal activities occur in response to external pressures. For example, the requirements of the Joint Commission on Accreditation of Healthcare Organizations (Joint Commission) and some external activities may depend on activities that are internal, such as reporting incidents to a state department of health.

Comment

We emphasize that the examples in this chapter are illustrative only; we do not intend to imply that they are exemplary or that, in practice, they perform as described. The reader is referred to Volume I, Chapter 9, for a discussion of the apparent strengths and limitations of many of the approaches enumerated in this chapter. Formal evaluations of the effectiveness of various methods are almost nonexistent; this fact must temper any conclusions and recommendations about specific approaches.

HOSPITAL

External Methods of Preventing Problems in Hospitals

Medicare Conditions of Participation

Hospitals are eligible to receive reimbursement from Medicare by meeting a set of Conditions of Participation. Under Section 1865 of the Social Security Act, hospitals that are *accredited* by the Joint Commission or the American Osteopathic Association are "deemed" to have met all the regulatory requirements specified in the Act, except for a rule concerning utilization, the psychiatric hospital special conditions, and the special requirements for hospital providers of long term care. Hospitals that are not so accredited for whatever reason can seek to meet the conditions by electing to undergo a state *certification* process.

Most hospitals that participate in Medicare do so by meeting the requirements of the Joint Commission. Approximately 77 percent of the 7,000 participating hospitals have received such accreditation; of this accredited group, only 13 percent have 50 or fewer beds. The remaining 1,600 unaccredited (but certified) hospitals are, for the most part, small rural institutions; about 70 percent of the unaccredited hospitals have 50 or fewer beds. Conditions of Participation and the certification process for hospitals are addressed in greater detail in Volume I, Chapter 5, and Volume II, Chapter 7.

The Joint Commission

The Joint Commission is undoubtedly the most important external influence on hospitals that seek its accreditation. Briefly, the Joint Commission's *Accreditation Manual* (Joint Commission, 1989b) is designed for use in hospital self-assessment and is the basis for the hospital survey, which for hospitals in "substantial compliance" occurs every 3 years. The surveys are scheduled at least 4 weeks in advance and are conducted by a physician, a nurse, and an administrative surveyor over a 3-day period using explicit scoring guidelines. After a concluding educational exit interview, hospitals may receive full accreditation or may be notified that accreditation is contingent on its carrying out a plan of correction. A hospital with contingencies may submit written evidence or may undergo a return site visit. It may then be fully accredited or, in due course, nonaccredited.

In 1978 the Joint Commission's Board of Commissioners decided to replace their prescriptive, structure-oriented standards with a standard requiring ongoing, hospital-wide monitoring of care. Nevertheless, structural standards designed to prevent problems and to ensure the capacity of the hospital to operate safely are still in effect. The *Accreditation Manual* (Joint Commission, 1989b) is organized around sets of "standards" defining requirements related to 24 hospital service areas, including the governing board, medical staff and nursing services, quality assurance, hospital departments, special care units (e.g., intensive care unit, burn unit), and hospital-sponsored ambulatory care services. Medical Staff Standards, for instance, emphasize clear definition and assumption of responsibility by the medical staff and review of physician credentials. Governing Board Standards specify the responsibilities of the governing board and the required content of hospital bylaws (two examples are shown in Exhibit 6.H1).

Other Accreditation Programs

Hospitals may also participate in other voluntary accreditation and certification programs. Among these are the College of American Pathologists certification of hospital laboratories.

According to information provided during site visits, military hospitals are surveyed by two external groups. In addition to a Joint Commission survey, for instance, Air Force hospitals have a 2-week survey process involving some 50 surveyors from the Office of the Air Force Inspector

EXHIBIT 6.H1 Example of Two Governing Board Standards

GB.1.14. The governing body requires that only a member of the medical staff with admitting privileges may admit a patient to the hospital and that such individuals may practice only within the scope of the privileges granted by the governing body, and that each patient's general medical condition is the responsibility of a qualified physician member of the medical staff.

GB.1.15. The governing body requires a process or processes designed to assure that all individuals who provide patient care services, but who are not subject to the medical staff privilege delineation process, are competent to provide such services.

SOURCE: Joint Commission, 1989b.

General. Regional military hospitals review smaller local hospitals of 25 beds or less. Care in military hospitals is also reviewed by an external civilian peer review group (Meyer et al., 1988).

State Licensing and Safety Requirements

Hospitals must comply with often extensive state legislation that regulates their structure and operations. These regulations pertain, for instance, to compliance with Life Safety Codes, explicit medical staff standards (Couch, 1989), and, more recently, risk management programs. For example, 10 states have enacted legislation or promulgated regulations requiring hospitals to implement risk management programs (GAO, 1989). In some states, a state survey of hospitals is conducted along with the Joint Commission. In other states the survey occurs on a separate cycle.

Other Hospital-Related Requirements

Various other external efforts have been legislated to protect the rights of hospitalized patients. First, hospitals are required to provide Medicare beneficiaries, at the time of their admission, with a notice regarding their right to appeal a discharge decision, presumably in an effort to forestall premature discharges. (See Volume I, Chapter 6, and Volume II, Chapter 8, on the Medicare PROs for more detail, as the PROs are required to monitor hospital performance in this regard.) Admitting physicians on the site visits repeatedly told us that their patients are unable to understand the notice.

Second, Congress enacted what is commonly called "anti-dumping" legislation by amending the Medicare statute in the Consolidated Omnibus Budget Reconciliation Act of 1985 (amending Social Security Act Section 1867, 42 U.S.C. Section 1395dd).[1] Under this legislation, hospitals with emergency departments are required to conduct a medical screening for any individual who comes to the hospital emergency room and requests examination or treatment for a medical condition (or has had such requested on his or her behalf). The hospital must provide for an appropriate medical screening examination to determine whether an emergency medical condition exists or to determine if a woman is in active labor. The hospital must provide for whatever further examination and treatment by the staff and other facilities of the hospital may be required to stabilize the medical condition or to treat the active labor, or it must provide for transfer of the individual to another medical facility in accordance with restrictions on transfer until the patient is stabilized.

As a third example, the Board of Registration in Massachusetts has been designated by the state as a centralized repository of quality-of-care information. Included in its functions (Code of Massachusetts Regulations, 243 CMR 3.01 to 3.16) is patient care assessment (PCA). A PCA unit requires each hospital semiannually to submit acceptable plans for patient care assessment; this requirement is in addition to hospital licensure, which is handled by a different agency. The PCA unit requires, for instance, that there be a PCA committee and coordinator, that an internal incident reporting system include procedures for "focused occurrence reporting," that major incidents be reported to the Board of Registration, and that policies and practices concerning patient complaints, informed consent, and patients rights be established.

Malpractice Insurance Underwriters

Hospitals insured by some insurance underwriters receive discounts for compliance with risk management standards established by the company. For instance, Virginia hospitals may receive a "basic risk management discount" on their premium from the The Virginia Insurance Reciprocal. This requires compliance with quality assurance and risk management functions, biomedical equipment, emergency power, medical and allied staff insurance, and competence-based appointment and privilege procedures. The hospitals are also eligible for three special discounts concerning anesthesia and surgical services, emergency services (relating to physician staffing and nursing policies and procedures), and obstetrical services (again relating to physician staffing and credentials, nursing staffing and credentials, facilities and equipment, and written policies about certain procedures).

International Efforts

Reerink (1989) compared quality assurance systems, in particular external efforts such as those implemented for the Medicare program in the

United States, with similar activities in other countries on the basis of materials provided by expert contacts in 20 countries in Europe, the Middle East, the Far East, Scandinavia, and North America. He found that descriptions of national quality assurance systems were generally meager and reflective of a near absence of well-developed national systems of assessment and assurance. Publications describe individual efforts by private institutions or practitioners. Some countries have implemented versions of hospital accreditation adapted from the Joint Commission approach (e.g., Kuwait, Saudi Arabia). The Netherlands has embarked on a systematic examination of the quality of health care through resource centers such as CBO (The National Organization for Quality Assurance in Hospitals), SDH (The Foundation for Skills Improvement in General Practice), and NZI (The National Hospital Institute) for nursing homes and mental health institutions. These are supported financially by providers and insurance companies and are encouraged, but not mandated, by the Dutch government (which is traditionally an outsider in health care matters).

Internal Methods of Preventing Problems in Hospitals

Medical Staff Standards

The Joint Commission's Medical Staff Standards (Joint Commission, 1989b) include bylaw requirements designed to prevent or minimize unwanted events. They also call for *departmental evaluation* of the clinical performance of each individual holding clinical privileges. Relevant findings from quality assurance activities are to be considered when the hospital reappoints medical staff or renews and delineates clinical privileges and may be used for feedback to the physicians. Typically conducted or coordinated by the medical staff office, activities in this area can involve tracking credentials, including licensure, training, and experience; tracking competence, including malpractice claim history, challenges to or relinquishment of licensure or registration; and monitoring physician performance, including such measures as numbers of procedures performed, average patient length of stay, complication rates, and findings of quality assessment committees concerned with blood and drug usage. The director of one clinic believed that the *departmental* evaluation of clinical performance is an especially fertile area for quality improvement.

In addition to specifying credentialing and reappointment requirements, some sections of the *Accreditation Manual* state that certain policies and procedures are required (e.g., policies for decontamination of personnel, equipment, and instruments). Other parts of the manual specify the requisite structural characteristics themselves. For instance, in the cardiac intensive care unit each bed must be equipped with monitoring equipment. In another standard, a defibrillator and resuscitative equipment must be available at the bedside when certain procedures are conducted.

Common Internal Organization Actions

Hospitals have incorporated numerous administrative and clinical systems to prevent problems. Examples of these include the following:

- staffing ratios, such as numbers of nurses per staffed beds;
- opportunities for continuing medical education and "inservice" educational programs for staff;
- limiting services offered to patients to those services for which staffing and volume are adequate (such as closing a wing or a special care unit, or not performing some procedures);
- safety precautions for patients at risk for medical complications such as falls or aspiration pneumonia (Exhibit 6.H2);
- safety precautions for the maintenance and operation of equipment and backup systems in case of equipment failure; and
- design of backup systems such as patient identification wrist bands, medication allergy flags on medical records, unit doses of medication, and policies requiring written (not oral) drug orders.

Risk Management

Risk management is more than controlling financial losses from a malpractice claim.[2] Risk management techniques are designed to prevent undesirable occurrences, where possible, and reduce the severity of those that occur. They are prospective interventions and thus should be seen as a system to prevent problems as well as interventions employed once an adverse event has occurred. From this point of view, risk management encompasses the activities of a broad range of personnel throughout the hospital. These may include the finance officer, security officer, legal counsel, personnel officer, biomechanical engineer, nursing director, chiefs of departments, medical director, quality assurance director, and, of course, the risk manager, whose responsibilities have usually been cast as pertaining principally to malpractice loss control.

In recognition of the mutual goals of quality assurance and the patient care component of risk management, a new Joint Commission standard requires an operational link between quality assurance functions and those risk management functions related to patient care safety and quality assurance. Although the goals of risk management and quality assurance are not entirely coincident, their integration is intended to maximize the use of limited resources, eliminate duplicative data collection, and help in devising solutions to problems. Complete integration of the two departments has been of concern to institutions because of the need to provide attorney-client protection for legal materials gathered for case investigation.

The intent of the evolving integration of quality assurance and risk management functions is to reorient risk management from a loss control function that takes place after the fact and is directed toward an individual case to one that might be considered "primary" risk management. That is, it helps to prevent adverse events from occurring and, by analyzing patterns, provides feedback to the organization about areas of weakness. In this sense, it is analogous to infection control.

External Methods of Detecting Problems in Hospitals

Medicare PROs

The efforts of Medicare PROs to detect quality problems by the use of a set of "generic screens" are possibly the broadest systematic approach to "external" problem finding (see Volume I, Chapter 6, and Chapter 8 in this volume for more details). Briefly, a nurse reviewer either on-site (at the hospital) or off-site (at the PRO offices) reviews medical records against a set of generic (non-diagnosis-specific) screens. Most records failing a screening criterion are then reviewed by a physician advisor. If the physician advisor believes that a quality problem likely exists, the attending physician or hospital may be asked for further information, depending on the content of that information. The provider may then be "put on intensified review," meaning that more cases from that hospital will be reviewed, or other corrective interventions may be invoked. Generic screening as practiced by hospitals is described more thoroughly in the section "Internal Methods of Detecting Problems in Hospitals."

Federal, State, Community, and State Hospital Association Data Bases

Types of data sets.[3] Large data sets include claims-based administrative data bases such as those for Medicare Part A and Part B claims. Roos et al. (1990) distinguish three types of data sets and the kinds of studies that are feasible with each. A Level 1 data base contains only hospital discharge abstracts and will permit aggregate studies of, for instance, in-hospital mortality rates and lengths of stay, either by geographic region or over time. A Level 2 data base contains, in addition, unique patient identifying numbers. It can be used to study, for instance, short-term readmissions and volume and outcome relationships at a hospital-specific level.

A Level 3 data base (the most comprehensive) also has information from

EXHIBIT 6.H2 Example of Hospital Interventions Concerning Nursing Interventions for Patients at High Risk of Falls

A. Patient and Family Education:

Orientation and instructions will be given to the patient and family to ensure safety during the period of hospitalization.

1. Orientation of patient and family to physical setting and facilities and hospital policies on safety measures.

   a) Introduction to staff and roommate
   b) Location of bathroom
   c) Location of waiting room
   d) Location of nurse's station
   e) Location of designated smoking areas for ambulatory patients and visitors
   f) Location of elevators and exits
   g) Visiting hours

2. Orientation and instructions of patient and family regarding use of beside equipment and safety devices:

   a) Use of call systems for nurse at bedside and bathroom
   b) Use of bed controls
   c) Use of siderails
   d) Use of assistive devices, i.e., walker, cane, prosthesis, shoes
   e) Use and location of light switches
   f) Use of telephone

3. Instructions for calling staff assistance:

   a) When to call for assistance, e.g.,
       —Assistance to use bathroom
       —Assistance to get out of bed
       —Assistance for bedside supplies not within immediate reach
       —When not feeling well
       —Assistance with use of assistive devices
       —Assistance to ambulate

B. Safe Environment

1. Bed

   a) Lock bed in lowest position
   b) Bedside equipment and supplies should be within patient's reach e.g., call light, bed pans/urinals, tissue paper, water, etc.
   c) Check that bed controls are all working, report any non-functioning controls
   d) Encourage use of siderails at bedtime and when appropriate

2. Lighting

   a) Ensure adequate lighting in room and hallway

   b)   Have overbed light within patient's reach
   c)   Provide appropriate lighting at night

3.   Furniture (mobile and fixed)

   a)   Place furniture for clear walkway
   b)   Check that bedside commode is in a locked position
   c)   Keep furniture in same arrangements if possible during hospitalization

4.   Floors

   a)   Keep walkway clear, i.e., cords, tubings, equipment, etc.
   b)   Keep floor dry
   c)   Wipe spillage immediately
   d)   Make sign "Wet Floor" visible
   e)   Avoid glossy floors
   f)   Use luminous signs to direct patient and visitors to physical facilities, i.e., bathroom and nurses' stations

5.   High Risk Patient Identification

   a)   Use luminous dot on Kardex and patient's bed and door
   b)   Verbal communication among staff of high risk patients to fall

6.   Bathroom

   a)   Keep bathroom light on
   b)   Have hand bar and assistive devices for use in the bathroom, i.e., raise toilet seat, grab bars, tub stool or seat
   c)   Keep bathroom floors dry at all time
   d)   Instructions on how to use bathroom call light
   e)   Have non-skid strips on tub and shower floors

C.   Pharmacologic Effects

1.   Follow pre-op procedures regarding use of siderails after administering pre-anesthetic meds.

2.   Inform patient and family of effects of medications.

3.   Inform patient and family of potential temporary post-operative psychologic changes.

4.   Schedule use of diuretics, cathartics, and cardiotonics for early in the day.

5.   Closely observe patients who are on the following medications: narcotics, sedatives, anti-histamines, psychotropics, hypnotics, tranquilizers, anti-depressants, hypoglycemic agents, anti-hypertensive, eye medication, and those that increase GI mobility, laxatives, and enema.

SOURCE: Columbia Presbyterian Medical Center, N.Y., used with permission.

health program enrollment files, including when individual eligibility begins and ends. This data base permits the highest-quality longitudinal studies, short- and long-term outcomes studies, and population-based (system-wide coverage) studies. Studies can include outcomes for "intervention-free" individuals and poor outcomes or other complications that are not recorded as part of the hospital stay. An example of such a study would be repeat surgeries performed at a hospital and by a physician different from those involved in the first procedure. The Health Care Financing Administration (HCFA) Medicare Automated Data Retrieval System (MADRS) files can now be used to examine linked Medicare Part A (hospital) and Part B (outpatient) utilization data at the person level (DHHS, 1989b).

Data sets can also be used to screen the processes and outcomes of ambulatory and inpatient care. Increasingly, they show promise for measuring continuity and for evaluating episodes of care that include several settings of care. A case in point is determining the percentage of patients who are identified as requiring further care but do not return or the percentage of all visits within an episode of illness made to the same provider (Weiner et al., 1989a). Another example is the proportion of diabetics receiving at least one blood glucose test each year by their regular physicians (Weiner et al., 1989b).

An important strength of Level 3 data bases is that they permit some assessment of population access to care and outcomes. Comparative studies should be able to identify possible areas of underuse. However, administrative data bases contain only contacts with the health care system, and, of these, only contacts that generate a claim. A person who is ill but has no encounter with the health care system produces no record. Copayments and other barriers to access may accentuate this bias and underestimate poor outcomes. Thus, such data bases can never be the sole source of quality information in either individuals or populations.

HCFA mortality rates. An example of the use of the Medicare Part A data base is the HCFA analysis of hospital-specific mortality data. The first public release by HCFA of data on hospital-specific mortality elicited bitter accusations of inaccuracy and highlighted the potential for misunderstanding of data that were not adjusted for severity. Since then considerable work has gone into the development of methods of adjustment; the model now includes such variables as hospital admission during the previous year and comorbid conditions. The data release scheduled for December 1989 will compare data from calendar years 1986, 1987, and 1988. These data highlight institutions that have significantly fewer or more deaths than expected in specific surgical or diagnostic categories. Multi-year data will provide comparisons over time to minimize the effect of chance variation. PROs have also been asked to review cases in these "outlier" hospitals.

Health service researchers have extensively analyzed the uses of mortality data as a quality indicator (Dubois et al., 1987a, 1987b; Daley et al., 1988a, 1988b; Greenfield, 1988; Jencks et al., 1988; Kahn et al., 1988; Chassin et al., 1989b; Dubois, 1989; Ente and Lloyd, 1989).

Small area variations analysis (SAVA). Both SAVA and studies of volumes of services are special aspects of the use of administrative data bases, and both have become major areas of research in their own right. SAVA can identify areas of high, average, and low rates of use of hospital services, but it cannot discriminate appropriate from inappropriate care. As a problem-detection method, SAVA should be regarded as a screening methodology for alerting analysts to areas where quality problems may be occurring, including areas of underuse, and for which more focused review should follow.

Volume of services (individual or organization). After reviewing the literature on the possible relation between volume of procedures done by institutions and the outcomes of those procedures, OTA (1988) concluded that good evidence exists that higher volume is associated with higher rates of good outcomes for a number of diagnoses and procedures. They cautioned, however, that the causal relation is by no means clear, with controversy remaining about whether higher volume permits the development of proficiency (e.g., in the surgeon or surgical team) or whether better practitioners attract a higher volume of patients. It is also not yet clear over what range of volume and under what circumstances the volume-outcome relation holds. Recent research has revealed that 24 percent of surgeons performing carotid endarterectomies did only one such operation in a year in the studied areas, and the authors note that few would regard that volume as sufficient to maintain skills (Leape et al., 1989). Accordingly, we were told of PRO pre-procedure review in one state that includes an inquiry about the requesting surgeon's complication rate and recommends that approval be conditional on his or her having amassed enough cases to provide morbidity rates.

Research on aggregate data has demonstrated their value for studying small area variations, length of stay, and variations in practice patterns and complications over time. Although work is under way to develop methods of risk adjustment, to improve linkages among data bases, and to validate and improve the accuracy of diagnosis and procedure codes, administrative data bases lack specificity in identifying quality problems for a given patient or for a particular episode of care. As a near-term strategy, they are best suited to directing quality assessment efforts toward topics, populations, or providers requiring further study.

Currently, Medicare data bases do not include clinical data, measures of patient need, or outcome assessments. Efforts to devise a uniform needs assessment instrument, to develop a uniform clinical data set (UCDS), and to include patient functional status could greatly augment the value of administrative data bases for internal and external quality assurance programs.

State and local hospital discharge data. Problems in care may also be detected by analyzing state and local hospital discharge data. Numerous state-level and purchaser-provider coalition initiatives are under way.

The better known include the Statewide Planning and Research Cooperative System (SPARCS) data base in New York, efforts by several state health-care cost-containment commissions to assemble, analyze, and disseminate data about health care (specifically on hospital care), and efforts by the Maryland Hospital Association to develop quality indicators to be used by hospitals to review their own performance.

The SPARCS data base was developed in 1977 to support the delivery of hospital care in New York (NAHDO, 1988). It is compiled from a Uniform Billing Code and a Discharge Data Abstract supplied for every discharge from all New York general hospitals. It can produce both standardized and customized reports on the type and severity of cases specific to a hospital or region and the charges associated with treating those conditions; it can be used by hospitals, researchers, local planning agencies, insurance companies, and local, state, and federal governments. The data base has also been used in research at the Department of Health Care Standards and Surveillance at the New York State Department of Health (NYSDOH) to identify cases for quality review (Hannan et al., 1989a; 1989b).

Twenty-eight states have enacted legislation for reporting hospital data. Pennsylvania and Colorado have spearheaded much of this work.

In Pennsylvania, the Health Care Cost Containment Commission's Data Council has required all Pennsylvania hospitals to install the MedisGroups software and to provide the state with case-mix-adjusted data on costs and outcomes. In June 1989 the Data Council published the *Hospital Effectiveness Report* (PHCCCC, 1989), the first report comparing average charges per case and the morbidity and mortality rates of central Pennsylvania hospitals by individual diagnosis-related groups (DRGs). The current and forthcoming reports are intended to help business and labor purchasers as well as the general public to make cost- and quality-informed choices.

The Pennsylvania Buy Right Committee is using the same data to educate its employer and hospital members. One member, ALCOA, is using the data to develop a "managed care plan of excellence," similar to a preferred provider organization (PPO) (Bader et al., 1989).

Since July 1986 the Colorado Data Commission has required hospitals with more than 50 beds to collect and report discharge data on their patients. In January 1988 it began to develop an extensive uniform clinical data set in conjunction with HCFA's UCDS project. Data reporting to the state has been delayed, however.

The Maryland Hospital Association's Quality Indicator Project preceded the Joint Commission's clinical indicator initiative. Developed as a voluntary hospital effort to provide interhospital quality-of-care data (Summer, 1987), it uses a limited number of data elements to be reported on 10 indicators:

1. hospital-acquired infections
2. surgical wound infections
3. inpatient mortality
4. neonatal mortality
5. perioperative mortality
6. cesarean sections
7. unplanned readmissions
8. unplanned admissions following ambulatory surgery
9. unplanned returns to special care unit
10. unplanned returns to operating room

The information from the data analyses is returned to participating hospitals for their "internal" use. Five national hospital systems have joined the data base, as have the Hospital Association of New York State, the Hospital Association of Rhode Island, and the New Hampshire Hospital Association (S.J. Summer, personal communication, 1989).

At a local level, the Rochester Area Hospitals Corporation (RAHC) has instituted a collaborative communitywide approach to controlling cost increases, the Hospital Experimental Payments Program. Recently, RAHC has focused on preventing any adverse effect on quality by distributing funds from a community risk pool. The distribution formula will be based on quality performance as adjusted for admission severity with MedisGroups software (Hartman, 1988).

Complaints

Patients or their families sometimes file complaints with a local, state, or federal agency with oversight responsibility for hospitals. One participant in the beneficiary focus groups mentioned the city health commissioner as the most appropriate place to seek recourse for a problem with hospital quality. State departments of health receive complaints regularly; for instance, NYSDOH maintains a 24-hour staffed telephone line and may respond to complaints by making unannounced investigations at hospitals.

During our site visits we were told that only a few complaints lead to identification of quality problems; nevertheless, an extensive amount of staff effort is directed toward following up complaints. On the other hand, at least one PRO visited in this study believed that patient (or other) complaints were a very useful problem-identification tool and that PRO review of patient complaints helped foster better relations with the patient community.

State Reporting Requirements

All states have reporting requirements and some states may have incident reporting requirements as well (Longo et al., 1989). Although unusual among states in its elaborate regulatory mechanism for detecting problems, NYSDOH requires that certain incidents be reported directly to the state. Reportable incidents are defined as (Title 10 of New York Codes, Rules and Regulations Section 405.8):

1. patients' deaths in circumstances other than those related to the natural course of illness, disease or proper treatment in accordance with generally accepted medical standards. Injuries or impairments of bodily functions, in circumstances other than those related to the natural course of illness, disease, or proper treatment in accordance with generally accepted medical standards and that necessitate additional or more complicated treatment regimens or that result in a significant change in patient status, shall also be considered reportable under this subsection;

2. fires or internal disasters in the facility which disrupt the provision of patient care services or cause harm to patients or personnel;

3. equipment malfunction or equipment user error during treatment or diagnosis of a patient which did or could have adversely affected a patient or personnel;

4. poisoning occurring within the facility;

5. reportable infection outbreaks (as defined in section 405.11 of the Code);

6. patient elopements and kidnapping;

7. strikes by personnel;

8. disasters or other emergency situations external to the hospital environment which affect facility operations; and

9. unscheduled termination of any services vital to the continued safe operation of the facility or to the health and safety of its patients and personnel, including, but not limited to, the termination of telephone, electric, gas, fuel, water, heat, air conditioning, rodent or pest control, laundry services, food, or contract services.

In 1988, hospitals reported nearly 9,000 incidents to NYSDOH. One-third were patient falls resulting in fractures. The remainder were primarily medication errors. Problems caused by laser surgery and fatal errors in administration of potassium were also identified. NYSDOH reviews about 15 percent of incidents onsite, typically where significant patient harm or unexpected deaths have occurred. Each year NYSDOH makes about 3,000 visits to its 272 hospitals, identifies about 2,000 quality problems, and issues about 40 enforcement actions.

Malpractice Claims

When malpractice claims are filed, hospitals may be named as the primary defendant or may be included in a list of defendants. A review by GAO (1987) of a sample of closed malpractice claims showed that 71 percent of the health care providers involved were physicians and about 21 percent were hospitals. In principle, court awards could be considered one way to detect problems in quality, and data on court decisions might be available through a state's Freedom of Information Act (OTA, 1988). The validity of such data for this purpose is very much in doubt, however.

Internal Methods of Detecting Problems in Hospitals

This sampler divides activities according to whether they are intended to prevent, detect, or correct problems, because the focus for each is distinct. In practice, these activities may be combined by hospitals as "integrated" programs of administrative organization, personnel, and data collection. A representative organizational chart shows the quality assurance function as a responsibility of the governing board and coordinated by a quality assurance department. This quality assurance function may be integrated in various combinations with utilization management, risk management, and infection control. The medical staff office typically handles credential and privilege requests and reappointment recommendations from individual departments. It receives, in addition, data provided to it by quality review committees. These committees may be departmental (e.g., surgery or nursing) or hospitalwide (e.g., blood usage or infection control). The organizational details, methods of data collection, and reporting systems are unique to each hospital.

Some hospitals implement proprietary programs designed to integrate these functions. Other hospitals purchase software to help with individual tasks such as severity measurement, credentialing, or incident tracking. Numerous vendors sell quality tracking software; although the use of such computerized aids is not yet widespread, it is increasing.

Possibly the best-known integrated system is the Medical Management Analysis system developed by Craddick (Craddick and Bader, 1983). It combines specialty-specific criteria, generic screens, and 100-percent concurrent review of medical records with utilization review and discharge planning. The program permits the hospital to track the findings of generic screening and monitoring activities, to follow corrective actions, and to develop profiles of practitioners.

A few hospitals have begun to implement a model of quality assurance based on the continuous improvement (CI) model (see Volume I, Chapter 2). Responsibility is to a greater degree dispersed, being vested in those who are closest to where care is performed. Although the CI model strongly emphasizes that final accountability for quality rests with the top leadership of the organization, each group is taught how to identify deficiencies in quality, how to analyze the details of the process, and how to redesign the process to reduce or eliminate errors (in CI terminology, "variations"). The activities included in the CI model must be coordinated so that self-evaluation and records of improvement also follow reporting and accountability requirements for accreditation. Two hospitals visited by the study committee, the Rush Presbyterian–St. Luke's Hospital in Chicago and the Hospital Corporation of America (HCA) West Paces Ferry Hospital in Atlanta, were implementing the CI model.

The listing that follows describes the component parts of quality assurance systems in hospitals and the Joint Commission requirements related to them. In the 1990 *Accreditation Manual for Hospitals* (Joint Commission, 1989b), the "Quality Assurance" standard states that for each facility,

> there is an ongoing quality assurance program designed to objectively and systematically monitor and evaluate the quality and appropriateness of patient care, pursue opportunities to improve patient care, and resolve identified problems. (p. 211)

Required medical staff functions include ongoing monitoring and evaluation of clinical departments or major clinical services (all medical staff, if nondepartmentalized), surgical case review, blood usage review, drug usage evaluation, pharmacy and therapeutics review, and medical record review. Required hospitalwide functions include infection control, utilization review, and review of accidents, injuries, patient safety, and safety hazards. These methods can be described as case-finding methods to identify individual patients who, on retrospective review, may have received suboptimal care. Case-finding as a screening method may be followed by focused review or further review by peers (or both) as described in more detail in the remainder of this section.

States may also enact statutory requirements. In New York State, for instance, hospital trustees, medical staffs, and administrators are held accountable for the quality of care rendered in an institution. The governing board must approve an integrated, hospitalwide quality assurance program and assign at least one member of the governing board to the quality assurance committee (Fisher, 1986).

Quality Assurance Committee

The quality assurance committee in some hospitals is a board-level committee. Minimally, its membership typically includes the following: the chief executive officer; the medical director; chairpersons of nursing, risk management, and quality assurance; and chiefs of the major clinical departments. Members of the governing board may also be members of the committee. The quality assurance committee receives summary reports from the various committees throughout the hospital, considers their findings, and recommends actions to correct problems not managed at committee or department level.

Quality Assurance Department

The quality assurance department provides direction and guidance to all departments and staff and coordinates the collection and monitoring of data and corrective actions. It also serves as an institutional resource for methods and information and as the locus for data analysis and reporting. Generic screening is conducted by nurse reviewers in the quality assurance department. This function may be coordinated with that of utilization review, discharge planning, and infection control.

We obtained data from an outside survey to learn more about resources and the organization of quality assurance activities in hospitals. Data were received from corporate offices of 13 multi-hospital systems and 58 individual member hospitals in 21 states describing the departmental structure, staffing, reporting arrangements, and time devoted to various quality assurance activities. The Appendix describes the survey methods and results in greater detail.

A striking finding was the very wide range of organizational arrangements and extraordinarily wide range of resources reported by hospitals. In hospitals with fewer than 100 beds, combined quality assurance, utilization review, and risk management functions were most frequently reported. In hospitals with 100 to 250 beds, quality assurance with utilization review was reported almost as frequently as the three-function combination, and in hospitals with more than 250 beds, the dual combination (quality assurance and utilization review) was most frequently reported (10 of 24 responding hospitals) (Appendix, Table 6A.6).

As might be expected, with increasing size of hospital (as determined by number of beds designated for medical and surgical services), the numbers of committees, charts reviewed, meetings, and personnel generally increase, but large ranges were reported. For instance, numbers of records reviewed concurrently averaged 587 per month in 3 small hospitals (range, 1 to 1,094 per month), 800 per month in 10 moderate-sized hospitals (range, 12 to

2,820), and 2,330 per month in 11 larger hospitals (range, 245 to 5,670) (Table 6.2).

Monitoring

The Joint Commission is moving toward substantial revision of the *Accreditation Manual*, developing its Agenda for Change using outcome monitoring and modifying its survey and accreditation methods (Joint Commission, 1987, 1989a). However, the standards described above are still in effect, and their influence on hospital activities is pervasive. "Monitoring and evaluation" is a 10-step review process (Exhibit 6.H3) to be applied to all medical staff quality assurance functions, hospitalwide quality assurance functions, and clinical and support service quality assurance activities. Monitoring is expected to be done by all clinical departments (such as nursing, nutrition, and social work) and by support service departments (such as the clinical laboratory, pathology, radiology, pharmacy, and central supply). Exhibit 6.H4 is an example of the results of such monitoring in several departments of one medical center.

Indicators for monitoring are written screens of acceptable practice, instruments that measure a quantifiable aspect of patient care (Lehmann, 1989). They are intended to be objective, measurable, and applied consistently to the review of care by nonphysician reviewers (O'Leary, 1988; Lehmann, 1989). The clinical indicators may be appropriateness protocols (based on adherence to condition- or procedure-specific standards), or they might be positive or negative health status outcomes. Monitoring is intended to signal the need for a more focused review, not to replace case review.

For monitoring, the Joint Commission distinguishes "sentinel events" and "comparative rate indicators." Sentinel events are serious complications or outcomes that should always trigger a more intensified review, such as a maternal death or the occurrence of a craniotomy more than 24 hours after emergency room admission. Comparative rate indicators, such as the death rate after coronary artery bypass graft or the rate of vaginal births after cesarean delivery, are rates over time or rates in comparison to other institutions that may trigger further review (Joint Commission, 1989d). Exhibit 6.H5 gives several illustrations.

Concurrent Review

Concurrent monitoring refers to the review of the process and outcome of care during the course of the hospital stay in order to identify potential and actual problems and reportable incidents. Data for assessment of severity of illness and suitability for discharge may also be monitored. Such concurrent screening may occur at admission and at periodic intervals during

TABLE 6.2 Quality Management Program Characteristics by Hospital Size

Hospital Size (No. of Beds)	Number of Indicators Screened						Number of Records Reviewed Per Month					
	For Physicians			Other Professionals			Concurrent			Retrospective		
	N	Mean	Range	N	Mean	Range	N	Mean	Range	N	Mean	Range
< 100	3	107	35–180	3	68	50–85	3	587	1–1,094	5	238	40–492
100–250	19	142	10–1,288	12	103	0–321	10	800	12–2,820	10	602	55–2,160
> 250	15	72	10–260	8	70	2–205	11	2,330	245–5,670	0		

SOURCE: Survey commissioned for the study, conducted by Mercy Health Services.

EXHIBIT 6.H3   Ten Step Monitoring and Evaluation Model of the Joint Commission

---

1. Assign responsibility for monitoring and evaluation activities;
2. Delineate scope of care provided by the organization;
3. Identify important aspects of care provided by the organization;
4. Identify indicators (and appropriate clinical criteria) for monitoring the important aspects of care;
5. Establish thresholds (levels, patterns, trends) for the indicators that trigger evaluation of the care;
6. Monitor the important aspects of care by collecting and organizing the data for each indicator;
7. Evaluate care when thresholds are reached in order to identify either opportunities to improve care or problems;
8. Take actions to improve care or to correct identified problems;
9. Assess the effectiveness of the actions and document the improvement in care; and
10. Communicate the results of the monitoring and evaluation process to relevant individuals, departments, or services and to the organizationwide quality assurance program.

SOURCE: Joint Commission, 1989b.

the hospital stay. One hospital visited reported 100 percent daily review of their hospital patients.

Generic Screening

Rutstein et al. (1976) first used the term "sentinel event" to describe adverse outcomes that can be especially closely linked with poor process of care. Each adverse event is chosen because it is thought to have a high probability of indicating poor quality and therefore warrants further review and possible intervention.

Generic screening is a method of identifying adverse, or sentinel, events by medical record review. Screens are "generic" in the sense that they apply broadly to the institution rather than to specific departments or diagnoses. Examples of generic screens are "unplanned repair or removal of organ," "severe adverse drug reaction," and "inpatient admission after outpatient surgery." Events subject to screening include those in which patient harm occurs (such as ocular injury during anesthesia care) and those with the potential for harm (such as equipment malfunctions or patient falls).

Generic screening, now widespread in hospitals, is a two-stage system of medical chart screening by nurse reviewers followed by implicit physician review. Data may be recorded on worksheets that are also used for admission, continued stay, and discharge review. Data may be collected within a designated period after admission (e.g., 48 hours), at periodic intervals (e.g., every 3 days), and after discharge, when all services provided have become part of the medical record (for an example see Exhibit 6.H6). Individual events that meet certain explicit criteria (sometimes called screen failures or variations) are further reviewed by a physician advisor. Direct action is taken if a quality problem is confirmed and individual action is appropriate (sometimes called adverse patient occurrences). Data are later aggregated (e.g., by time, service, shift) to determine trends.

If it is done at frequent intervals and if data are reviewed and collated promptly, screening for adverse events can result in immediate action. When potentially dangerous conditions exist, response can be timely enough to prevent further harm to an individual patient and to other patients exposed to similar risks. If data are retrieved by well-trained reviewers and combined with other tasks such as utilization review and discharge planning, screening supports coordination of care and efficient use of resources. Well-developed screening criteria sets could be generalizable to many sites and could provide benchmark data for comparison across sites and over time.

Generic screen data applied by internal quality assurance programs are most frequently reviewed long after the patient has been discharged. As most commonly used, then, they are not helpful for concurrent interventions. Their value for patient care thus depends on dissemination of data on patterns of problems, but the study committee was unable to assemble evidence that this occurs in hospitals.

Screening for adverse occurrences may also be department-specific rather than facilitywide. Exhibits 6.H7 and 6.H8 show some department-specific screens provided during site visits.

Surgical Case Review

Surgical case review addresses the indications or justification for all invasive surgical and diagnostic procedures performed in inpatient and ambulatory care settings (Longo et al., 1989). For cases in which tissue is removed, surgical review includes a comparison of the surgeon's pre-operative diagnostic findings and the post-operative pathology findings. A discrepancy requires further case review to determine whether the surgery was justified.

Some surgical procedures (e.g., cardiac catheterization, angioplasty, angiography, and pacemaker insertion) do not result in removal of tissue, and other surgical procedures (e.g., endoscopy, bronchoscopy, and fine-needle biopsy) may not result in removal of tissue. Surgical review for these cases in one model (Longo et al., 1989) includes (1) criteria development, (2) retrospective case screening by nonphysician reviewers, (3) review by surgical

EXHIBIT 6.H4 Selected Examples of Medical Center Quality Assurance Activities, Quarterly Report (August–October, 1988)

| | | PROBLEMS/ISSUES/PROJECTS | |
	Monitoring Activities	Conclusion	Recommendations/Actions
Pathology	1. STAT turnaround time	The threshold for STAT turnaround time is 60 minutes, the threshold was not exceeded. The average time (July, Aug, Sept) was 57 minutes.	Monitor monthly
	2. Percentage of STAT orders greater than 60 minutes	Threshold exceeded.	Results forwarded to QA
Department of Radiology	Double reading evaluations	100 radiographs were randomly reviewed which had been performed, the minor discrepancies were noted, which did not impact on the patient care.	None
Radiology, Diagnostic	1. Repeat/Retake Analysis a. Outpatient	9-10 Aug 88, 858 films exposed, 129 repeats or 15.03%.	Exceeded threshold of 10%
	b. Inpatient	20-23 Sept 88, 1706 films exposed, 84 repeats or 4.92%.	Well below threshold of 10%

Radiology	Double reading evaluation	75 radiographs reviewed, only 3 minor discrepancies noted, did not impact on patient care.	None
	Radiology request form legibility evaluate	Below the established threshold of 10%.	None
	Radiology request form completeness review	Aug error rate is 16%, Sept 13.3%, Oct-11% exceeded threshold of 10% - note July rate was 14.7%, over the 10% threshold.	Results will be forwarded to QA.
	Radiology report distribution review	Aug, Sept, Oct all exceeded the threshold of 5 days except Aug with 4.88 days. Sept average was 21.33 days, Oct average was 17.85 days.	
Dept of Emergency Service	Tracking ambulance transfers	ER personnel continue to have difficulty tracking ambulance transfers using computer retrieval. The transfer of patients must be tracked and audited for QA/RM.	Effective immediately (Aug 88) Ambulance transfer of patient will be converted to an occurrence screening.
Dept of Medicine	1. Defective Bone Marrow Biopsy Needle	A defective bone marrow biopsy needle resulted in a broken needle remaining in the iliac crest of a patient, requiring a surgical procedure to remove the needle.	A report has been sent to investigate. Hematology-Oncology will continue to follow this to resolution.

EXHIBIT 6.H4 continues

EXHIBIT 6.H4 Continued

PROBLEMS/ISSUES/PROJECTS

Monitoring Activities	Conclusion	Recommendations/Actions
2. Lack of outpatient peritoneal dialysis capability.	Dr ___ is working to obtain staffing for this critically needed dialysis modality. There has been significant progress regarding this issue. Solution may occur in near future.	Continue interaction with nursing service.
3. Lack of acute dialysis. Evaluation of this issue shows that the ICU personnel have traditionally been responsible for maintenance of the acute peritoneal dialysis machine cycler and associated equipment. Recently the machine cycler, tubing, and dialysis solutions were found nonfunctional, not available, or expired, leaving us without this capability.	Purchasing and requisition forms are being submitted for the purchase of two new Travenol Peritoneal Automated cyclers. Dialysis fluid should be stocked at all times in CNS. There should be frequent inservices by the nursing service on implementation of acute peritoneal dialysis.	Continued diligence in following purchase order problem will be reviewed by Dec. 88.
1. Lack of screening mammogram service.	Manpower restrictions, prevent the Dept. of Radiology from	Exploration of other avenues to facilitate

Radiology Service	revealed no present or future plan to reinitiate screening mammography.	providing screening mammography service. Yearly screening is the standard of care and should be recommended for all eligible patients.	access to screening mammography service.
Rheumatology Service	A beeper is needed for the clinic.	The doctor covering the clinic is not always in the clinic because of other responsibilities yet needs to be available for related problems.	This issue is to be referred to the division level.
Internal Medicine Service	Screening Mammography	The lack of screening mammography is compromising our health maintenance program and places us in an untenable position should a patient in the Internal Medicine Clinic develop breast cancer. Screening mammography is clearly the standard of care in the community. It is anticipated that we will suffer medicolegal consequences unless this situation is corrected.	Will generate a memo requesting department and division support. Also seeking additional support from other services such as Hematology-Oncology.
Mental Health Inpatient	1. Inadequate clearance both psychiatric and medical of patients prior to transfer for inpatient psychiatric admission.	In spite of no further occurrence screens, this continues to be a potentially significant QA/RM problem.	Will continue to monitor.

SOURCE: Provided by a site visit medical center and used with their permission (abbreviations and other details as in original).

EXHIBIT 6.H5 Examples of Clinical Indicators
_____

Clinical Outcome Indicators (Comparative)[a]

The rate of development of wound infections after clean or clean-contaminated surgical procedures. Possible threshold for review: 2.5 percent.

Each patient with a systolic blood pressure on admission greater than 150 mm Hg or diastolic pressure greater than 95 mm Hg has his or her blood pressure measured and recorded in the medical record at least twice during the 24 hours following admission to the inpatient unit.
Possible compliance threshold: 98 percent.

Clinical Outcome Indicators (Sentinel)

Unplanned readmissions to a hospital shortly after inpatient surgery.

Mortality among patients treated in the hospital for injuries sustained immediately prior to treatment when death occurs within thirty days of injury or during a hospitalization that was precipitated by the occurrence of the injury.

Failed intubation during anesthesia.
Severe adverse drug reactions.
Ocular injury during anesthesia care.
Patient transfer from post-surgical unit to operating rooms.

Nursing QA Monitors (Sentinel)

Joint in central venous line not taped to prevent separation.
_____
[a]SOURCE: Joint Commission, 1989e

review committee of those cases failing to meet criteria for justification, and (4) documentation in minutes of findings, conclusions, recommendations, actions, and follow-up.

Blood Usage Review

Review of blood usage includes assessment of justification for transfusions, review of transfusion reactions, approval of policies on transfusion, monitoring transfusion services, and blood product ordering (Longo et al., 1989). As in surgical review, screens are developed based on criteria for justified transfusion episodes (Exhibit 6.H9). The clinical review nurse may screen for blood usage while doing utilization review. Cases failing screens are forwarded for review by the blood usage review committee.

Drug Usage Evaluation

Drug usage review has been broadened from what was once the review of antibiotic use only. It includes review of the indications and justifications for drug use, appropriate monitoring of drug levels, and correct dosage and route (e.g., oral or intravenous). Drugs for review might be high-volume or high-risk drugs or those considered important by the medical staff for other reasons such as unusual toxicity or potential for interaction with other drugs (see Exhibit 6.H10 for an example of cardiology drug review).

Pharmacy and Therapeutics Review

In addition to medical staff, pharmacy personnel, nursing personnel, and hospital administrators are likely to be involved in pharmacy and therapeutics review. Along with approving pharmacy policies and procedures and maintaining the hospital formulary, the pharmacy and therapeutics review committee also reviews serious untoward drug reactions.

Medical Record Review

Medical record review is conducted by a medical record review committee. It consists primarily of the review of records—such as admission history, operative notes, and discharge diagnosis for DRG assignment—of discharged patients to determine the timeliness of completion of various elements of care.

Focused Review

Focused review of care may take place when occurrence screening or clinical indicators warrant further evaluation. Unlike the retrospective audits of traditional quality assurance approaches, focused review is usually intended to be a prospective review, aimed at a particular topic or practitioner, and it remains in place until actual performance reaches a level of expected performance (Longo et al., 1989). Examples of topics for focused review might include infertility workup or hysterectomy in the obstetrics-gynecology (OB-GYN) department, workup of newly diagnosed diabetics in an internal medicine department, cholecystectomy in a department of general surgery, and streptococcal endocarditis in a department of infectious disease. Focused review utilizes principles of criteria development, data collection, analysis, and dissemination to the relevant clinical departments or staff committees (Longo et al., 1989). One hospital in New York City, for instance, conducts a chart review of all patient deaths within 24 hours of death, or within 72 hours when an autopsy is performed.

Peer Review

Peer review as a formal process is part of the functions listed previously. Once screens or monitors indicate further review is necessary, medical records are reviewed by a physician advisor in the clinical department or in the

EXHIBIT 6.H6 Example of Integrated Patient Care Monitoring - Data Source Document for Quality Assurance, Risk Management and Utilization Review

---

Adm. Date _____   Age _____   Sex _____   Physician Code _____   Ins. _____

Patient Code _____   Service Code _____   Adm. Unit _____

D/C Unit _____   D/C Date _____   Final Diagnosis _____

Appropriate Admission   Yes _____   No _____   Comments_____

Appropriate Cont. Stay   Yes _____   No _____   Comments_____

Appropriate D/C   Yes _____   No _____   Comments_____

Appropriate D/C Planning   Yes _____   No _____   Comments_____

Mortality   Yes _____   No _____   Anticipated _____   Not Anticipated _____

Possible Cause _____   Autopsy Ordered Yes _____   No ____

Generic Screens   None _____   Type_____

Complications   None _____   Type_____

Surgery: None _____   Meets Criteria
Date   Surg.   Surgeon   Consent   Note   Rept.   Yes   No   N/A
____   _____   _____   _____   ____   ____   ___   ___   ___
____   _____   _____   _____   ____   ____   ___   ___   ___
____   _____   _____   _____   ____   ____   ___   ___   ___

Procedures: None _____   Results   Meets Criteria
Date   Procedure   Physician   Consent   WNL   ABN   Yes   No   N/A
____   _____   _____   _____ ____   ____   ____   ___   ___
____   _____   _____   _____ ____   ____   ____   ___   ___
____   _____   _____   _____ ____   ____   ____   ___   ___

Medical Record Review: Meets Criteria   Yes _____   No _____   Phys. 1/Var._____
Admit ____   H&P____   Prog. Notes _____   Consults _____   Phys. 2/Var._____
Blood Utilization: Consent Yes _____   No _____   Phys. 2/Var._____
None _____   Total Units   Criteria #   Variation#
PRBC's   _____   _____   _____
Whole Blood _____   _____   _____
Platelets   _____   _____   _____
Plasma   _____   _____   _____

Date   Time   Date   Time   Date   Time

Medical Staff Appropriateness Monitoring Dept. _____   Monitor _____
Meets Criteria: Yes _____   No _____   N/A _____   Variation #_____
Comments:_____
_____
_____

EXHIBIT 6.H6 continues

quality assurance department. The physician advisor reviews the record and may ask the responsible physician to discuss the case or to provide further information. Sometimes immediate intervention is warranted to ensure that the patient is given appropriate care.

In contrast to the earlier methods described (which might be seen by practitioners as fairly mechanistic), peer review is generally reserved for

EXHIBIT 6.H6 Continued

CARDIOPULMONARY Test/Procedures	Meets Criteria Yes No N/A	Variation #	Comments

PHYSICAL THERAPY Test/Procedures	Meets Criteria Yes No N/A	Variation #	Comments

PHARMACY Test/Procedures	Meets Criteria Yes No N/A	Variation #	Comments

UTILIZATION REVIEW

QA Coord.	Date	Diagnosis	Description	Discharge Planning

QA Coord.	Date	Phys. Called	Purpose

Outcome _____

Actual L.O.S. _____   < or > DRG Days _____   Comments if > _____
_____

Transfer   Yes ____   No ____   To _____   Reason _____

Transfer. Form Complete   Yes ____   No ____

SOURCE: Pasadena Bayshore Medical Center, Pasadena, Texas, used with permission (abbreviations and other details as in original).

the last stage, in which a "comparable" physician passes judgment using his or her sense of the entirety of the medical care. This approach offers an opportunity for more evidence to be brought forward and thus a chance to recognize not unreasonable decisions; peer review generally reinforces a strong collegial sense of the complexity and uncertainties in the case.

After reviewing the record, the physician advisor may decide that the quality problem was not practitioner-related. The problem could have resulted from an unforeseeable patient complication, such as an allergic reac-

EXHIBIT 6.H7 Examples of Department-Specific Indicators

INTERNAL MEDICINE SCREENS
    Review of medication errors or major adverse drug reactions with serious
        potential for harm or resulting in special measures to correct (intubation,
        cardiopulmonary resuscitation, gastric lavage)
    Management of patients with primary diagnosis of hypertension:
        Blood pressure recorded daily, and once on both arms
        Blood urea nitrogen or creatinine, done once
        Electrocardiogram, done once
        Fundoscopy, done once
        Radiologic exam of chest, done once
        IVP or other renal/endocrine screening measures, if appropriate
        Electrolyte profile
    Management of acute renal failure:
        Monitoring of blood urea nitrogen, creatinine clearance
        Serial quantification of urine output
        Provide dialysis or refer patient for dialysis when creatinine clearance is less
            than 10 cc/min, serum creatinine is greater than 7 mg. %
        Document patency of urinary tract
        Document presence of adequate blood supply to kidneys (i.e. renal isotope
            study, etc.) when clinical situations dictate
    Review cases with cardiac catheterization complications:
        Contrast media reaction
        Evidence of arteriothrombosis following procedure
        Hematoma or excessive bleeding at injection site
        Circulatory impairment of the extremity
        Cerebrovascular accident during or within 24 hours of the procedure
        Medication error, requiring intervention
        Dissection of artery during acute PTCA requiring intervention
        Equipment malfunction/failure/disconnection that results in or has the
        potential to result in patient injury
CRITICAL CARE UNIT SCREENS
    Review of readmissions to the unit within 48 hours after transfer
    Complications occurring after central line insertion
    Review of reintubations within 24 hours of extubation
    Equipment failure
        Ventilator malfunction
        Defibrillator malfunction
        Intravenous (IV) pump failure
        Pacemaker battery pack failure
    Compliance with protocols for use of wrist restraints
    Compliance with protocol for Swan Ganz
    Compliance with NRM policy
    Review of incident reports
    Review of all deaths in critical care units
FAMILY PRACTICE INDICATORS
    Physical exams are done on chemical dependency patients
    Appropriate treatment recommendation are made for chemical dependency pa-
        tients
    Failure to obtain consultation when indicated:

Patient has shown no progress
Patient's condition has deteriorated (exclude if terminal on admission)
Dismissal of primary physician by patient or family
Unsubstantiated diagnosis eg. no appropriate x-rays, lab, other test to confirm diagnosis
IFMC [PRO] quality of care issues
Unnecessary admission to the hospital
Inappropriate admission to unit
Quality of care monitors for patients with acute stroke (including embolus, transient ischemic attack, occlusion of pre-cerebral artery):
    Presence of radiologic exam of central nervous system
Quality of care monitors for adult patients with pneumonia:
    Chest x-ray is present
    Smear and culture of sputum and/or bronchial secretions
    Culture and sensitivity studies with antibiotic therapy
    Appropriate bacterial investigation prior to starting antibiotic therapy
Quality of care monitors for patients with abdominal pain, etiology unknown:
    Documented plan of action for diagnostic investigation (e.g., complete blood count, urinalysis, serum amylase, rectal and pelvic exam, barium contrast studies, intravenous pyelogram, KUB, chest x-ray, surgical procedures)

PSYCHIATRY SCREENS
If the patient is admitted to the psych unit by a physician who is not a psychiatrist, a psychiatric consultation must be obtained within 24 hours
A comprehensive treatment plan by staffing must be done with the physician in attendance on each patient, describing problems, goals, and estimated dates of achievement
Initial staffing within 60 hours and weekly staffing review thereafter
Progress notes must be completed at least every 48 hours
Renewal of seclusion and restraint orders every 48 hours
Social history will be on the chart within 48 hours after admission to the unit
Review of all suicides or attempted suicides
Transfer from a psychiatric unit to a medical, surgical, or intensive care unit when primary care becomes medical (oxygen, IVs, fever more than 48 hours, draining infections, cardiac monitoring)
Patient on suicide precautions within 2 days of discharge will be reviewed by Psychiatry Section
Patients discharged against medical advice will be reviewed
Patients with assaultive behavior or assaulted patients will be reviewed

EMERGENCY MEDICINE SCREENS
Correlation of clinical and radiology results
Compliance with chest pain protocol
Review of patients whose emergency room stay is longer than 4 hours
Review of all deaths in emergency room and deaths within 48 hours after admission
Review of patients who leave against medical advice
Review of patient who leave before being seen
Management of patients with renal colic/ureteral stone

SOURCE: Iowa Methodist Medical Center, used with permission (abbreviations and other details as in original).

EXHIBIT 6.H8 Example of Surgical Review Screens

{ } Outpatient   { } Inpatient

ACCOUNT # ——————
DATE   ——————

—————— 1. Improper or no informed consent for procedure performed
—————— 2. Preexisting acute condition (e.g. respiratory infection, conjuncti-
             vitis, etc.)
—————— 3. Patient classified by anesthesia Class III or above
—————— 4. History and physical not on chart
—————— 5. Lab repeated morning of surgery
—————— 6. Presurgical testing incomplete or not ordered
—————— 7. Wrong patient operated on*
—————— 8. Wrong procedure performed*
—————— 9. Unplanned removal or repair of an organ or body part not cov-
             ered in consent form* (Exception: incidental appendectomy,
             biopsy of an organ)
—————— 10. Foreign object or material found in or left in wound*
—————— 11. Incorrect needle, sponge, or instrument count or omission of a
             count required by hospital policy
—————— 12. Patient operated on for repair of a laceration, perforation, tear or
             puncture of an organ subsequent to performance of an inva-
             sive procedure*
—————— 13. Adverse results of anesthesia
—————— 14. Intubation resulting in injury*
—————— 15. Nerve damage noted postoperatively
—————— 16. Cardiac/respiratory arrest
—————— 17. Acute myocardial infarction during surgery or in PAR
—————— 18. Patient injured during transfer to or from the OR*
—————— 19. Any unusual or untoward incident (s)
—————— 20. Surgery more extensive than anticipated
—————— 21. Complication (s) of treatment or care
—————— 22. Patient/family complaints
—————— 23. Medication error
—————— 24. Break in sterile technique
—————— 25. Instrument/Equipment breakage or malfunction
—————— 26. Cancellation of surgery after patient's arrival or OR suite
—————— 27. Antibiotics given parenterally
—————— 28. Surgery started after 1300 (Same-Day), 1600 (OR)
—————— 29. Late discharge
—————— 30. Left Same-Day Surgery Unit against medical advice
—————— 31. Unplanned admission to hospital/SICU
—————— 32. Oxygen therapy { } Routine { } Special Order
—————— 33. This is an unplanned return to surgery
—————— 34. Death

*Requires Incident Report

Comments: ——————————————————————————————
——
——

SOURCE: Iowa Methodist Medical Center, used with permission (abbreviations
and other details as in original).

EXHIBIT 6.H9 Example of Indications for Transfusion of Whole Blood in Adults

---

1. Hypovolemia due to surgery, trauma, gastrointestinal or other blood loss documented by <u>one</u> of the following:
   a. Fall in blood pressure >20% or fall in systolic blood pressure to <100 mm Hg.
   b. Pulse > 100 per minute.
   c. 750 ml or greater estimated blood loss.
   d. Orthostatic change in blood pressure or pulse.
2. Continuous blood loss (or anticipated blood loss) at a rate greater than 100 ml/ 15 min.
3. Already received 10 units RBC's.
4. Massive transfusion (>10 units in 24 hours).

SOURCE: St. Luke's Episcopal Hospital, used with permission (abbreviations and other details as in original).

tion to diagnostic contrast media, or it might represent a "systems" problem, such as a failure to receive a laboratory report in timely fashion or unavailability of equipment. This information is useful for tracking problems in a department or on a hospitalwide basis; problems of this nature may be more appropriately linked to administrative and policymaking groups than to individual practitioners.

If the case is practitioner-related, the physician advisor may seek additional review from others in the same or a related specialty, the appropriate departmental or other committee, the department chair, or the medical director.[4]

One hospital described the tasks of peer review as the following: First, a physician advisor decides whether an adverse patient occurrence has taken place.[5] If the physician reviewer determines that the standard of care was met, the case is dropped. Second, if questions persist, a medical care evaluation committee can determine that the standard of care was or was not met (most prudent physicians given the same set of circumstances, would or would not have managed the situation in a similar fashion), or that it is questionable (other practitioners might have managed the case differently with presumably a better outcome, but there was no clear breach of the standard of care). The attending physician may attend the meeting, but not during voting. The department chairman attends as a nonvoting member. Third, the committee decides which persons, departments, or systems were most closely associated with the event. Fourth, the committee designates a severity score. Fifth, incidental findings that have a direct bearing on the patient's care are recorded.

Various systems for assigning levels of severity were described by hospitals. One guide proposes four severity categories (Longo et al., 1989):

EXHIBIT 6.H10 Example of Cardiology Drug Review

Ward _____

Privileged staff _____ Resident _____

	YES	NO	COMMENTS/NA
1. **Treatment Criteria** (Any NO=Departmental Review)			
a. Presentation consistent with acute MI *and*			
b. EKG evidence of acute MI *and*			
c. Recent onset of symptoms (less than 6 hours)			
2. **Contraindications** (Any YES=Departmental Review)			
a. Active internal bleeding			
b. History of cerebrovascular accident			
c. Receiving other thrombolytic therapy			
d. Recent intracranial or intraspinal trauma or surgery			
e. Intracranial neoplasm, AVM, or aneurysm			
f. Known bleeding diathesis			
g. Severe uncontrolled hypertension at the time of therapy: Systolic greater than 200 Diastolic greater than 110			
h. Recent (less than 10 days) traumatic CPR			
i. Recent (less than 10 days) severe trauma			

predictable events within standards of care, unpredictable events within standards of care, marginal deviation from standards of care, and significant deviation from standards of care. The severity scores may be used in profiling practitioner performance for reappointment and for documentation toward any further action to be taken. Results of review may be presented or distributed in summary form at departmental medical staff meetings.

In the mid-1980s, Congress recognized that one of the more important ways that the quality of health care could be assured was through vigorous peer review activity; it also acknowledged that peer review, as conducted by hospitals and medical societies, was encumbered by the perceived threat that antitrust and defamation actions could be brought against the organizations and their individual members. In response to this serious drawback to peer review, Congress enacted the Health Care Quality Improvement Act.[6] This act provides for the immunity of professional review bodies, their members and staff, persons under contract to such bodies, and persons par-

EXHIBIT 6.H10 Continued

Section 1. Occurrence Description (To be completed by person reporting occurrence) Include reviewer initials.

Section 2. Initial Review by QM Department

    Not provider related   To department for review   Copy to _____

Section 3. Departmental Review (Include results of professional review)

    A. Findings:

    B. Conclusions:

    C. Recommendations:

    D. Actions:

        /_____ / Provider related   /_____ / Not provider related

        _____ Predictable occurrence within standard of care

        _____ Unpredictable occurrence within standard of care

        _____ Occurrence related to marginal deviation from standard

        _____ Occurrence related to significant deviation from standard

Name/titles of providers responsible for occurrence

Name and signature of reviewer   Date

Department head signature

Section 4. QM Disposition, Recommendation, Actions, and Follow-up:

_____ To credentials file   _____ To be trended   Copy to _____

QM Coordinator   QM Physician Advisor

SOURCE: Longo et al., 1989, used with permission.

ticipating or assisting in professional peer review from liability under the laws of the United States and of any state, so long as specified standards are met.

The Health Care Quality Improvement Act of 1986. The Health Care Quality Improvement Act (HCQIA), Title IV of P.L. 99-660, was enacted in November 1986 to "encourage professional peer review in order to restrict the ability of physicians and dentists to move their practices from one state to another without disclosure or discovery of previous substandard performance or unprofessional conduct." It is scheduled to be implemented in April, 1990. Part A is mainly concerned with peer review; Parts B and C, which relate to reporting of disciplinary actions, are discussed in the section on ambulatory care, later in this chapter.

Part A of the HCQIA provides professional review entities and physicians participating in the peer review process immunity from private civil antitrust suits (with a few exceptions) arising from review actions that have been "undertaken in good faith by health care entities and professional societies." This protection is believed to be critical to successful quality assurance, the basis of which lies in peer review and review of credentials. The peer review specifications for protection under this act are very explicit; action must be taken in the furtherance of quality health care, after a reasonable effort has been made to obtain the facts, following adequate notice of action and hearing procedures, and with the belief that the disciplinary actions are warranted by the facts. Several individuals and groups are covered under the antitrust immunity provisions of this Act. They include professional review bodies (i.e., a health care entity, the governing body or committee of a health care entity, and any committee of the medical staff when assisting the governing body), individuals, and those persons providing information to professional review bodies.

Patrick v. Burget appeared to many members of the medical profession, including the American Medical Association (AMA), to pose serious limits to the degree of protection from antitrust liability (and its treble damages awards) provided by the HCQIA (Holthaus, 1988).[7] The plaintiff, Dr. Patrick, claimed that doctors on a hospital peer review committee criticized the care he provided his patients, sought to terminate his hospital privileges at the only hospital in the community, and acted against him because he was in competition with them. An initial judgment went in Dr. Patrick's favor. The appellate court, however, then found the defendants not liable on antitrust grounds, although it noted that they had engaged in "shabby, unprincipled and unprofessional activities" against Dr. Patrick. The court grounded its decision on the exemption from antitrust laws of state regulatory authorities and of private parties enforcing state policies through activities "closely supervised" by state officials. In an 8-0 ruling, the U.S. Supreme Court reinstated a $2.2-million award initially won by Dr. Patrick. The Supreme Court ruled that despite the fact that Oregon law requires reviews for medical competence, the process is not so closely supervised by state authorities to qualify for the "state action" exemption. The court further noted that the defendants were not protected by the HCQIA because that act insulates only those peer review activities conducted in the reasonable belief that they are in furtherance of quality health care.

In the wake of *Patrick v. Burget*, there was a question of just how vigorous non-Medicare peer review should be. Since the ruling, it has become clear that its impact was not as devastating as first feared (Cross and Berman, 1988; Holthaus, 1988). In *Bolt v. Halifax Hospital Center et al.* the U.S. Circuit Court of Appeals answered a question left open by *Patrick*: if the state courts retain the power to overturn a peer review decision, are peer review bodies and their members shielded from federal antitrust scrutiny under the state action doctrine? The court ruled that:

> judicial review cannot constitute active state supervision [required for application of the state action doctrine] unless it is available on an established basis and is of a sufficiently probing nature. To be sufficiently probing, the scope of judicial review must first of all encompass the fairness of the procedures used in reaching the decision. Furthermore, it must involve consideration of whether criteria used by decision makers were consistent with state policy and whether the decision had sufficient basis in fact. Our review of Florida case law convinces us that such review is available in Florida courts.

This decision, which technically applies only to the 11th district federal courts, appears to protect peer review under the state action doctrine if it is subject to judicial review to determine whether it incorporates due process and is performed in accordance with the state's law. The *Bolt* ruling also provides, according to one authority, that state judicial review of peer review will meet state action doctrine requirements "even under circumstances where judicial review is not required in every case" (Holthaus, 1988, p. 34).

Another case that may prove of some importance in protecting non-Medicare peer review from antitrust liability is *Mitchell v. Howard Memorial Hospital.* In *Mitchell,* the 9th Circuit Court of Appeals ruled that peer review actions by the 38-bed Howard Memorial Hospital did not significantly affect interstate commerce and thus found the hospital exempt from liability under those statutes. Antitrust laws apply only where interstate commerce is affected. Although the hospital did carry on interstate commerce, the court said the volume of such commerce was not substantial. The effect may be that peer review bodies at small hospitals or at hospitals in isolated, rural areas may be protected under the Commerce Clause.

These cases make it clear that non-Medicare peer review has not been severely impaired by the *Patrick* decision. In general, peer review can be carried out in most cases without fear by members of the risk of liability.

Case Conferences

Case conferences are primarily educational meetings in which physicians review the care of difficult cases. The case may be presented because it was unusual or complex, forced difficult management choices, or had an adverse outcome. The discussion may cover a great many topics such as the value of new technologies, approaches to care that might have been more conservative, clinical findings that were overlooked, or an ethical dilemma presented by the case.

The Morbidity and Mortality (M&M) conference is a department-based conference that occurs after autopsy, typically after a surgical procedure. The course of illness and diagnostic, autopsy, and pathology findings are presented and discussed by the attending physician and pathologist.

Case conferences are highly valued by clinicians as an effective method of learning. They are conducted in a nonjudgmental atmosphere and are considered clinically pertinent. They accord with medical training in that they focus on individual cases.

Autopsy Findings

Although the proportion of hospital deaths that are accompanied by autopsy has declined greatly in recent years (from 50 percent in the 1940s to 14 percent in 1985) (Geller, 1983; MMWR, 1988), unexpected findings at autopsy are still considered to be an excellent way to refine clinical judgment and identify possible misdiagnosis. Landefeld and Goldman (1989, p. 42) summarized numerous studies that show that in 5 to 10 percent of cases, "treatable, major unexpected findings have been discovered that, if known premortem, would probably have improved the patient's chance of survival. Other major unexpected findings were revealed in another 10 percent of cases." Autopsies can provide information on the rates of and reasons for discrepancies between clinical diagnoses and postmortem findings.

Utilization Review

Quality and utilization review functions are sometimes linked to minimize duplicative review of the medical record (as noted earlier with respect to activities of a quality assurance department). Patients with extended lengths of stay in comparison to norms are likely to have experienced some adverse occurrence (PRO, personal communication, 1989). Similarly, patients who remain in the hospital longer than medically necessary because of placement problems are at risk of adverse events in a hospital environment that is geared to acute, short-term care.

Software designed for utilization review such as the ISD-A Review System[8] (InterQual, 1987) is widely used to assess intensity of services, severity of illness, and appropriateness of discharge. Each instrument consists of a series of criteria that are applied, regardless of the patients' diagnosis, to determine whether inpatient care is justified. The relevant information comes from the medical record, and the instrument is used by nonphysician reviewers.

The Appropriateness Evaluation Protocol (AEP) was developed in Boston in the late 1970s and early 1980s and has been revised by Gertman and his colleagues (Gertman and Restuccia, 1981). The AEP assesses the appropriateness of timing and level of care for adult and noninfant pediatric patients. If any of 16 admission criteria are met, the admission is deemed appropriate. If any of 20 day-of-care criteria are met, that day is deemed appropriate (Payne, 1987).

Both internal and external groups have developed increasing interest in severity-of-illness software that is used to predict resource use and to assess the case-mix of the hospital. These software products include the Computerized Severity Index (CSI), Disease Staging, MedisGroups, and Patient Management Categories. The APACHE II system focuses on physiologic measures of patients treated in critical care units. Such software is sometimes claimed to provide quality-related information (Aronow, 1988). For instance, MedisGroups (MediQual, 1986) suggests that an increase in patient severity level between the time of admission and a later time (say the 6th or 10th day after admission) may indicate a problem in quality that would merit further review. It does not, however, claim to measure quality per se.

Discharge Planning

Quality assurance and discharge planning are sometimes integrated as well. Review forms for concurrent screening may include discharge screens to indicate when patients are ready (or not ready) for discharge. When discharge screens are not met the case is referred to the attending physician.

Infection Control

The Centers for Disease Control have estimated that 5 percent of all patients admitted to a general hospital in the United States will develop a nosocomial infection (Haley et al., 1987). These rates are even higher for patients who are very ill, have had invasive procedures, or who are immunologically compromised. Hospital infection control programs have been established to prevent and to promote early identification and control of infections, and they are required by the Joint Commission as a hospitalwide function. Infection control is the earliest and most well developed program of epidemiological surveillance in hospitals. Historically, the goals of infection control have included "public health" programs and policies designed to prevent the spread of infection, including isolation and waste disposal policies. The programs recognize discrete patient infections when they occur and are designed to identify wider infectious outbreaks and to trace their causes. This may require investigation and alterations in traffic patterns, storage policies, ventilation patterns and air exchange rates, and laboratory practices. For example, staff at one site visit hospital related the experience of tracing a series of infections to an ice bucket used during surgery.

In addition, infection control programs, under the direction of an infection control officer, are responsible for employee health programs and staff education (for further information see the *Accreditation Manual* Infection Control Standard [Joint Commission, 1989b]). Some states, such as New York, require that infection control activities be integrated with the hospital quality assurance program. Many quality assurance programs have done so because they consider it good practice; moreover, in many small hospitals the coordinator of quality assurance has many responsibilities including that of infection control specialist (Longo et al., 1989).

With the adoption of the outcome screening approach to other areas in the hospital, some hospitals have moved from "whole house surveillance" (tracking the occurrences of all infections) to more targeted review. Nosocomial infections are detected by a trained reviewer during concurrent and retrospective generic screening of the medical record by diagnoses listed, symptoms recorded in progress notes, or positive laboratory slips. Another way to detect an infectious outbreak is to review antibiotic use.

Reports to the infection control committee include rates of infection by site (e.g., urinary tract, respiratory, skin) and by service so that significant trends and patterns can be identified. Other hospitalwide data that may be summarized include rates of communicable and other reportable diseases and measures of employee exposure such as needle stick injuries and Hepatitis B vaccines given.

Risk Management

Asserted claims may be seen as an end point in a continuum of a grievance process. Intermediate (or alternative) steps taken by the patient may be filing a complaint, switching physicians, or refusing therapy. The aim of hospital risk management is to reduce financial losses and adverse publicity and to prevent reoccurrence of a similar event. The first step is often the implementation of an early warning system, the most traditional being the incident reporting system.[9] Health professionals are expected to report certain kinds of events to the risk management office. Although this reporting system is intended to include major events, such as surgical mishaps, incidents have traditionally been underreported and have involved largely "slips and falls" and "medication errors" that may have little clinical consequence. The American College of Surgeons estimated in 1985 that only 5 to 30 percent of major mishaps are reported on traditional incident forms (cited in GAO, 1989, p. 15). In fact, the development of occurrence screening was originally a research tool to move beyond incident reporting to determine how frequently adverse events with potential legal liability were occurring. Now occurrence reporting and generic screening are seen to serve the purposes of both quality assessment and risk management; however, more work is needed to determine their reliability, validity, and cost-effectiveness for both applications (Morlock et al., 1989; OTA, 1988;).

Patient and Family Grievance Systems

Some hospitals have patient representative or ombudsman programs as a response to patient or family grievances. The role of the patient care representative is frequently that of loss control on behalf of the hospital. During site visits, hospitals did not stress this activity as serving a quality assurance function.

Patient and Employee Satisfaction Surveys

Most hospitals use some form of patient assessment survey. Because questionnaires are frequently distributed to patients at the time of discharge, however, response rates are typically very low. The Hospital Corporation of America has made surveys a central part of its effort to implement the continuous improvement model; their patient satisfaction questionnaire contains 11 patient judgment scales (Exhibit 6.H11).

Employees and attending staff are also the subject of surveys about patient care issues. At the time of our site visit, for example, the Cleveland Clinics were conducting a staff survey.

Patient Complaints

Reviewing complaints can be a method of detecting as well as correcting problems in care. Responding to complaints can have two valuable effects. It indicates to patients that the organization takes problems seriously, and it may prompt intraorganizational reforms that would not have been suggested by formal quality assurance mechanisms.

Observation

Observation is an unusual activity of formal quality assurance programs. The former medical director of an Air Force hospital described one innovative approach. He routinely assigned new staff to keep diaries of problems in patient care during their first month, and he required other staff to spend some of their first month observing the delivery of care and interpersonal process in patient care areas throughout the hospital. Proposals for resolving observed problems were presented to a staff meeting.

EXHIBIT 6.H11 Example of Elements in a Patient Satisfaction Survey Instrument for Hospitals

---

1. Admissions (i.e., efficiency of the admitting procedure, preparation for admission, attention of admitting staff to patient's individual needs).
2. Daily care (i.e., consideration of patient's needs, coordination of care, helpfulness and cheerfulness, sensitivity to problems).
3. Information (i.e., ease of getting information, instructions, informing family or friends).
4. Nursing care (i.e., skill of nurses, nurses' attention to patient's condition, nursing staff response to patient's call, concern and caring by nurses, information given by nurses).
5. Physician care (i.e., physician's attention to patient's condition, coordination of care, availability, concern and caring, skill, and information given by physicians).
6. Auxiliary staff (i.e., quality of laboratory staff, x-ray staff, physical therapy staff, intravenous therapy staff, transportation staff).
7. Living arrangements (i.e., privacy, restfulness, condition of room and hospital building, availability of parking, visitor arrangements).
8. Discharge (i.e., discharge procedures and instructions, coordination of postdischarge care).
9. Billing (i.e., explanations to patients about costs and handling of hospital bills, efficiency of billing process).
10. Total process (i.e., composite measure based on the scores of the nine previously listed process quality scales).
11. Allegiance (i.e., intention to use hospital again, likelihood of recommending hospital, whether patient has bragged about hospital to others).

SOURCE: Nelson et al., 1989, used with permission.

Note on Individual-Case Methods

Several methods of case-by-case problem detection have been developed and implemented in health care settings, such as autopsy and case conferences as previously described. Other approaches have administrative or even legal purposes, such as patient complaint and incident reporting systems. Still others might be considered monitoring devices to identify poor practitioners with the use of lengthy external processes. These include PRO sanctions, disciplinary actions by state medical boards, and malpractice settlements.

Two associated problems limit the value of case-by-case systems as problem detection methods. First, they have not in the past been aggregated and classified consistently so that patterns of quality-related problems can be found. Second, they are usually not linked to quality assurance efforts or even to a common reporting pathway (e.g., to the governing board), so they do not support analysis of patient problems, play a role in an integrated system of educational feedback, or otherwise help in "closing the loop" (Nelson, 1976).

External Methods of Correcting Problems in Hospitals

PRO Actions Regarding Physicians and Hospitals

The formal PRO sanction process is discussed in detail in Volume I, Chapter 6, and in Chapter 8 of this volume. Before a sanction recommendation is forwarded to the Office of Inspector General (OIG), PROs have a number of steps available to them involving interaction with the physician and the development of remedial actions.

The process is begun when the PRO identifies and confirms a relatively isolated but serious case of medical mismanagement or a pattern of problems and after a panel of peer physicians has evaluated the care by reviewing inpatient and outpatient records and has asked the attending physician by means of a Letter of Inquiry to respond to the allegations. If the response is unsatisfactory, the peer group develops specific charges and lists identified deficiencies in care that are the subject of sanction activity; that activity might include corrective action only or might eventually result in forwarding a sanction recommendation to the OIG. Dettmann and Simmons (1989, p. 3) describe the "prototype physician most likely to be susceptible to the sanction process" as,

> . . an overworked generalist working in isolation who does not have time to keep up by reading journals or who attends meetings in a perfunctory or disinterested manner. On the other hand, the prototype physician who is least likely to be subject to the sanction process would be a specialist with frequent contact with and oversight by professional colleagues including, perhaps, a residency program, taking time to read and write articles, presenting papers at local and regional meetings, participating in didactic educational programs, and maintaining a practice that allows adequate time to thoroughly study and digest the clinical aspects of his patients' situations.

It has also been pointed out that isolation may be a result not only of geography but also language, culture, or substance abuse.

If the practice issue is considered to be amenable to education and if the physician is receptive to this approach, a corrective action plan is developed, approved, implemented, reported to HCFA, and tracked for later evaluation. Corrective actions were stressed by PROs we visited as providing a much needed alternative to expulsion from the Medicare program or exoneration.

Corrective action may take various forms such as mandatory consultation for certain kinds of cases (often by telephone) or other corrective approaches that have been called focused continuing medical eduction (CME). The Texas Medical Foundation has been attempting to match the intensity of efforts to the level of risk to patients. A "low-risk case" is one involving a pattern of oversight, inattention to detail, but little risk. A moderate-risk situation is one where errors in judgment have been identified in two or more cases. A high level of risk is one where there is an apparent error in judgment and a lack of knowledge posing a significant risk to the patient. (An example was a physician who 2 days in a row gave insulin to an 83-year-old patient to stimulate her appetite.) One PRO described a problem involving moderate patient risk and the related intervention; in this case, a physician who repeatedly misused antibiotics but for whom a CME course had not been effective. The PRO required that he consult a handbook on antimicrobial therapy before prescribing any antibiotic and document in each case the most likely infective organism, the handbook's recommended drug of choice, and if not used, why this drug was not being prescribed.

Other focused CME approaches include self-education or self-assessment assignments. These might include Advanced Cardiac Life Support, the Surgical Education Self-Assessment Program of the American College of Surgeons, the Medical Knowledge Self-Assessment Program of the American College of Physicians, the Georgia Academy of Family Physicians Education Foundation (a self-assessment and continuing education course for family physicians), the Peer Assistance Recovery Program sponsored by the American Academy of Family Physicians, and other programs sponsored by specialty societies.

Sometimes physicians are referred to their hospital quality assurance committee for corrective action plans. One physician who discharged a patient prematurely was given pertinent journal articles. In addition, because of the potential patient risk he was the subject of focused review by his hospital for 90 days and was required to review 100 records of patients who had failed PRO generic screens.

Enrollment in local miniresidency programs, in continuing education courses, or in courses in a local medical school are another approach. In describing a newly developed six-stage remedial CME program in the Wisconsin PRO, Dettmann and Simmons (1989) identify the most likely departments for CME as those of family practice, medicine, surgery, OB-GYN, and pediatrics. For clinical continuing education (a miniresidency), the chief residents in these departments would be responsible for the one-on-one teaching. The PRO may help to locate a physician to take over the enrollee's practice temporarily during the miniresidency. Still other focused CME approaches are suggested literature reading, such as chapters in *Scientific American Medicine*. Subject areas for educational interventions most often include electrolyte management, choice of antibiotics, general cardiology, use of pacemakers, pre-operative preparation, surgery on an unstable patient or with unrecognized complications, and other areas of diagnosis and management (Dettman and Simmons, 1989).

The number of hours, type of CME, and amount of time permitted for completion depend on the level of severity and risk the PRO considers likely. For instance, for patterns of low-risk problems, 10 hours of specified CME in 6 months and 40 hours of general CME in 1 year would have to be completed. In contrast, for a pattern of high-risk deficiencies, 50 hours of PRO-specified CME would have to be completed in 6 months. The PRO must monitor performance on an intensified basis during and after completion of the corrective action plan by, for example, pre-admission and pre-procedure, concurrent, and pre-discharge screening. The PRO may also notify the state medical board and appropriate hospital committees.

Some PROs prefer to develop and monitor corrective actions themselves. Other PROs see themselves as catalysts and stress the considerable advantage in involving the physician's hospital as a way of reinforcing internal quality assurance activities and CME coordinators. They also point out that some problems go well beyond the single physician identified and may involve protocols and changes in rules. The issue of whether the PRO must notify the hospital, may notify the hospital, or is prohibited from notifying the hospital at stages before sanction recommendations are forwarded, however, has been an ambiguous one, with PROs differing substantially in their interpretation of HCFA rules.

Actions by State Entities

The Massachusetts Board of Registration has developed prescription practice guidelines for practitioners. It has also encouraged speciality societies to develop practice guidelines for use in hospitals. Two examples are in anesthesiology and neonatal monitoring. The board monitors corrective disciplinary actions undertaken by hospitals, such as monitoring or proctoring of a surgeon or limiting privileges, through periodic reports to the board. If the board believes that the hospital is not acting in good faith, it can fine the hospital. The board retains the prerogative to restrict, suspend, or revoke licensure.

Internal Methods of Correcting Problems in Hospitals

Event-Based Actions

Problems in care are corrected in a myriad of ways throughout hospitals. Most of these are case-oriented, informal, and involve some form of colleague notification. For example, a nurse, fellow clinician, the chief of a clinical department, a residency director, a laboratory technician, or pharmacist might become aware of a specific problem in the care of a patient and intervene by a telephone call, note, or in person. Hospitals also have patient representatives (also called ombudsmen) who may be contacted by a patient or the patient's family. Such problem detection and resolution is case-based, however, and is not generally considered to be part of a quality assurance program because of its "invisibility" internally and externally, and such an activity is typically not recorded, aggregated, or analyzed for possible further action.

Practice Pattern-Based Actions

Corrective action directed at individual practitioners based on a pattern of poor process or outcomes varies in intensity. The quality assurance committee may review an enlarged sample of a given physician's records to validate a pattern of poor care, or an individual instance may result in some corrective action. At its most informal and noncoercive, it may take the form of reminders and exhortation by the medical director, chief of a department, or chairman of a quality assurance committee. These individuals, acting on behalf of the medical staff and in response to identified patterns of poor outcomes, may also invoke a variety of more serious actions. These can include requiring entrance in a residential impaired-physician program, remedial education in the form of courses or conferences, restriction of privileges, proctoring when certain procedures are performed, or mandatory consultation for specific kinds of cases such as admission to the intensive care or cardiac care unit (ICU or CCU) for certain diagnoses. In more extreme cases, admitting privileges may be withdrawn from the individual. Such an action, of course, entails very careful procedures to ensure fairness and avoid adverse legal action (Meyer, 1989). Continued monitoring of actions is necessary following any of these actions (except withdrawal of admitting privileges).

One hospital staff member described interventions as involving only the department chairman if the problem was minor. This might then result in sending a letter to or further monitoring of the physician involved. In the case of a "major" problem, the medical director would be alerted and corrective actions might include education and required consultation.

The study committee heard a great deal during site visits about gathering data on adverse events and clinical performance for the purpose of review and reporting. However, few examples were provided about how that information is given back to the providers on an ongoing basis. Indeed, it seems that attending or staff physicians typically hear very little about quality assurance activities unless there is a problem in the care they provide, nor are they typically involved in, or particularly interested in, the work of the quality assurance program. One hospital reported that it had involved physicians by providing salary and status to physicians who were involved in quality review, and they tried to make peer review part of the academic process in the clinical department meetings in their teaching hospital.

Organization-Based Actions

Some problems identified in the hospital are of a more general nature and reflect a breakdown in the systematic approach to patient care. Problems of this kind that were identified for us during site visits include: routine delays of several weeks in receiving autopsy results; a perception that surgical specialists did not call in medical specialists soon enough; a dispute between the departments of medicine and surgery on appropriateness standards for endoscopy; inordinate delays in initiating drug therapy due to pharmacy problems; delayed admission to the ICU, and an increasing patient/nurse ratio in the ICU resulting in demonstrably increased morbidity; long trips for patients with head injury for magnetic resonance imaging tests; and delayed patient discharges because plans for prostheses were not made early on and because the forms were difficult to complete. These problems may be caused by diffusion of or improperly delegated responsibility, inappropriate allocation of resources (e.g., equipment, personnel), or lack of timely data for patient care. Other problems in clinical care reflect a lack of updated knowledge or insufficient attention to the use of drugs or other technologies; for instance, inappropriate antibiotic prescribing or safety procedures in caring for patients with infectious disease. All these topics may be addressed at departmental meetings or hospital conferences. Policies may be changed, formalized, or restated in newsletters or other circulars. Information comparing their own performance to others in the department may also be distributed to physicians.

Staffing responsibilities, work patterns, and communication avenues may be changed. Many organizational factors may influence the effectiveness of quality assurance efforts. Particularly important may be the collaborative nature of medical practice. Knaus et al. (1986) studied treatment and outcomes of care in ICUs and hypothesized that differences in outcomes could be attributed to differences in clinician interaction and coordination, especially among doctors and nurses in such areas as continuity through primary care nursing, routine discussions of patient treatment, and staffing capacity.

Findings from quality review may also be used for facility planning by identifying the need for space, equipment, or staffing or the need to change current procedures or priorities. For recommendations to be carried out and result in improvement there must be a thorough understanding of the causes of the problem, appropriate interventions, and potential barriers to change, and there must be sufficient authority to bring about change at the appropriate level in the organization. That is, a departmental problem may be corrected within the department, but a cross-disciplinary problem may require action at the level of top management, the medical director, or the board of directors or trustees. Further, the level of detail or aggregation of data needed for appropriate interventions will differ depending on whether the actions are directed at individuals, groups of practitioners, or across an entire facility. Identification of problems and implementation of these changes entail reevaluation as part of the overall quality assurance process.

Although many hospitals still track progress on identified problems with manual systems, some have developed or purchased software to track progress on quality indicators from identification through assessment of contributing factors, corrective actions, and monitoring. In some cases these indicator tracking data bases are integrated with other quality assurance subsystems such as credentialing, risk management, incident reporting, and generic screens.

Continuous Improvement Approaches

Another approach to organizational change is embodied in the "continuous improvement" model as described in Volume I, Chapter 2. Organizations that have implemented this model may convene a task force or team to examine review findings, the expectations of customers, and needs of suppliers, and to delineate all the steps in a process to understand the most promising places for improvement.

For example, West Paces Ferry Hospital, an HCA hospital in Atlanta, Georgia, is studying more efficient use of its operating rooms by decreasing delays between scheduled operations. An eight-page flow diagram identified all the steps taken by patients and hospital personnel to ready the patient and operating room for surgery. An observational study of 100 cases demonstrated the proportion of delays and average time contributed by delays related to the surgeon, patient, equipment, or staff. Although 45 percent of the delays in the operating room were a result of surgeon unavailability, the team determined that patient availability (29 percent of all delays) presented the greatest potential for successful improvement. This led to an examination and redesign of the pre-admission process and to a physician and patient education program to increase the percentage of patients who are pre-admitted. The hospital found that from the start of the study in October 1988 to July 1989 (after the intervention period) the percentage of patients pre-admitted rose from 14 percent to over 75 percent (information provided at site visit and cited with permission).

AMBULATORY CARE

Preventing Problems in Ambulatory Care

Methods of preventing quality problems in ambulatory care focus on both individuals and organizations. Efforts aimed at the former include licensure and certification for physicians in solo and office-based group practice as well as credentialing and privileging activities (similar to those in hospitals) in ambulatory care facilities such as clinics, independent practice association (IPA) HMOs, and staff-model HMOs. Efforts aimed at facilities themselves include accreditation and licensure, state department standards, and Conditions of Participation for Medicare risk-contract HMOs and competitive medical plans (CMPs).

External Methods of Preventing Problems Directed at Individuals (Physicians)

Credentials, Licensure, and Specialty Certification

Credentials are given considerable weight as methods of assuring high quality. The process is used (1) by state boards in granting licenses to practice, (2) by specialty and subspecialty boards in granting certification, (3) by hospital committees in reviewing applications to the medical staff, and (4) by payers in determining eligibility to be paid for services (Chassin et al., 1989a). Two areas of credentials, licensure and board certification, are emphasized by these groups.

Physician Licensure[10]

Each state has statutes regulating the practice of medicine through physician licensure. Most of these laws define the practice of medicine and prohibit those who are unlicensed from engaging in it. State medical practice acts are administered by state boards of medical examiners. Those who apply for licensure are judged on the basis of their education, postgraduate training and experience, results on licensing examinations, and moral character. Applicants for licensure must be graduates of schools of medicine or osteopathy accredited by the Liaison Committee on Medical Education, with special provisions being made for graduates of foreign medical schools. A postgraduate internship of 1 year is required by approximately three-quarters of the states, and applicants must successfully pass a licensing examination. All states currently use the Federation Licensing Examination, prepared by the National Board of Medical Examiners (NBME) for the Federation of State Medical Boards. Most states will also accept the so-called National Boards, also prepared by NBME or by the National Board of Examiners for Osteopathic Physicians and Surgeons. These examinations are administered in three stages as students progress through their education (Havighurst, 1988).

Some states have reciprocity agreements, whereby licenses granted by them are recognized in other states. Other states require that an applicant go through the procedures specified in their medical practice acts regardless of being licensed in another state (Havighurst, 1988).

The Health Care Quality Improvement Act of 1986

Part B of the HCQIA establishes a National Practitioner Data Bank (NPDB) for collection of several types of information. First, information concerning disciplinary action by state medical and dental boards regarding the license of a physician or dentist must be reported to the data bank. Second, all malpractice payments made by any entity on behalf of licensed health care practitioners as a result of a court judgment or an out-of-court settlement must be reported to the data bank. Third, reporting is required for all adverse actions taken against a physician's or dentist's clinical privileges that lasts more than 30 days and for the surrender of privileges as an agreement not to investigate further. Finally, professional societies must report "their adverse actions taken against the membership of a physician or dentist when they have reached that action through peer review (due process) and when they assess practitioner competency and/or professional conduct."

A 5-year $15.9-million contract has been awarded through a competitive bidding process to UNISYS to establish and operate the NPDB. The data bank, expected to be operational in 1990, will be overseen by the Division of Quality Assurance and Liability Management, Bureau of Health Professions, in the Health Resources and Service Administration, Public Health Service. No retroactive information will be entered into the data bank.

After the NPDB becomes operational, all hospitals must consult it when a physician, dentist, or other licensed health care practitioner seeks to join the staff or receive clinical privileges. Other health care entities and state licensing boards may query the data bank when they need information "to achieve their mission." Hospitals are also required to consult the data bank every 2 years regarding all physicians and health care professionals on staff. Individuals have access to their own records in the NPDB. UNISYS is also required, as part of its contract, to provide a research service program "through which aggregate data stripped of identifiers will be available to interested parties."

Part C of the HCQIA contains detailed definitions pertinent to Parts A and B. (Part A pertains mainly to peer review and was discussed earlier in the section on "Internal Methods of Detecting Problems in Hospitals.") It also requires various reports to the Congress (e.g., a review of small malpractice awards), and it encourages participation by other federal agencies in the data bank.

Specialty Certification and Recertification

The American Board of Medical Specialties (ABMS) recognizes 23 specialty boards that certify physicians as medical specialists in carefully delineated areas of practice. Several other entities also certify physicians, but because the ABMS system is so dominant, "board certification" is generally taken to mean certification in a medical specialty by a board recognized by ABMS (Havighurst and King, 1983).

For a specialty board to achieve "accreditation" status, it must be sponsored by a professional group, such as a specialty society, and by the appropriate scientific section of the AMA. All the boards are evaluated for recognition according to the ABMS "Essentials for Approval of Examining Boards in Medical Specialties." Each board thus requires similar levels of training and experience.

The residency program must be approved by the Accreditation Council for Graduate Medical Education (ACGME), an organization composed of members of ABMS, the AMA, and other concerned organizations. Together with appropriate specialty boards, ACGME develops accreditation standards for each specialty residency program. These are regularly modified in conjunction with changing specialty board requirements and must be approved by the AMA's Council on Medical Education (Havighurst and King, 1983). Ultimately, candidates must also pass comprehensive examinations administered by the specialty board.

Candidates for board certification must receive and complete specialty training in an approved graduate medical program, the length and extent of which varies somewhat among the specialties. A majority of physicians in the United States identify themselves as specialists, but only about one-half are certified by an ABMS board. The number seeking certification has grown and continues to grow rapidly. Almost all physicians newly entering practice now seek some sort of certification. Of those who designate themselves as specialists, an increasing number are actually board certified.

External Methods of Preventing Problems Directed at Institutions

Accreditation

Ambulatory facilities can seek accreditation on a voluntary basis from the Accreditation Association for Ambulatory Health Care and from the Joint Commission's Accreditation Program for Ambulatory Health Care. The National Committee on Quality Assurance (NCQA) offers accreditation to HMOs. The Joint Commission has also just begun to offer accreditation for managed care organizations. To date, these forms of voluntary accreditation have been used only infrequently. The Joint Commission currently accredits over 300 ambulatory programs, chiefly hospital-sponsored programs, government-sponsored programs, and ambulatory surgery centers (Couch, 1989).

In 1989 the Joint Commission released an updated manual *Ambulatory Health Care Standards Manual*. The voluntary accreditation program is not available to solo practitioners; its primary application is for the ambulatory care clinics, ambulatory surgery centers, college or university health programs, community health centers, emergency care centers, group practices, HMOs, primary care centers, and urgent care centers. Hospital-sponsored fee-for-service and managed care outpatient facilities that are operated under the same governing board must be accredited at the time of the hospital accreditation process during their next scheduled accreditation visit.

The Quality Assurance Standard for ambulatory care requires that "an ongoing quality assurance program [exists that is] designed to objectively and systematically monitor and evaluate the quality and appropriateness of patient care, pursue opportunities to improve patient care, and resolve identified problems (Joint Commission, 1989c, p. 3)." The program must be focused on several issues—that is, prevent, detect, and correct problems. The Joint Commission encourages each provider to develop its own indicators of quality for the respective clinical care area. Examples of some possible indicators in the ambulatory care setting were suggested by Flanagan (1985). These include allergic reactions to immunization or allergy injections, miscarriage, high cholesterol levels, patients receiving more than two antibiotics, overlooked pregnancy in radiology, patients unable to leave an ambulatory surgery facility 2 to 4 hours postoperatively, or patients seen twice within 72 hours and subsequently admitted.

NCQA was formed in 1979 to perform quality-of-care reviews for the Office of Health Maintenance Organizations (OHMO) in the Department of Health and Human Services (DHHS). More recently it was restructured to assure independence of the HMO industry. The survey process includes an assessment of the organization's quality assurance program, interviews with key staff, review of appropriate records, and review of a sample of medical records. Surveyors include physicians who themselves are from the HMO community. The survey process results in a decision for full approval, provisional approval (subject to modifications), or denial.

External Methods of Preventing Problems Directed at Prepaid or Managed Health Care Plans

Federal HMO Act

The HMO Act of 1973 required that HMOs seeking federally qualified status meet certain standards of organizational structure, benefit levels, and financial stability, and that they have an organized medical structure capable of providing clinical services that, in turn, are subjected to quality review. They must have an ongoing quality assurance program with an emphasis on health outcomes. During the 1980s, however, federal budget reductions precluded OHMO from continuing to contract for quality reviews.

State HMO Regulations

State regulations cover many aspects of HMO services, financial arrangements, grievance procedures, and quality assurance programs. In Kansas, for instance, a new law requires independent, on-site quality-of-care inspections at least once every 3 years. In California, the Knox-Keene Health Care Service Plan Act of 1975 (Section 1370, Title 10, California Administrative Code) stipulates licensure requirements for some 60 health care service plans serving 8 million Californians. Included in that act is a requirement for internal quality-of-care review systems: "Every plan shall establish procedures in accordance with department regulations for continuously reviewing the quality of care, performance of medical personnel, utilization of services and facilities, and costs."

A recently proposed revision of Section 1300.70 specifies that the act is intended to apply to all plans (group, staff, or IPA models or combinations) to ensure the provision of a minimally acceptable level of health care. It emphasizes flexibility in meeting act requirements, but it also indicates that service components such as accessibility, availability, and continuity must be addressed as well as the appropriate provision and utilization of services (including speciality care and preventive health care). It specifies assurance that a minimum acceptable level of care is being delivered to all enrollees, that quality-of-care problems are identified and corrected, that physicians are an integral part of the quality assurance program, that appropriate care is not withheld or delayed, and that the plan does not "exert economic pressure to cause . . . health care providers or institutions to render care beyond the scope of their training or experience."

Accreditation for PPOs

Accreditation is available for preferred provider organizations (PPOs) through the American Association of Preferred Provider Organizations. Criteria in eight areas have been proposed: the breadth of the PPO's managed care network; provider selection criteria; payment levels and incentives; utilization management program; quality assurance program; capability of the PPO's management and administrative staffs; legal structure; and financial solvency (DiBlase, 1988).

Legislation Related to Negative Financial Incentives

Some states have shown increasing concern with the potentially negative effects on quality secondary to financial incentives to overuse of services. Particular attention is directed at referrals to physician-owned facilities such as home health agencies, diagnostic imaging centers, or "emergicenters." They are also concerned with the incentives to underuse, particularly in risk-sharing arrangements in managed care. Massachusetts, for instance, has legislation pending to require "disclosure of any [financial] incentives under which doctors operate." Prompted by a case of alleged underprovision of care, during its 1989 session the Delaware legislature introduced a bill banning all financial incentives in HMOs that have the potential of creating conflicts between the doctor's financial interests and the health interest of patients (Hallowell, 1989).

Internal Methods of Preventing Problems in Ambulatory Care

Efforts to prevent quality problems in ambulatory care lie almost exclusively in the province of organized group practices, especially prepaid systems. Organizations providing ambulatory care have many ways to structure the delivery of care so that it is provided safely and effectively. These include credentialing systems and probationary periods for new practitioners, policies and procedures, patient risk assessment and education programs, preventive care guidelines, clinical reminder and follow-up systems, and continuing education for health care practitioners.

Credentialing

HMOs and clinics may have extensive credentialing systems for practitioners. In addition to the minimal proof of licensure, Drug Enforcement

Administration number for prescribing controlled substances, board status, and malpractice insurance coverage, some also employ a probationary period for new physicians during which they engage in increased evaluation. For instance, the Cleveland Clinics view their probationary period as a major feature assuring quality. After the successful completion of the probationary period, the physician is offered full (voting) partnership. An HMO in Spokane uses senior physicians to monitor and assess the quality of care provided by newly hired physicians after 6 months. The plan monitors hospitalizations (e.g., admission justified by diagnosis, length of stay, timeliness of admission), consultations and referrals, record documentation (e.g., clarity, conciseness), and overall strengths and weaknesses of the physician (Berman, 1988).

Group Health Cooperative of Puget Sound includes in-depth reference searches both by telephone and in writing, review of risk management information, practice audits, and answers to key questions about style of practice and customer service. Interviews include examination of the applicant's personal and professional background and his or her ability to perform key procedures. Applicants are reviewed by multispecialty regional medical staff executive committees and by a regional review committee that includes medical and administrative staff and consumer members. After an initial appointment, a 2-year probationary period ensues during which physicians are reviewed quarterly by department chiefs and at 6-month intervals by regional medical staff executive committees.

Health Insurance Plan (HIP) of New York requires that physicians who are not board certified when they join the group become so within 5 years. Performance review of probationary and regular medical staff includes at least annual, and in some topics monthly, review of six areas of performance; these include (1) professional competence, (2) quality of service/patient relationships, (3) personal productivity/practice management, (4) resource use/economic efficiency, (5) peer and coworker relationships, and (6) contributions to the organization/community (Perry and Kirz, 1989).

PPOs may also use a screening process to determine which practitioners to designate as "preferred providers." For example, CIGNA emphasizes appropriate provider selection and credentialing and has proposed minimal criteria for credentialing and selection as follows (Goodspeed and Goldfield, 1987):

- a minimal length of postgraduate training
- valid license to practice
- board certification
- hospital privileges
- satisfactory malpractice history
- absence of disciplinary action by state medical board.

One group-model HMO visited described a selective contracting process used to select specialty care, in this case an ophthalmology group. Included among a number of other factors used for selection was information on aggregate outcomes of cataract surgery 2 months after surgery compared with patients' baseline conditions. For other groups, so-called selective contracting was based on geographic coverage rather than any measures of quality.

Continuing Education

Many practices include provisions for continuing education in their contracts or partnership agreements. One small internal medicine group practice emphasized the value of regularly taking the American College of Physicians *Medical Knowledge Self-Assessment Program.* It is published every few years and is currently in its eighth edition.

Other Structural Requirements of Practices

In addition to setting criteria for training and competence for practitioners, an IPA-model HMO may designate required structural features of the office environment and conduct site visits. For example, U.S. Healthcare requires that offices be open at least 20 hours and 4 days per week, keep appointment books that demonstrate reasonable access times for urgent and routine appointments, have acceptable after-hours coverage, and maintain private examination rooms with specified minimal equipment (Exhibit 6.A1) (Stocker, 1989).

Practice Guidelines and Algorithms[11]

In medicine, and particularly in organized ambulatory care practices, guidelines and algorithms serve many uses, but primarily they are intended to be educational. They may specify appropriate and inappropriate uses of medical interventions, act as reminders for relatively simple tasks (e.g., a vaccination timetable), or serve as shorthand adjuncts for complex clinical decision making. For this last use they are sometimes called patient care algorithms. In all these applications, practice guidelines can help to forestall the occurrence of problems in patient care. In modified formats, they can also be used for retrospective quality review.

Patient management guidelines can be viewed as translating a medical text into a visual (or computerized) format. The use of branching reasoning and flow diagrams allows for great complexity and logically complete presentations. Well-constructed guidelines can allow for patient preferences to be elicited or taken into account.

EXHIBIT 6.A1 Example of Office Standards for IPA-Model HMO

Each primary medical office must:

A. Be clean, presentable, and have a professional appearance.
B. Have a waiting room with at least five chairs.
C. Have a sign containing the names of all physicians practicing at the office or a sign identifying it as a medical office. The office and the sign must be visible and identifiable when open.
D. Be adequately staffed for patient load as determined by the Executive Committee. There must be an assistant available for specialized examinations.
E. Have at least two examining rooms which are clean, properly equipped and provide privacy for the patient. The office must provide an examining table with stirrups, an otoscope and an ophthalmoscope. The equipment must include a blood pressure cuff.
F. Have an EKG machine (except pediatric offices).
G. Have a clean, properly equipped bathroom easily accessible to the patient.
H. Have adequate plans for managing growth of patient load.
I. Be approved by a U.S. Healthcare site visit.

SOURCE: U.S. Healthcare, used with permission.

Numerous groups, including medical specialty groups, have formulated such guidelines. They are also frequently developed by interested clinicians within health care facilities and by health services researchers. In these cases they take on a variety of formats, depending on their highly individualized use. Exhibit 6.A2 is a flow diagram developed at Harvard Community Health Plan for care of women with dysuria; Exhibit 6.A3 is an example of health care screening guidelines used at the Ochsner Clinic; and Exhibit 6.A4 is a data base form devised to help HMO practitioners track age-specific preventive care and counseling needs.

Clinical Reminder Systems

Clinical reminder systems are computerized methods used in some managed care plans, clinics, and office practices to remind clinicians of preventive tests that should be performed, of laboratory monitoring that is due for patients with chronic disease, and of potential drug interactions (McDonald, 1976; Barnett, 1977; Barnett et al., 1978, 1983; McDonald et al., 1984; Tierney et al., 1986, 1988). For example, one practice visited during the site visits—the Woodburn Internal Medicine Associates of northern Virginia—has demonstrated consistently improved compliance with their own cancer screening guidelines with the use of a computerized data base and

EXHIBIT 6.A2 Example of Practice Management Algorithm

ACUTE DYSURIA IN THE ADULT FEMALE (A)

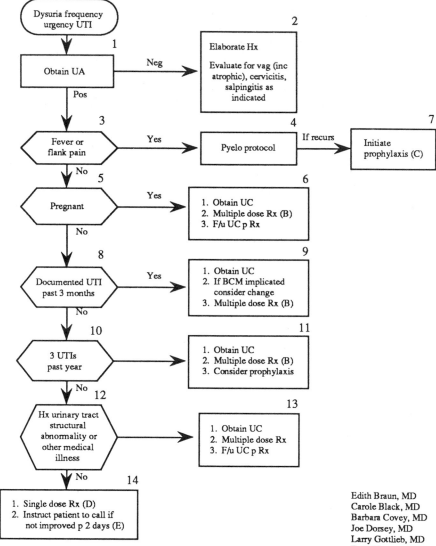

Edith Braun, MD
Carole Black, MD
Barbara Covey, MD
Joe Dorsey, MD
Larry Gottlieb, MD
Talia Herman, MD
Beth Ingram, PA
Carl Isihara, MD
Mon Kim, MD
Tom Lawrence, MD
Carmi Margolis, MD
Marvin Packer, MD
Barbara Stewart, MD

HCHP clinical guidelines are designed to assist clinicians by providing an analytical framework for the evaluation and treatment of the more common problems of HCHP patients. They are not intended either to replace a clinician's clinical judgement or to establish a protocol for all patients with a particular condition. It is understood that some patients will not fit the clinical conditions contemplated by a guideline and that a guideline will rarely establish the only appropriate approach to a problem.

EXHIBIT 6.A2 Continued

ACUTE DYSURIA IN THE ADULT FEMALE

A. A primary goal of this algorithm is to separate women with acute uncompli-
    cated UTI that can be treated with single dose antibiotic therapy from women
    with complicated UTI that will require further evaluation or longer duration of
    therapy. Therefore, women who have symptoms longer than 2 or 3 days,
    women who have fever or flank pain, pregnant women and women with fre-
    quent recurrences or other underlying medical problems need to be eliminated
    from this algorithm. Initial steps in their management are suggested at branch
    points of this algorithm, but other algorithms will be necessary to more fully
    address the management of these groups of patients.

Stamm, W., Causes of the Acute Urethral Syndrome in Women, NEJM 1980; 303;
409-415.

B. Choices for multiple dose Rx include 7-10 day course of:

1. Trimethoprim sulfa DS BID (contraindicated in pregnancy, known G6PD
    deficiency or allergic Hx).
2. Amoxicillin 250 mg po tid (1st choice in pregnancy).
3. Nitrofurantoin 50 mg QID (alternative for patient with multiple allergies
    or pregnant patient with Hx Pen allergy).

C. Prophylaxis is usually continued for 6 months.

Options for prophylaxis include:

1. Trimethoprim sulfa 1/2 regular strength tab, QHS.
2. Nitrofurantoin 50 mg QHS (in pregnant patient or patient with Hx T/X
    allergy or known G6PD deficiency).

Ronald, A. and Harding, G., Urinary Infection Prophylaxis in Women, Annals Int.
Med. 1981; 94(2) 268-269.

D. Options for single dose Rx include:

1. Trimethoprim sulfa DS 2 tabs x 1.
2. Amoxicillin 3 gm po x 1.

Kamaroff, A., Acute Dysuria in Women, NEJM 1984; 310; 368-375.

E. Patients who have failed single dose Rx should be considered to have upper
    tract infection and treated per pyelo protocol.

SOURCE: Harvard Community Health Plan, used with permission (abbreviations and other details as in original).

EXHIBIT 6.A3 Example of Health Care Screening Standards

Complete Physical Exam (to include rectal exam)	— Initial visit; yearly after age 50
Blood Pressure	— Every 3 years after age 18 Every 1 year with family history of hypertension
Complete Blood Count (Coulter)	— Initial age 18 or greater every 1-3 years in menstruating females and after age 50
Urinalysis	— Initial visit
Fasting Blood Sugar	— Initial visit
Electrocardiogram	— Baseline; female age 50, male age 40
Chest X-ray	— Determined by attending
Cholesterol, Triglycerides	— Initial age 18, repeat: every 1 year, 200–240 mg/ml with unfavorable dispoprotein analysis; every 2 years 200–240 mg/ml with favorable dispoprotein analysis; every 5 years less than 200 mg/ml
Breast Exam	— Physician-every 1 year after age 35 Self-every one month after age 20
Hemoccult	— Every 1 year after age 40; 35 if a family history of colon cancer
Flexible Sigmoidoscopy	— Beginning at age 50 every year x 2, then every three years
Testicular Self Exam Instruction	— Initial visit
Eye Examination	— Initial screening at age 4* then every 10 years 40; every 2-3 years age 40-50; every 1–2 years age 50 or greater
Immunization	— Tetanus and diphtheria every 10 years
Mammograms	— Baseline age 40 and every other year 40 to 50 and every year after 50
Pediatric IM Schedule	— See attached
Pap/Pelvic	Pap (assuming the cervix is present) — Initial at 18 or onset of sexual activity — Every 1 year if ≤ 35 years — Every 1-3 years if > 35 years — Every 1 year if ≥ 40 years and uterus has been removed Vaginal/Vulvar Exam — Every 3–5 years after total abdominal hysterectomy with bilateral salpingo-oophrectomy

---

*Eye examination at age 4 is defined as a screening examination

SOURCE: Ochsner Medical Institutions, used with permission (some abbreviations and other details modified from original).

EXHIBIT 6.A4 Example of Age-Specific Data Base Check-Off Form for Use During Periodic Exams, Intercurrent Acute, and Follow-up Visits

ADULT HEALTH SCREENING AND HEALTH
MAINTENANCE FLOW SHEET Recommendations of the Quality Assurance Program
of the GWUHP as adapted from
recommendations of the American Cancer
society. Canadian Task Force and the
review by Frame and Carlsen.

AGE 60 YEARS AND ABOVE — DATE OF EXAMINATION AND CORRESPONDING AGE

HISTORY AND PHYSICAL EXAMINATION:

	60	61	62	63	64	65	66	67	68	69	70	71	72	73	74	75	76	77	78	79	80	81	82	83	84	85	86	87	88	89
Blood Pressure q visit																														
Height once																														
Weight once																														
Visual acuity near/far c glasses: q 2 yrs																														
FUNDOSCOPY q 4 years age 50-70 if cup/disk ration is < .5 no tonometry if indeterminate do tonometry, if > .5 or tonometry elevated send to Ophth. Fundoscopy and Tonometry q 2 yrs >70																														
HYPOTHYROIDISM postmenopausal q 2 yrs																														
BREAST EXAM q years																														
PELVIC EXAM q 3 years																														
RECTAL EXAM q 2 years																														
SIGMOIDOSCOPY q 3-5 years																														
• ORAL q 2 years: smoking/ETOH																														
• THYROID q year irradiation history																														
• SKIN q 2 yrs. if high risk: sun exposure fair skin, fam. hx melanoma																														
Other:																														

IMMUNIZATIONS:

dT q 10 years																														
Pneumovax once only - all > 65 yrs																														
Influenza q year - all > 65 years																														
• Hepatitis B one series only																														
Other:																														

COUNSELING:

Women Only: Self breast exam q year																														
Osteoporosis Prevention																														
Report postmenopausal bleeding																														
Men and Women: frequency discretionary Seat belts																														
• • Use of alcohol, drugs and tobacco																														
Nutrition: obesity, lipids, cancer																														
• • Eating Disorders																														
Exercise																														
• • Sexually transmitted disease																														
Sexual dysfunction																														
• • Depression/Stress/Bereavement																														
Pre-retirement evaluation																														
Family/Social Support																														
Financial/Housing/Transportation																														
Other:																														

LABORATORY:

Tine q year unless positive																														
PAP q 3 years																														
Cholesterol q 5 years																														
Hct q 3 years																														
Mammogram q year																														
Hemoccult cards x3 q year																														
• STS																														
Other:																														

Key: X = normal. ✓ = done/ordered

*HIGH RISK ONLY
**The presence of a check indicates this topic was addressed. It does not imply the presence of a problem, past or present
'Data for screening guidelines for people over 70 years of age are scarce and protocol should be individualized

© 3 87 George Washington University Health Plan

SOURCE: The George Washington University Health Plan, used with permission.

reminders (Hattwick et al., 1981). Clinical reminder software called PROMPT (Physician Reminder of Medical Protocol Tasks), which is in the public domain, is newly available for use in practices where COSTAR (Computer-Stored Ambulatory Record) is used (NCHSR, 1989).

Member Education and Outreach

Some HMOs consider their most valuable and effective method of preventing quality problems to be appropriate, thorough, and timely orientation of new enrollees. During our site visits to HMOs with Medicare risk contracts, several HMOs emphasized the importance of such orientation programs, in particular for the elderly. These HMOs felt that "access" problems were best prevented by educating enrollees about "how to use the system"—what to do during emergencies, what to do if dissatisfied with the primary care physician, and what to do to see a specialist. HMOs may also contact new enrollees (before they seek care) and offer preventive care to asymptomatic enrollees with underlying health problems, behavioral risk factors, or incomplete immunization status (Berman, 1988; Luft, 1988). One HMO reported that they have frequent "open houses" for new Medicare patients and that they call new Medicare enrollees to get a medical history before their first appointment and to make sure they have sufficient supplies of their prescriptions.

Patient Education

Staff-model HMOs have developed extensive patient education programs for members who are at high risk for problems, complications, or poor outcomes. These may include patients with newly diagnosed diabetes, members with hypercholesterolemia, those with obesity, enrollees identified as under stress, or members seeking to stop smoking. For example, the Kaiser Foundation Health Plan of Mid-Atlantic States has implemented an education program for asthmatic patients and their families.

Geriatric Programs

Some HMOs, such as the Kaiser Foundation Health Plan of the Southern California Region, have formed multidisciplinary task forces to review and develop policies specifically for care of their elderly members. A geriatric nurse practitioner evaluates the home environment when needed and oversees long term care for its enrollees. Group Health Cooperative of Puget Sound similarly puts a considerable emphasis on specialized programs for its elderly members.

Case Management

HIP emphasizes its case management program to help ensure the most appropriate handling of complex problems, scheduling of referrals, follow-up of abnormal tests, and general monitoring of care by one person. For the elderly, several HMOs noted the difficulty of having to negotiate the HMO system and the value of case management in this regard.

Mission Statement

Some ambulatory practices have developed mission statements that describe their priorities and commitment to providing quality care. These are used chiefly to introduce and remind practice partners and employees of the concepts of high-quality care, especially the interpersonal aspects (Exhibit 6.A5).

External Methods of Detecting Problems in Ambulatory Care

PRO Review of HMOs and CMPs

Before HCFA awards a Medicare risk contract, it requires an HMO or a CMP to have an internal quality assurance plan. In addition, PROs (or entities known as Quality Review Organizations [QROs]) have been required, effective January 1987, to review the quality of care rendered in HMOs and CMPs and to place emphasis on appropriate treatment and setting, access and timeliness of services, and the potential for underutilization of services based on three levels of review. (See Volume I, Chapter 6, and Chapter 8 of this volume for a more complete description.)

PRO medical record review is required for five main areas of care. First are hospital admissions for 13 sentinel conditions, such as serious complications of diabetes, certain malignancies, and adverse drug reactions. For these, both prehospitalization and posthospitalization ambulatory care is reviewed against criteria developed by the PRO. Second is a random sample of inpatient admissions. Third are samples of readmissions within specified time periods. Fourth are nontraumatic deaths in all health care settings. A fifth area is focused review of ambulatory care, for which PROs were given 6 months to develop a methodology. Finally, beneficiary complaints are also monitored, and PROs must perform community outreach activities for risk-contract enrollees similar to those for fee-for-service beneficiaries. Each PRO is responsible for developing a focused review methodology and clinical screening criteria for reviewing sentinel conditions; as of mid-1989, several PROs were in the process of implementing review instruments developed by an industry-PRO task force.

EXHIBIT 6.A5 Example of Office Group Practice Mission Statement

---

Our goals are, in order of priority:

I. To provide the best possible medical care.

    1. We will know what optimal care is.

        A. Through in house review, CME, and goal setting.

        B. Through periodic special courses and training.

    2. We will care for the entire patient: body, feelings, mind, and spirit.

        A. Body -
        The sine qua non of our life and practice, we place first priority on healing and caring for physical problems.

        B. Emotions and feelings -
        We know disease means dis-ease, feeling bad, and we recognize and treat the discomfort that each patient feels, whether or not we find also a physical disease.

        C. Mind -
        We care that the patient understands what he or she must know and do in order to become or stay healthy, and we try to understand what the patients' problems mean to them.

        D. Spirit -
        We know that each of our patients will die one day, as will we. We respect the mystery of their, and our life and death, and know we have responsibility as their physicians to help them cope with profound, and at times ultimate problems. Where we can appropriately help patients deal with ethical or spiritual issues we will try to do so.

    3. We will stress preventing problems whenever possible.

    4. We will monitor our patients and ourselves to maintain optimal care.

        A. By systematic supervision and evaluation of our care.

        B. By targeted individual follow-up.

II. To make sure our patients are happy with our care

    1. We will provide a patient centered, unified practice style which always stresses reassurance, respect for persons, and privacy.

        A. Reassurance. Whatever the problem, we will try to reassure the patient:

            1. That we are in control, and there is no emergency.

            2. That whatever happens we will do all we can to help them cope.

        B. Respect for persons

            1. We believe our patients are partners in their care, and that they have much to teach us. We will always listen carefully to them and try to learn from them and understand what they think and feel about their problems.

            2. We care for our patients, and therefore their convenience is important to us. We will try not to waste their time by poor scheduling or keeping them waiting unnecessarily.

    C. Privacy
       1. We will respect their privacy and avoid activities, discussions or communications which might compromise their privacy.
       2. We will try to provide an atmosphere of peacefulness and quiet whenever patients are in the office.
  2. We will try to provide what the patient wants in addition to what we think the patient needs.

    A. To the extent that this is compatible with providing optimal medical care, we will try to satisfy both needs and wants.
    B. When there is a conflict between what the patient wants and what we think they need, we will respect the patients right to differ with us. We will discuss these differences with the patient, and if necessary with each other to try to resolve the conflict.

III. To make sure the Corporation is healthy and happy

  1. We will strive to be optimally managed.
    A. We will always be plan based: we will know what we want to do, and measure how well we do it.
    B. We will make a priority of efficiency, striving to minimize waste, or duplication.
    C. We will manage the corporation to make it profitable.
  2. We will work as a team.
    A. We will respect each others talents and differences and work to complement and help each other so the overall practice goals are met.
    B. We will recognize that teamwork is essential, and that each member of the team is important. So far as is practical we will strive to have a non-hierarchial management style.
    C. We will try to provide responsibilities, working conditions, and salaries for each employee which will help them best perform and enjoy their work.

SOURCE: Woodburn Internal Medicine Associates, Ltd. Used with permission.

State HMO Review

State requirements for HMO inspection vary widely. Typically, states conduct annual or other periodic on-site inspections. For instance, Kansas law requires independent, on-site quality assessment at least once every 3 years. New York law requires all HMOs to have internal quality assurance programs, and state on-site inspections occur every 6 months. In Florida, monitoring responsibility is shared between two state departments; the Insurance Department oversees financial and operational matters and the Department of Health and Rehabilitative Services reviews and monitors quality of care. The state requires ongoing internal quality assurance, specifies minimum quality standards, and conducts quality reviews every 3 years. California inspects HMOs every 1 to 2.5 years. Several states, including Pennsylvania and Kansas, have enacted legislation to allow HMOs in their states to select one of several accrediting groups, such as NCQA, to conduct the survey for the state. The NCQA survey includes a review of several hundred medical records; in the case of IPAs, this activity specifies at least 10 records from each primary care practitioner to be forwarded to a central location.

Under the "squeal law" in Massachusetts, hospitals, clinics, HMOs, and nursing homes are required by statute (Massachusetts General Laws c.111, Sec. 53B) to report all disciplinary actions against physicians. In addition, health care providers—including physicians, dentists, registered nurses, as well as hospitals, clinics, HMOs, and nursing homes, and any of their employees—must report to the Board of Registration "any physician who has acted in such a way that there is reasonable basis to conclude that the physician would be subject to disciplinary action by the board" (PCA Today, 1987, p. 4). The board has been designated the central information center in Massachusetts, to which insurance agencies, courts, and the PRO are to report problem physicians.

Other External Review

At least four groups have conducted research projects to review care provided by Medicaid-certified HMOs. These are reviewed below in the section "Historical Efforts and Research Projects Applicable to Internal Quality Assessment Efforts."

The Michigan Project is one example of a collaborative effort to review care. This study involves the United Automobile Workers, the major automobile manufacturers, and the HMOs they offer as health benefits. The project plans to monitor four components of care: satisfaction with care, process of care using explicit criteria, provision of services in mental health and for substance abuse, and accessibility. The project intends to use these data to assess performance of the HMOs and to provide each HMO with comparative data to judge its own performance.

Medical Malpractice and the HCQIA

When patients believe they have suffered a medical injury, they or their representatives may file a claim against a practitioner or provider. This claim may accompany or be followed by a lawsuit. For medical malpractice claims to be established in court, the patient must prove that: (1) the practitioner owed him or her a duty of care; (2) a particular standard of care was due; (3) the practitioner failed to meet that standard of care; and (4) as a result, the patient sustained an injury.

It is widely believed that a practitioner who has been found liable for malpractice in a court action, particularly where he or she has repeatedly been found so liable, is a provider of inadequate quality care (OTA, 1988). Against this background, Congress passed the Health Care Quality Improvement Act of 1986 and established the National Practitioner Data Bank [see description under "External Methods of Preventing Problems Directed at Individuals (Physicians)"]. The intent of Congress was to "restrict the ability of incompetent physicians to move from state to state without disclosure or discovery of the physician's previous damaging or incompetent performance" (Sec. 402). Both hospitals and HMOs will be required to consult the data bank when making decisions on extending privileges to physicians.

Recent work by Schwartz and Mendelson (1989) indicates that physician-owned insurance companies may play a role in detecting and deterring negligent behavior that may relate to malpractice. Physicians in these companies often review care provided by members and advise the underwriter on decisions about insurability and conditions of coverage. These conditions are comparable to sanctions that might be applied by hospitals, such as restrictions on practice and requirements for supervision.

Internal Methods of Detecting Problems in Ambulatory Care

Methods to identify quality problems that can be used by prepaid, managed, or fee-for-service organizations, clinics, and practices fall into several categories. Some are off-the-shelf, proprietary "quality assurance" programs. Others are organization-specific, internally developed systems, which in principle could be adopted by (or generalized to) other practices and organizations. Still other methods have been developed through research efforts; in some cases these have been incorporated into existing quality assurance efforts and in other cases they simply have the potential for further application. As with hospitals, ambulatory health care organizations try to integrate their quality assurance activities, although, given both the diversity and the relative immaturity of approaches in this field, measurement is for the most part an "eclectic enterprise" (D. Berwick, quoted in Fintor, 1988, p. 216). Selected examples of these types of efforts are described in the remainder of this section.

Historical Efforts and Research Projects Applicable to Internal Quality Assessment Efforts

With the growth of managed care, recent efforts to enroll Medicare patients in HMOs, and rapidly increasing numbers of procedures being performed on an ambulatory basis have come increasing concerns about ambulatory care quality assurance. Interest in the field is not, however, de novo. A sizable literature since the 1960s and particularly the early 1970s records efforts to develop and validate methods of timely, effective internal review (Williamson, 1977; Williams and Brook, 1978; Logsdon, 1979). Despite many years of research and operational effort, however, progress has lagged behind that in the hospital environment because of several very difficult features of ambulatory care (see Volume I, Chapter 8).

Assessment methods developed through research or demonstration projects could be (and in some cases have been) adapted for use by internal programs. This is especially the case when and if they do not require large, externally derived data bases. Some of the leading research efforts of the past decade are briefly described here.

Health accounting. In the early 1970s, Williamson (1971, 1978; Williamson et al., 1975) advanced a program called "Health Accounting," which has many similarities with current trends in continuous improvement methods. In measuring "achievable benefit not being achieved," Williamson was the first to use patient reports, to compare intended results with results obtained, and to look systematically for underuse by sampling an enrolled population for missed and misdiagnosis such as recognition and follow-up of hypercholesterolemia and hypertension. In one instance of the application of this method, adult members of an HMO were tested for undiagnosed depression; those who had already been diagnosed and had received treatment were contacted for a follow-up self-assessment of their progress, and corrective action was implemented for both groups as appropriate (Schroeder and Donaldson, 1976).

Ambulatory Care Medical Audit Demonstration Project (ACMAD). Palmer et al. (1984, 1985) conducted a randomized controlled trial of eight pediatric and eight medical practices in Boston to investigate if physician involvement in quality assurance and technical assistance improved patient care. Physician-led task forces selected tasks for improvement and helped to design and review criteria. Tasks for the medical practices included follow-up of low hematocrit, annual Pap smear and breast examination, follow-up and control of high serum glucose, and monitoring of digoxin levels. Control groups received no interventions, whereas experimental groups were told of improvement efforts, offered journal articles and criteria for compliance with the task chosen, and given feedback of performance. Significant improvement occurred in two of eight tasks and marginal improvement in one task. Improvement did not correspond to those tasks believed by physicians to have the greatest health consequences if not met. Lack of improvement, however, was correlated with the need for delivery system changes beyond the immediate control of the individual practitioner.

College of Family Physicians of Canada. The Committee on Practice Assessment of the Ontario Chapter, College of Family Physicians of Canada (CFPC) (Borgiel, 1988; Borgiel et al., 1985) conducted a pilot research effort during 1987 to develop a practical, economical, and acceptable method of practice assessment appropriate for use in office practice of family physicians. Its conceptual base was the notion of "tracers" (Kessner et al., 1973), in which general conclusions about care provided by the practitioner or facility are drawn on the basis of tracer, indicator, or representative conditions and problems that are intensively studied. The CFPC computerized process evaluation focused on chart review for a set of tracer conditions to evaluate routine care for common ailments.

The CFPC process included self-administered questionnaires completed by physicians, on-site computer algorithm evaluations by nurse reviewers, and patient satisfaction questionnaires. The physician questionnaire sought information in the following categories: (1) structural characteristics relating to the doctor's training, work schedules, and practice features, as well as level of satisfaction with his or her present practice; (2) office facilities, including accessibility (availability of local transportation, technologies such as X-ray and laboratory); (3) after-hours coverage; (4) community services available and use of them by the practice; (5) referral and consultation patterns; (6) hospital practice; (7) medical records; and (8) education and research activities.

The computerized process evaluation focused on chart review for a set of tracer conditions to evaluate routine care for common ailments. Conditions were selected to meet certain requirements: (1) general agreement on the presence of a minimal standard for diagnosis; (2) diagnosis did not require use of sophisticated equipment, and the tracer condition could be diagnosed easily and objectively by the average family physician; and (3) an understanding of the effects of nonmedical factors on the tracers. The chart review assessed chart format, prevention, use of drugs, resource utilization, and compliance with clinical criteria. Finally, the patient questionnaire measured satisfaction with the doctor-patient relationship, access to care, unmet health needs, after-hours coverage, preventive medicine counseling, and satisfaction with the facility.

Although the study is still in a pilot phase, it provides a promising method of ambulatory office-based assessment. It also has potential for selecting doctors for participation in managed care organizations and for physician recertification (Chassin et al., 1989a). Moreover, the computerized algorithms developed for this study have continued to be adapted and extended.

Some 280 screens cover about 85 percent of all primary care diagnoses, including condition-specific history and physical examinations, laboratory tests, therapies, and patient education (M. McCoy, personal communication, 1989).

Studies involving Medicaid enrollees. Four research studies have developed and applied methods of quality assessment for Medicaid eligibles. In California, the Prepaid Health Research, Evaluation and Demonstration Project (PHRED) (Leighton, 1981) took place in the late 1970s. It included an extensive effort to clarify the methods that could be used to monitor the quality of care in HMOs contracting to provide care to Medicaid eligibles. The demonstration used a set of criteria[12] thought to be necessary to evaluate the care and compared the validity, completeness, and cost of two ways to gather quality-of-care data. One approach used condition-based samples of medical records ("Selective method"); the other used administrative data[13] ("Monitoring method"). The selective method used a portable microcomputer to guide the abstracting of only relevant data items from a sample of medical records by trained abstractors. Results indicated that the system was relatively inexpensive, feasible, and flexible for detecting likely problems in quality of care.

The monitoring method sought to determine if routinely gathered administrative encounter data from three participating HMOs could be analyzed using computer logic to recognize unusual instances or patterns (which then might be followed by medical record review). The encounter form included diagnostic, procedure, and drug information as well as provider and enrollee identification. Results indicated that great care needed to be taken in validating the criteria set and interpreting apparent "exceptions" that might be due to data problems, misunderstanding of the protocol, or conflict with the sites' internal medical protocols. The study design provided little opportunity for follow-up review of exceptions or opportunity to evaluate any changes in medical practice. The California Department of Health Service judged the monitor approach both feasible and desirable and moved to make it available for voluntary use by prepaid contractors. The project evaluators could not make an overall determination that either method was superior. They recommended consideration of the appropriate uses of both for internal and external quality assurance efforts, with the choice depending on, for instance, the regulatory style of the external body, the previous history of the HMO, and the HMO's internal quality assurance program.

The PHRED project also applied the staging approach (Gonnella et al., 1976) to quality assessment in ambulatory care settings; ambulatory staging definitions were developed for 22 conditions including alcoholism, otitis media, pharyngitis, sinusitis, urinary tract infection, and viral pneumonia.

This was an attempt to go beyond its previous uses for hospital review to examination of stages of ambulatory conditions that might focus evaluation of quality. Application to the demonstration sites was unsuccessful because of incompleteness in recording hospital and other information and limitations in the medical record clinical content. However, the investigators concluded that the concept was valid and would have utility if applied to better medical records.

The Joint Commission, in collaboration with the Ohio Department of Health Services (Card and Lehmann, 1987; P.D. Phillips et al., 1989), used medical record audits of outcomes, preventive and diagnostic services, therapeutic procedures, and follow-up to assess the effectiveness of the Ohio HMOs' quality assurance process. Investigators audited a sample of medical records of both Medicaid and non-Medicaid patients focusing on 13 clinical conditions, classified as either high-volume, high-risk, or problem-prone. Staff conducted quarterly site visits and reviewed reports of corrective actions based on findings of audits.

The Nationwide Evaluation of Medicaid Competition Demonstrations (RTI, 1988) was a major HCFA-funded demonstration project involving Medicaid HMO enrollees. One aspect of the study involved quality of care. The investigators used three methods to evaluate quality of care: (1) chart review of the process and outcomes of health care in ambulatory and hospital inpatient settings; (2) analysis of the structure of the HMO quality assurance program; and (3) self-assessed health status, health behavior, care-seeking activities, and patient satisfaction among elderly enrollees.

A final project measured quality of care rendered through the Arizona Health Care Cost Containment System (AHCCCS), a capitation-based alternative to traditional Medicaid coverage (SRI, 1989). The study included four conditions: well-child care, otitis media, prenatal care, and pregnancy. Audits of outpatient medical records in physicians' offices and inpatient hospital records of AHCCCS beneficiaries were compared with those of a control group of traditional Medicaid beneficiaries. The tracer methodology employed demonstrated significant differences in care between the two groups. For instance, completeness of well-child examinations was consistently better in AHCCCS. Compliance with immunization standards in both groups was well below standards set by the American Academy of Pediatrics at 19 months of age (20 percent and 16 percent of children, respectively, had up-to-date immunization records), but compliance rates tripled by 37 months of age. Use of the tracer conditions necessarily limited the evaluation to enrollees in urban counties who had received care and to children with long periods of continuous enrollment.

The investigators in both the RTI and AHCCCS studies noted the limitations in validity, reliability, and completeness of claims data. They further noted that fragmented care and the rates of conformity with standards under both experimental and control systems fall far short of standards and indicated serious problems in utilization, especially in immunization status.

National Medicare Competition Demonstrations. The National Medicare Competition Demonstrations evaluated the quality of care received by Medicare beneficiaries who enrolled in HMOs compared to fee-for-service groups. Panels of expert physicians developed record review criteria for routine elements of care such as medical history taking, screening and follow-up of abnormal tests, and management of two chronic conditions—diastolic hypertension and diabetes mellitus. Exhibit 6.A6 shows the criteria set used for review of follow-up visits for a patient with hypertension.

Administrative data base studies. Several groups have used Medicaid or similar data bases to review patterns of care and to identify inappropriate practices (Avorn and Soumerai, 1983; Ray et al., 1985; Roos et al., 1989). For instance, Lohr (1980a, 1980b) studied the misuse of injectable antibiotics among New Mexico Medicaid recipients and documented how a combination of education interventions and sanctions targeted at a small number of outlier practitioners by the New Mexico Experimental Medical Care Review Organization (a peer review organization that antedated Medicare PROs) reduced the inappropriate use of these therapies.

RAND HMO study. The RAND Corporation is conducting a major study of HMO quality indicators. It is an effort to develop quality-of-care as well as premium and benefits information that can be used by consumers (presumably corporate purchasers) to make purchasing decisions. With the guidance of a consortium of HMOs, the researchers have identified tracers covering preventive, acute, and chronic care for HMO members of various ages. Measures have been sought that (1) would not penalize nonhospital care, (2) would provide information about overuse and underuse, (3) are appropriate for conditions for which morbidity or mortality are preventable, and (4) are appropriate for conditions whose health effects can be mitigated by care. Three such measures are lowering serum cholesterol by 27 percent (for patients in the top quintile), decreasing the number of smokers by 10 percent, and increasing thrombolysis therapy for 20 percent of eligible patients. Although the study group does not envision these measures being "mandated" by regulators, it does see them as a model of external evaluation that uses positive performance measures rather than adverse outcomes.

Components of Ambulatory Care Quality Assessment Programs

Process measures for detecting problems in ambulatory care. Problems in ambulatory care can be identified by examining processes of care or by

EXHIBIT 6.A6 Example of Criteria Set for Retrospective Ambulatory Record Review for Patients with Diagnosis of Hypertension

HYPERTENSION - FOLLOW UP

I. Definition of Control
- 1a. Systolic blood pressure < 90mm Hg + age ± 5, and/or
- 1b. Diastolic blood pressure < 90mm Hg unless notation of why not (e.g., notation that patient not tolerating more aggressive therapy).

II. History
1. Change in mental status (new depression, confusion, weakness, fatigue): all drugs except calcium channel blockers should be discontinued or dosages decreased.
2. Acute gouty attack — discontinue thiazide
3. Any acute arrythmia — discontinue thiazide.

III. Physical Examination
1. Blood pressure (in two postural positions on at least one half of total visits)

Laboratory
1. If on thiazide with weakness or confusion, obtain serum sodium and potassium
2. If on thiazide and arrythmia, obtain serum potassium
3. If bradycardia (45 beats/minute or below) do electrocardiogram or decrease Inderal and recheck pulse within 24 hours
4. After initiating therapy with a thiazide diuretic, serum sodium and potassium should be obtained within 30 days and at least every six months
5. Patients receiving methyldopa (Aldomet) should have a liver function (serum enzyme) test: lactic dehydrogenase (LDH), aspartate amino transaminase (SGOT), alanine amino transaminase (SGPT) and Hct or Hgb at least once a year.

Other
1. Electrocardiogram for any new anginal pain (defined as radiating to left arm and/or new chest pain on exertion or "pain typical of angina").

IV. Treatment
1. If the blood pressure is not under control
   a. There is evidence of a change in drug regimen in an effort to achieve control
   b. Next visit within three months.

V. Obtain Consult from Board Eligible Internist (unless present provider is an internist) if:
1. Abnormal renal echogram/renal scan suggest obstruction
2. Extended lack of control (diastolic blood pressure > 110 mmHg after three months while under therapy).

VI. Indications for Immediate Hospitalization
(Same as Hypertension - Initial Diagnosis and Work-up)

SOURCE: Retchin et al., 1988.

following outcomes of care. Approaches more oriented to the process of care are noted here; those relating to outcomes follow.

Process studies review the provision of care according to many categories. Among them are diagnosis, patient symptom or complaint, abnormal test result, type of therapy, and need for preventive care. Sources of information vary widely. They include the insurance billing form, visit logs or appointment books, laboratory or pharmacy data, records of emergency room visits, outpatient encounter forms, standard medical charts, and computerized patient management data bases. HMOs also monitor appointment availability, telephone access, and waiting time in the reception areas compared to internal standards.

Profiling. The process (or outcomes) of care can be analyzed in aggregate to identify patterns of practice and outlier practitioners or sites of care; typically, claims data are used for such profiling of utilization patterns (generally high-use patterns, although low-use patterns are possible areas of concern as well). The use of claims data, or encounter and utilization data in HMOs that do not generate claims, has been reviewed by Steinwachs et al. (1989) and Weiner et al. (1989a). Profiles can array access (visit rates), preventive care, diagnosis and treatment, continuity of care, and adverse outcomes such as complications.

Monitoring and clinical quality indicators. Just as hospitals are in the process of developing and refining quality-of-care indicators, the search for efficient ambulatory indicators has been launched. Group Health Cooperative of Puget Sound uses a framework recommended by the Joint Commission in looking at systemwide and departmental indicators. These include complications of outpatient colonoscopy and endoscopy and gastrointestinal bleeding that requires more than 2 units of blood. Primary care physicians may monitor some areas of care on an ongoing basis; among the topics are frequency of consumer complaints, immunization status of enrollees, and availability of master problem lists (Perry and Kirz, 1989).

Retrospective evaluation of process of care. Process studies review the provision of preventive, acute, and chronic care. Retrospective review of records using explicit criteria is the classic approach to assessing quality. Criteria and standards may be developed by a consensus of experts using their knowledge of literature and their clinical experience as guidance. Volume I, Chapter 10 discusses issues in the development, validation, and evaluation of criteria for evaluating patient care.

Both Palmer et al. (1984) and Greenfield (1989) have described the development of what are generally considered to be well-constructed algorithms for ambulatory patient care evaluation. These have been used to evaluate a range of medical situations: compliance with preventive and well-child care; relatively simple interventions such as management following an abnormal Pap smear and treatment of streptococcal sore throat or middle ear infection; and more complex care of patients presenting to the emergency room with chest pain (Greenfield et al., 1981). Other topics include evaluation of child abuse, follow-up evaluation of positive tests of blood in the stool, and adequacy of evaluation of microhematuria (small amounts of blood in the urine).

Using an abstracting form developed for review, quality assessors cull information from the medical record and judge the quality of that care, usually against explicit process-of-care criteria. Sometimes the level of compliance with criteria is given a score; in other formats care is simply rated as acceptable or unacceptable. Although some criteria sets are poorly constructed, others, such as patient management guidelines, may use branching criteria and an inclusive range of options in an attempt to approximate closely the clinical decision-making process.

Peer review. The evaluation of medical care by peers generally occurs in one of two situations. It can follow the identification of worrisome patterns of practice during claims review or other profiling, or it can follow the identification of some adverse outcome of care. Traditional peer review has also been used to review charts chosen according to some sampling process, such as by diagnosis, type of visit or hospitalization, or random sampling (Rubin, 1975).

During the peer review process, attention is paid to the adequacy of the master problem list, the patient history, diagnostic and therapeutic process, counseling, follow-up plans, continuity, and documentation. Various techniques can be used to make the quality assessment process more rigorous than unguided implicit review. For instance, the quality program might use two reviewers (and even a third in the case of discrepancies) and a guided or explicit format for review. Findings of these reviews can be presented in a formal report or given in a more informal discussion approach (Warner, 1989).

Outcome measures for detecting problems in ambulatory care. Outcome data are attractive for quality assessment because they address the primary goals of health care. These include cure, repair of injured or dysfunctional organs, relief of pain or anxiety, rehabilitation of function, and prevention or delay of the progression of chronic disease. They are ultimate criteria of judging the quality of care; as such they have great face validity for both patients and caregivers. Sources of outcome data include administrative data bases (e.g., deaths; complications of treatment, such as wound infection or postoperative pulmonary emboli; readmissions), medical records (e.g., infections, return to the operating room), questionnaires and interviews about health status, and surveys of patient satisfaction.

Sentinel events. Rutstein et al. (1976) first advanced the idea of using sentinel occurrences to target ambulatory review; this approach has been incorporated directly into the use of sentinel hospital admissions to target ambulatory HMO review by PROs (see Chapter 8 in this volume). The Minnesota Project, a joint study of three HMOs and the Minnesota Department of Health, modified the PRO list of 13 sentinel hospital admissions to review preceding ambulatory care (Solberg et al., 1987). Exhibit 6.A7 shows the screen developed for ambulatory review of patients admitted in diabetic acidosis. The Ochsner Medical Institutions also have a list of 17 sentinel events to trigger review of ambulatory care (Exhibit 6.A8).

Mortality and morbidity review. Unexpected deaths and complications of treatment are a variant of sentinel events that can be applied to ambulatory care. Some HMOs conduct reviews of these problems; for example, Health Care Plan in Buffalo, New York, has a standing morbidity and mortality review committee.

Health status. Health status measures related to patient outcomes include disease-specific clinical endpoints of care (e.g., physiological or anatomical health outcomes), a broad set of generic measures of functional and emotional status, and well-being (see Volume I, Chapter 2).

The RAND Health Insurance Experiment developed a large series of health status measures (physical, social, mental) (Brook et al., 1984); some were used to review ambulatory care for experimental enrollees in both HMO and fee-for-service settings. Since then, increasingly refined health status measures have emerged that apply to both chronic and acute illness (Lohr, 1988). Health status measures that might be appropriate for office practice include patient functioning (physical, role, and social functioning), emotional health, and various other quality-of-life variables.

These types of measures are not in wide supply, although they are available (Nelson and Berwick, 1989). One set was developed to use in the Medical Outcomes Study (MOS), which is investigating outcomes of care in different types of outpatient practice settings (Stewart et al., 1989; Tarlov et al., 1989). This study has shown promising interim results using one version of the MOS "Short Form" instrument (Stewart et al., 1988), a generic measure of functional status, to demonstrate different functional "profiles" for patients with chronic disease (e.g., hypertension, coronary heart disease, diabetes, and depression) that might be useful as benchmarks for evaluating care.

One innovative set of visual charts to measure dimensions of health status is called COOP charts. Selected items in these charts tap areas of physical, mental, role, and social functioning (Exhibit 6.A9). The COOP charts are being tested for use in ambulatory practice (Nelson et al., 1987; Nelson and Berwick, 1989) .

Outcomes such as patient health status measured at some transitional point in care can help to evaluate preceding care in another setting; that is, health status at the time of admission to the hospital or admission to home health care tells something about the previous steps of patient management. Similarly, periodic health status measurement can provide information about differences in observed health status compared with expected status.

Patient reports. Patient reports refer broadly to interviews and surveys of patients conducted either at the time care is provided or later, by telephone or by mail. Surveys can include potential patients, such as HMO members who have not used care. Interview and survey content can include patient *reports* about the process of care (both technical and interpersonal) and outcomes of care, as well as *ratings* about the quality of those aspects of care and about the patient's satisfaction with the encounter.

Surveys can address such aspects of patient experience as access to care, amenities of care, interpersonal and technical aspects of care, health status, understanding of instructions, experience in comparison to expectations (including a judgment of outstanding as well as poor care), and unmet needs. Detailed satisfaction surveys are fielded by many HMOs and, increasingly, by hospitals. In addition to compiling assessments of care received in primary care facilities, some surveys also include questions about specialists' offices, affiliated hospitals, and patient education programs.

Patient reports can provide information about (1) underuse (such as perceived lack of access, underdiagnosis, or undertreatment), (2) interpersonal aspects of the care received, and (3) values and preferences in relation to decisions about care. All three aspects of quality measurement are lacking in most problem-detection methods. Including a request for open-ended response in patient surveys can be an important way to identify unexpected problems and useful suggestions. Satisfaction questionnaires that are sufficiently sensitive to specific elements of care and to change over time can be a valuable way of documenting improvement and excellence.

Assessments can be used to compare sites if data are properly adjusted for differences in populations and expectations. Assessments are commonly used internally by organizations (although they are not necessarily fielded by or used by the quality assurance program), and only rarely by external groups. Recently a great deal of work has gone into the development of valid and reliable patient assessment instruments (Davies and Ware, 1988). The Group Health Association of America, the HMO industry's trade association, has made available to its members a well-designed satisfaction

EXHIBIT 6.A7 Example of Ambulatory Record Review for Patient with "Sentinel" Hospital Admission for Diabetic Acidosis

SCREENING QUESTIONS

DIABETIC ACIDOSIS

PT. NAME _____ CLINIC _____

PT. ID NO. _____ BIRTHDATE _____ SEX _____ AGE _____

EFF. DATE OF HMO ENROLLMENT _____ PRIM. M.D. _____

HOSP. _____ ADM. DATE _____ DISCH. DATE _____

CONSULTANT _____

PRIM. DX. _____

SEC. DX. _____

SURG. PROCEDURES _____

CODES: 250.1, 250.2, 250.3, 251

DEFINITION: All hospitalizations for diabetic acidosis with lab reports indicating blood sugar >250 mg. dl, arterial ph≤ 7.30 or venous $CO_2 \leq 12$ and ketonuria or ketonemia.

DATA TO BE COLLECTED REGARDING OUTPATIENT CARE: YES   NO

1. Was there a physician visit related to this diagnosis outside the hospital within 10 days prior to admission? (s   same day) Date _____   ____   ____

2. Was patient seen in ER within 10 days prior to admission? (s   same day) Date _____   ____   ____

3. Was there telephone contact related to this diagnosis within 10 days prior to admission? (s   same day)   ____   ____

4. Was diagnosis of ketoacidosis made more than 24 hours prior to admission?   ____   ____

5. Was patient a known diabetic?   ____   ____

6. Was there a history of any of the following within 10 days prior to admission? If yes, circle: a) infection; b) change in diet; c) trauma   ____   ____

7. Was there a history of any of the following within the 10 days prior to admission? If yes, circle: a) weight loss; b) abdominal pain; c) polyuria; d) dehydration   ____   ____

8. Was patient on insulin prior to admission?   ____   ____

9. Was patient seen in outpatient setting for diabetes in last 6 months? Date last seen _____   ____   ____

10. Were blood sugars monitored by patient or clinic within 30 days prior to admission? (s   same day)   ____   ____

11. Was patient on home glucose monitoring or had they been instructed in glucose monitoring?   ____   ____

12. Was there follow up care within 10 days after discharge? If yes, circle where it occurred: a) clinic; b) nursing home; 3) home health care; d) other _____   ____   ____

13. Was there evidence of patient noncompliance with treatment plan (e.g. drugs, diet, follow up visits)? If so, comment _____   ____   ____

14. Was there a readmission or mortality within 30 days after admission? Date _____ Diagnosis _____   ____   ____

15. Were there other admissions related to this diagnosis within 6 months before or after this admission? Date(s) _____ Diagnosis _____   ____   ____

| | Check if comments on back   B 1 82

11

EXHIBIT 6.A7   Continued

INSTRUCTIONS

"Primary M.D." is the physician who had seen the patient most frequently during the preceding year.

"Consultant(s)" are the one or more physicians, other than the primary care physician, seen either before hospitalization or during preceding year.

Record "yes" or "no" answers from information in either inpatient or outpatient record.

When Emergency Room (ER) is used, the term includes both hospital ER and urgent care clinics outside of hospitals.

When a question asks whether there was a documented history or symptom, record "yes" if there is documentation in chart to answer question in the affirmative; or "no" if there is documentation in chart to answer question in the negative or absence of data requested by the question.

Comments:

EXHIBIT 6.A8 Example of Outpatient Clinic Sentinel Events

OCHSNER MEDICAL INSTITUTIONS
QUALITY ASSESSMENT DEPARTMENT

17 SENTINEL EVENTS

Principal Diagnosis	Qualifiers	Denominator on Trending Report
Prematurity	Born in house Before 37 weeks Exclude intentionally induced within 30 days of Clinic visit	# of OB deliveries
Pulmonary embolism/infarct	Must have been seen in the Clinic within 30 days	none
Cellulitis	Lower extremities No operative procedures	none
Hypokalemia	Serum level <3 mEq/1 Diuretic therapy prior to hospitalization	none
Ruptured appendix	Supported by Pathology report Seen in the Clinic/ Emergency Department within 10 days of admission	# of appendicitis cases, to include non-ruptured

GI catastrophies
  GI hemorrhage
  Chronic stomach ulcer with hemorrhage
  Chronic stomach ulcer with hemorrhage and perforation
	With transfusion	none

Endometrial cancer	History of uninterrupted estrogen therapy for one year Total abdominal hysterectomy as principal or OR procedure	none

Principal Diagnosis	Qualifiers	Denominator on Trending Report
Breast cancer	Stage II, III/IV Breast surgery	none
Cervical cancer	Abnormal Pap smear III, IV, V Pap smear within a year	none
Asthma	Clinic visit within one month	# of clinic patients seen for Dx asthma during the review period
Diabetic acidosis	none	All patients with insulin-dependent diabetes seen in the hospital during the review period
Severe preclampsia and eclampsia	none	# of OB Clinic patients seen in the clinic during the review period
Gangrene	Only extremity Comorbidity diagnosis of peripheral vascular disease	# of clinic patients seen during period with a peripheral disease
Ruptured ectopic pregnancies	none	# of new OB clinic patients seen in the clinic during the review period
Drug toxicity and/or reaction	none	none
Cancellation/delay in surgery	Ambulatory care concern	none
Other: Review that indicates admission to the hospital resulted from ambulatory care management	none	none

SOURCE: Ochsner Medical Institutions, used with permission.

EXHIBIT 6.A9 Example of Health Status Measure

PHYSICAL CONDITION

During the past 4 weeks . . .
What was the most strenuous level
of physical activity you could do for at
least 2 minutes?

Very heavy, e.g.

    Run, fast pace
    Carry heavy bag of
      groceries upstairs

Heavy, e.g.

    Jog, slow pace
    Climb stairs at moderate
      pace

Moderate, e.g.

    Walk, fast pace
    Garden, easy digging
    Carry heavy bag of
      groceries

Light, e.g.

    Walk, regular pace
    Golf or vacuum
    Carry light bag of
      groceries

Very light, e.g.

    Walk, slow pace
    Drive car
    Wash dishes

SOURCE: Trustees of Dartmouth College/COOP Project, 1986, used with permission.

instrument that can be used for enrollee and patient satisfaction surveys (Exhibit 6.A10). The increasing availability of such instruments may bring a degree of standardization of methods and instruments to the health care field for use by the Medicare program as well as by internal quality assurance programs.

Complaints and incidents. Although only rarely described in our site visits, some HMOs have developed complaint coding systems and incident reporting systems to monitor problems in delivery of care and to track their resolution. Examples of ambulatory incidents include: abusive or bizarre behavior, cardiac arrest, drug reaction, bruises and burns, and equipment malfunctions.

Continuous improvement. The availability of medical records and laboratory results, timely access to patient services such as specialty care or routine appointments, and tracking and follow-up evaluation of special cases are ubiquitous concerns in ambulatory facilities. Increasingly, such facilities are attending to the continuous improvement model, which emphasizes participation of locally involved practitioners in the examination and redesign of the many complex steps required in health care. Exhibit 6.A11 uses one of the analytic tools, a "fish bone diagram," to display the possible reasons for failure to institute urgent antibiotic therapy.

Organization-Specific Programs

General approaches in prepaid or managed care settings. Quality assurance program activities in HMOs include guideline development, criteria-based record review, generic screening, patient surveys, and complaint review. They also involve analysis of access and system problems, such as waiting time in the reception areas, dropped phone calls, and rate of repeat X-rays because of poor film quality. Methods chosen depend on the resources and the sophistication of the data system of the HMO. HMOs with computerized medical record systems or clinical information in their management information systems can undertake more extensive review, but most HMOs depend on manual data collection.

General approaches in staff- and group-model HMOs. The Harvard Community Health Plan has a computerized clinical information system (COSTAR) and one of the more extensive programs of quality measurement we encountered. Its program focuses on eight areas:

1.   outcomes, in particular health status outcomes
2.   technical processes including scheduled preventive and screening processes

EXHIBIT 6.A10 Selected Items from an HMO Satisfaction Survey

THINKING ABOUT YOUR OWN MEDICAL CARE, HOW WOULD YOU RATE THE FOLLOWING? . . .

	Poor	Fair	Good	Very Good	Excellent
Access to Care					
Access to speciality care if you need it	1	2	3	4	5
Access to medical care in an emergency	1	2	3	4	5
Length of time spent waiting at the office to see the doctor	1	2	3	4	5
Availability of medical information or advice by phone	1	2	3	4	5
Finances					
Protection you have against hardship due to medical expenses	1	2	3	4	5
Technical Quality					
Thoroughness of examinations and accuracy of diagnosis	1	2	3	4	5
Skill, experience, and training of doctors	1	2	3	4	5
Communication					
Explanations of medical procedures and tests	1	2	3	4	5
Attention given to what you have to say	1	2	3	4	5
Advice you get about ways to avoid illness and stay healthy	1	2	3	4	5
Interpersonal Care					
Personal interest in you and your medical problems	1	2	3	4	5
Respect shown to you, attention to your privacy	1	2	3	4	5
Amount of time you have with doctors and staff during a visit	1	2	3	4	5
Outcomes					
The outcomes of your medical care, how much you are helped	1	2	3	4	5
Overall quality of care and services	1	2	3	4	5

SOURCE: Adapted with permission from Group Health Association of America, Inc. © 1988 by GHAA/D&W. Potential users are encouraged to write GHAA, 1129 Twentieth St., N.W., Suite 600, Washington, D.C. 20036 for the complete instrument and users manual.

Exhibit 6.A11 Example of Quality Control Methods Used to Analyze Ambulatory Care Process in Industrial Control Model (Fish Bone Diagram)

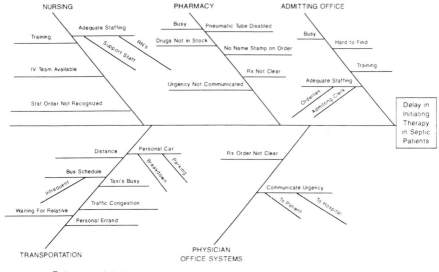

Delay in antibiotic therapy

SOURCE: Batalden and Buchanan, 1989, used with permission.

3. access, such as emergency care and telephone access,
4. interpersonal care,
5. integration of care among multiple care providers,
6. physical facilities (e.g., cleanliness and privacy),
7. staff morale, and
8. variation that allows for flexibility to meet needs of individual patients.

Computerized record reviews use over 60 variables to conduct retrospective and prospective reviews of process, outcome, and patient satisfaction (e.g., well-baby, hospital, and telephone encounters; access to appointments; rate of colon cancer screening; pharmacy waiting time). Four central areas are given priority because of their high potential as problem areas: poor access, failure to communicate, unclear areas of responsibility, and failure of proper supervision (Fintor, 1988).

The quality management program of Group Health Cooperative of Puget Sound (GHC) includes the rigorous credentialing and performance assessment efforts described earlier, departmental case reviews, departmental and systemwide clinical indicators, and multidisciplinary and regional review committees. GHC also emphasizes consumer criteria for care; these outline 52 expectations for service-related aspects of care such as access to emergency services, waiting times for routine appointments and specialty referrals, and courtesy and behavior of professional staff. The office of quality-of-care assessment provides technical support at the regional and departmental level, staffs committees, maintains and provides cross-site statistics, manages the flow of information to councils and the governing board of GHC, and responds to external reviewers (Perry and Kirz, 1989).

General approaches in IPA or PPO settings. "Quality assurance" in IPAs is complicated by several factors: dispersed delivery sites; sites that may participate in many HMOs; variation in medical record format between sites; and lack of a history of quality review. Quality review in IPAs has generally consisted of claims review of utilization patterns (e.g., rate of specialty referrals, hospital admissions, length of stay, pharmacy), pre-procedure review, and second opinion programs; all are methods to identify overuse (Koizumi and Sorian, 1988). One IPA reported to us that it now expects medical directors to have direct interaction with its physicians concerning quality-of-care issues (presumably rather than writing a letter).

Because IPAs (like staff- and group-model HMOs) have an enrolled population, they have access to registration and claims data for developing profiles of practitioners and reviewing patient care across many sites of care. For instance, computerized pharmacy reports can be used to monitor drug prescribing patterns and drug incompatibilities. The potential exists to assess health needs and accessibility for nonuser enrollees. As a case in point, U.S. Healthcare, an IPA-model HMO with approximately 1 million members in six states, assesses and provides its physicians with aggregate information about their own practices. It conducts member surveys and reviews 20 office records per year in each office looking at two standards of practice. Standards are chosen to meet five criteria; they must be noncontroversial, measurable against an expected compliance level, auditable by a trained college graduate with a high level of accuracy and reproducibility, important enough to make a difference in the delivery of medical care, and have the potential for improvement based on current levels of performance (Stocker, 1989). The "quality assurance rating" provided to practitioners, which is included as part of a financial incentive formula, includes member satisfaction measures from surveys, rates of patient transfers, results of medical record audits, and managed care philosophy (Schlackman, 1989).

Likewise, PPOs are administrative entities of great variety with geographically dispersed providers and little institutional or group loyalty. Recently, some PPOs report that they require member physicians to provide access to medical records for quality of care and utilization review and to agree to possible disciplinary measures in their contracts (Goodspeed and Goldfield, 1987). Some PPOs have begun to emphasize quality and cost-effectiveness, to use systematic peer review, and to develop risk-adjusted outcome indices, ambulatory care treatment standards, and clinically based measures of appropriate care (Boland, 1987). Other performance measures, such as postoperative complications and patient satisfaction, are expected to be increasingly available (Goodspeed and Goldfield, 1987). For practitioners with unusual utilization data or unusual numbers of specific diagnoses, retrospective review of office records can be conducted. Selected indicators derived from claims data analysis can be used to develop aggregate quality indicators for screening for early detection of disease (e.g., mammography, stool occult blood screening, or Pap smears).

General approaches in fee-for-service settings. Some quality assessment methods are applicable to large group practices. The collection of indicator data (including access indicators), patient surveys, and review of complaints are applicable to all types of office practice in both the prepaid and fee-for-service sectors. Outpatient clinics also use combinations of methods such as access, clinical indicators, and generic screening.

For instance, the 60 outpatient clinics of the University of Chicago Hospitals group use a single data collection tool to acquire information on indicators that address both servicewide and clinic-specific concerns. The indicators include seven volume indicators, screens for complications possibly caused by misdiagnosis or mismanagement (Exhibit 6.A12a), and clinic-specific indicators (Exhibit 6.A12b) (Oswald and Winer, 1987). Administrative responsibility for managing the system is delegated in part to each of the medical center's quality assurance coordinators and physician directors. Each clinic is responsible for conducting a quality review annually on *all* patients seen during two 1-week periods.

Although quality assurance programs tend to be the most well developed in large clinic settings, even very small practices sometimes develop programs. For instance, the Pike Street Clinic in Seattle, which serves mainly low-income elderly in the immediate area, has voluntarily developed a Medical Practices Committee. It draws on outside medical expertise (for instance, colleagues from a nearby hospital) for help in developing criteria and conducting chart review. Among the issues addressed are compliance with screening guidelines and review of ambulatory records of hospitalized patients to determine whether the admission might have been avoided.

In another example, a four-person practice in Fairfax, Virginia, has devised a multifaceted approach to quality assurance. A computerized data base flags preventive care needs based on patient age and sex. The four physicians meet every day, review each other's charts, and cross-read X rays. Once a month they have "doctors rounds" that function as a journal club. Nurses alert the doctors when patients call in for prescription renewals, and they review the records of patients who fail to keep appointments. They emphasize continuing medical education; the corporation pays for 2

EXHIBIT 6.A12a Example of Procedures and Complications for Monitoring

PROCEDURES AND COMPLICATIONS FOR MONITORING

CLINIC	PROCEDURES	COMPLICATIONS
Gynecology	Cervical biopsy	Excessive bleeding
	Endometrial biopsy	Perforation and/or excessive bleeding
Obstetrics	Amniocentesis	Premature rupture of membranes and/or premature labor
Orthopedics	Joint injections	Allergic reaction
	Casts	Swelling, pain, or coldness of extremity
Cardiology	Anticoagulation therapy	Bleeding episodes
Gastroenterology	Endoscopic procedures	Perforation and/or bleeding
Pulmonary Medicine	Management of acute asthma attack in outpatient department	Need for inpatient admission outpatient department management
Hematology/ Oncology	Bone marrow aspiration	Excessive bleeding/lidocaine reaction
	Lumbar puncture	Lidocaine reaction
Surgery	Breast biopsy	Excessive bleeding at site
	Incision and draining	Recurrence of abscess post incision and drainage
	Kidney biopsy (post-transplant patients)	Excessive bleeding
Ophthalmology	Applanations	Corneal abrasion
	Fluorescein angiograms	Reaction to dye
General Medicine	Phlebotomy	Prolonged bleeding at site, inability to draw, syncope
Rheumatology	Gold injections	Nitroid reactions
Ear, Nose, and Throat	Fiberoptic nasopharyngoscopy	Airway obstruction, infection
	Myringotomy	Infection, impaired hearing

SOURCE: Oswald and Winer, 1987, used with permission.

weeks of professional meetings each year. Finally, as recommended by the American Society of Internal Medicine, they routinely send laboratory samples to the College of American Pathologists to check their laboratory test results.

Commercial Systems

Medical Management Analysis. Craddick's Medical Management Analysis (MMA) system, originally designed for use in hospitals, has been adapted for ambulatory use. It is being tested by Kaiser Foundation Health Plans, Oakland, California, in two sites—Hawaii and North Carolina (Johnsson, 1988). The outpatient design focuses on certain "high-risk" ambulatory

EXHIBIT 6.A12b Example of Clinic-Specific Screening Criteria

CLINIC-SPECIFIC CRITERIA

CLINIC	CRITERIA	STANDARD
Cardiology	Percent of patients receiving antihypertensives whose potassium levels are below normal.	0%
Gastroenterology	Percent of patients over age 50 without hemoccults for past year.	0%
	Percent of patients over age 50 without proctoscopy or flexible sigmoidoscopy during past five years.	20%
Obstetrics and Gynecology	Performance of Pap smear not documented (exception: hysterectomy).	0%
	Performance of breast exam not documented.	0%
	(Population includes all gynecology patients who are new or returning for an annual visit, and all pregnant patients.)	
Pulmonary	Tuberculin testing performed on all new patients (exception: where physician notes contraindication).	100%
Hematology/ Oncology	Temperature and weight taken on all patients at every visit.	100%
Nephrology	Weight and blood pressure taken on all patients at every visit.	100%
Psychiatry	All patients on neuroleptics screened for tardive dyskinesia at least monthly. All patients and/or family members educated regarding symptoms of tardive dyskinesia and need to report same.	100%
	All patients on lithium have lithium blood levels drawn at least every three months.	
General Pediatrics	Percent of patients (15-24 months of age) who have been screened for anemia.	100%
	Percent of patients (15-24 months of age) who have had a tine test.	100%
	Percent of patients (24 months of age) who have had 4 diphtheria-pertussis-tetanus vaccines, 4 oral polio vaccine, 1 measles-mumps-rubella vaccine.	100%
	Percent of patients (24 months of age) with height and weight recorded in the chart.	100%
Pediatric Neurology	Percent of seizure patients receiving Tegretol and/or Depakene (anticonvulsants) for whom complete blood count with differential and liver function tests have been documented within the last 6 months.	100%
Ophthalmology	Percent of patients who were refracted out of all patients where this examination was indicated.	100%
Adult Neurology	Percent of all patients having positive syphilis serology test results who received appropriate follow-up and antibiotic therapy.	100%
General	Percent of patients with verified hypertension, (i.e., blood pressure >140/90 taken on three occasions during a two month period) who received physician assessment and follow-up.	100%

SOURCE: Oswald and Winer, 1987, used with permission.

visits, particularly unplanned revisits that might represent complications or incorrect management of problems. Examples would be an unplanned visit to the clinic or to the emergency room after a previous emergency room visit or hospitalization.

AmbuQual. The AmbuQual system, a proprietary system for ambulatory care review in clinics and HMOs, was developed at Methodist Hospital of Indiana (Benson et al., 1987). AmbuQual bases its review of care in the ambulatory setting on 10 "care parameters," although it has now developed some 150 indicators to measure 40 aspects of care.

Weightings of the relative importance of each of the 10 care parameters were assigned by 48 Joint Commission ambulatory facility surveyors as follows:

practitioner performance	1.92
appropriateness of services	1.39
patient compliance	1.25
support staff performance	1.11
accessibility	0.91
continuity of care	0.90
patient risk minimization	0.70
medical record system	0.68
patient satisfaction	0.59
cost of services	0.54

These weights imply, for instance, that the impact on patients' health of "appropriateness of services" is twice that of "risk minimization" activities, and that "practitioner performance" has approximately 3.5 times the importance of "cost of services."

Patterns of Treatment. Software marketed by Current Review Technology (CRT) uses ambulatory claims data to review the amount and type of physician services compared to diagnosis-specific norms. Thus, this approach requires accurate and complete diagnostic and procedural coding on insurance claims. Although marketed as a utilization review tool, it can be used for quality assessment by identifying inappropriate care, primarily overuse of services by a small percentage of aberrant practitioners (Chassin et al. 1989a).

External Methods of Correcting Problems in Ambulatory Care

Clearly, activities related to changing behaviors of physicians and other practitioners in the hospital setting are available for correcting problems of clinicians in their ambulatory care roles. Options not described in earlier sections of this chapter are briefly noted here.

State Disciplinary Action (Licensing Board)

In most states, the same board that grants licenses to applicants is also invested with the authority to discipline physicians deemed to be unfit to practice. Possible disciplinary actions include probation, limitations on practice, fines, reprimands, letters of censure, letters of concern, collection of the costs of proceedings, and revocation of license. Usual grounds for disciplinary actions are professional incompetence or misconduct. Violation of state-specific medical practice acts provide specific grounds as well, including drug abuse and the incorrect prescribing of medication (AMA, 1986; Grad and Marti, 1979).[14]

State medical boards may require physicians to enter an impaired clinician program, or they may require continuing education in areas of deficiency. In some states the publishing of the disciplined physician's name in the newspaper is a powerful option.

PRO/HCFA Actions Related to HMOs and CMPs

Medicare risk contracts require HMOs to have procedures for addressing and resolving enrollee complaints such as problems in service delay. Enrollees may also appeal to the Secretary of DHHS if they believe services have been denied improperly or that charges were excessive for services received (if the amount involved exceeds $100) (Merlis, 1988). PRO interventions in response to quality problems discovered on PRO review include moving the HMO to intensified review status and removal from the program (see Volume I, Chapter 6, and Chapter 8 in this volume).

Other Indirect Interventions

In addition to state sanctions and penalties directed toward individual practitioners, indirect interventions include those based on assumptions about competition and market forces, such as information release and public disclosure. Publication (or fear of publication) of malpractice data or publication, such as in California and Pennsylvania, of the names of disciplined physicians might lead some patients to change providers. Data collection and dissemination efforts by state data commissions or business coalitions might lead to nonrenewal of contracts or to selective contracting by state Medicaid or private third-party payers.

Any number of other methods to change physician practice have been developed or recommended over the years. These include voluntary physician self-audit systems for CME (Sanazaro, 1983; Sanazaro and Worth, 1985) and restructuring the reimbursement system in order to change financial incentives to overuse or underuse, and so neutralize incentives.

The Maine Medical Assessment Program relies on specialty-based study groups to analyze practice variations in nine specialty areas: orthopedics, OB/GYN, urology, internal medicine, pediatrics, ophthalmology, family practice, general surgery, and substance abuse. Statewide and regional meetings provide practitioners with feedback on practice patterns. For instance, observed hysterectomy rates dropped to "expected" levels in both urban and other areas following the feedback process. The orthopedics-neurosurgery group found a very high rate of laminectomies (a surgical procedure to correct damaged spinal discs) in four geographic areas. After feedback and discussion regarding the appropriateness of surgical intervention, surgical rates dropped to the state average the following year (MMAF, 1989). Many health analysts believe this approach has great promise as a physician practice "change agent."

Internal Methods of Correcting Problems in Ambulatory Care

As with external methods, intraorganizational approaches to corrective action mimic those of hospitals, and they are not discussed in detail here. The chief difference is that the average hospital has a considerably stronger hand in requiring formal action than does the average office-based practice. In small practices, problem correction lies solely with the members of the practice; to the extent that habits die hard, that a significant hierarchy of professional reputation exists in the practice, or that financial constraints are important, internal efforts at change may be difficult to implement. Only in the larger prepaid or multispecialty clinics is the range of options and organizational leadership likely to be similar to that of hospitals and thus easier to put into place.

Corrective actions in HMOs are probably most comparable to those in hospitals. Wilner et al. (1978) have described several kinds of problems and possible intervention strategies developed for an HMO (Exhibit 6.A13). HMOs may, for instance, provide their physicians with information about their practice patterns (with much the same philosophy that guides the Maine project). They may also develop problem tracking reports with corrective actions indicated. To respond to patient complaints, HMOs often define grievance procedures that include several levels of appeal and that may culminate in a formal grievance hearing; this in turn may prompt a change in practitioners' performance (Exhibit 6.A14). At a more serious level, HMOs frequently include in their contracts with physicians a "terminate without cause" clause, which allows them to terminate or not renew contracts without having to have any elaborate process to justify it.

HOME HEALTH CARE[15,16]

A variety of factors have made the topic of quality measurement and assurance for home health care an especially relevant topic. Perhaps the

EXHIBIT 6.A13 Example of Possible HMO Intervention Strategies in Ambulatory Care

Problem Type	Possible Intervention Strategies
No problem	No active intervention indicated, but repeat retrospective audit or pilot study periodically
Provider knowledge or skill	Retrospective feedback on group and individual performance, followed by educational or training session; peer group pressure
System design	Modification of impacting systems in terms of: policy, procedures, staffing, delineation of responsibility, and/ or output
Provider oversight	Computer-generated flags or concurrent reminders geared to individual patient care situations; peer group pressure
Patient noncompliance	Patient education; outreach; system modification
Provider commitment to standards	Peer group pressure; reassessment of standards; conference with department chief or medical director

SOURCE: Wilner et al., 1978.

most central concerns are that the elderly needing and receiving in-home care are particularly vulnerable to inadequate care and that current public regulation is poorly equipped to assure the quality of in-home services. As the American Bar Association (ABA) notes in its "Black Box" report (ABA, 1986, p. 1):

> Consumers and their families face an utterly confusing array of changing services, a dearth of information on which to base expectations, and little control over what happens. Even more significant is the in-home location of services that makes their actual delivery essentially invisible and, therefore, largely beyond the easy reach of public or professional scrutiny.

Concerns flow from five related factors. First, although home health care generally enjoys a good reputation, serious questions have arisen about the quality of home health care. Second, state and federal quality assurance systems, where they exist, have at best worked imperfectly, while peer and professional reviews have also been inadequate. Third, the drive to contain program costs may have an adverse impact on quality of care. Fourth, the growth of the proprietary home health sector and of unlicensed agencies may negatively affect quality of care. Finally, the nature of home care means that minimal professional supervision of direct care will occur at the same time that there is heavy reliance on nonprofessional caregivers who work with vulnerable clients.

EXHIBIT 6.A14 Example of Grievance Plan for Group Model HMO

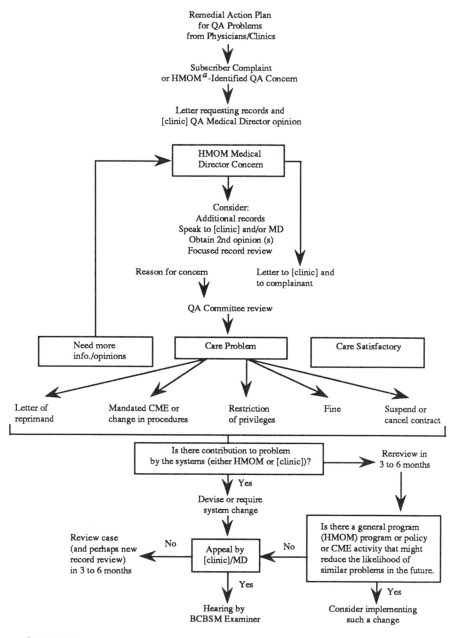

[a]HMO Minnesota
SOURCE: Blue Plus (Blue Cross and Blue Shield of Minnesota), used with permission.

The provision of such critical services to frail consumers warrants monitoring in any setting. The issue is especially sensitive when the services are provided at some distance from the clinical backup provided in a clinic or hospital, when supervision and quality review are distant, and when care providers may not be sufficiently or appropriately trained to provide such care (McAllister et al., 1986). Moreover, although aides do not typically provide the same proportion of care in the home as in nursing homes, they still provide a significant portion of care, even in Medicare-certified agencies. Indeed, the ABA (1986) study found an increasing trend to use aides for tasks formerly handled by nurses.

Publicly funded home care for the elderly involves federal, state, and local responsibilities. The federal government partially funds home care services through Medicare, Medicaid, the Older Americans Act (Title III), and the Social Services Block Grant (Title XX of the Social Security Act). The primary responsibility for service delivery and quality assessment, however, lies with the state (Macro Systems, 1988).

External Methods of Preventing Problems in Home Health Care

Medicare and Medicaid Conditions of Participation

As with other areas in which it is a major payer, the federal government has established standards for the type and quality of home health services provided to Medicare beneficiaries (Hawes and Powers, 1987). A provider who wishes to be reimbursed by either Medicare or Medicaid must be certified as being in substantial compliance with federal standards before being authorized to receive such payments. With Medicare, agencies must actually be certified. For Medicaid, agencies must merely meet the requirements for certification, but need not actually be certified. As with nursing homes, the responsibility for regulating agencies is shared. The federal government sets the standards (and pays for the survey); the states are responsible for monitoring and surveying the agencies and determining whether they are in compliance with the standards.

When surveying home health agencies for certification, state health department staff use a survey instrument developed by HCFA that measures basic compliance with the federal Conditions of Participation. These conditions address the following:

- compliance with state and local laws
- organization of services and administration
- requirements for professional staff
- acceptance of patients, plan of treatment, and medical supervision
- provision of skilled nursing services
- provision of therapy services

- requirements for medical social services
- availability of home health aide services
- maintenance of clinical records
- ongoing evaluation.

The standards are largely structural, with some process requirements, and they do not address patient outcomes. They also do not contain basic requirements for the training and competency of aides. The survey consists of a checklist of procedural and structural requirements that a surveyor can complete from agency records.

The survey process for visits to home health clients has been criticized for being announced in advance to providers or timed so predictably as to be easily anticipated. Critics argue that such a process allows poor providers to change their performance dramatically for the brief period around the date of the survey, and, therefore, that it does not yield an accurate picture of the care provided. When conducted as part of the survey and certification activities, home visits are scheduled in conjunction with the home health agency visit to a client. Although this may facilitate observation of care, there is some legitimate question as to whether the care provided under observation will accurately replicate routine care. Further, few observers believe such a process facilitates an open exchange with the client or a family caregiver about any problems with the agency (Harrington, 1988).

Although federal survey procedures require the surveyor to conduct a minimum of three home health care visits to clients as part of the survey process, results of a study of home health regulations in California and Missouri reveal that home visits are frequently not conducted (Harrington, 1988). Thus, in practice, interviews with patients and their families and observation of care have not been part of the survey. In addition, there is no independent assessment of the accuracy and completeness of the agency's initial patient assessment and care plan, nor, as noted, is there regulatory attention to patient outcomes.

More recently, home health agency surveys have become even more circumscribed. As a result of several factors, including federal budget reductions, state licensing and certification agencies appear to be limiting surveys primarily to those agencies about which they receive complaints. Reports from California indicate that in 1987–1988, only about 10 percent of the Medicare-certified home health agencies actually faced yearly surveys (Harrington, 1988). However, a survey conducted by the National Association for Home Care (NAHC) reported that 82 percent of respondents (typically Medicare-certified, nonprofit, free-standing agencies) reported annual on-site surveys (NAHC, 1986).

Practitioners employed by home health agencies must be certified in order to be reimbursed by Medicare. Conditions of Participation require licenses of health professionals. Effective January 1, 1990, unlicensed individuals such as home health aides must complete a training and competency evaluation program.

OBRA 1987 Mandates on Home Health Quality and Regulation

The Omnibus Budget Reconciliation Act (OBRA) of 1987 (P.L. 100-203) made sweeping revisions of both nursing home and home health Conditions of Participation (now called requirements), the survey process, and enforcement mechanisms for Medicare and Medicaid. New home health requirements were published in August 1989. Much of the new home health survey process and enforcement remedies are similar to the changes in nursing home regulation, which in turn derive from the recommendations of the IOM Committee on Nursing Home Regulation (IOM, 1986).

The new home health requirements create a patients' bill of rights, specify notification and disclosure of agency ownership, require that home health agency personnel be either licensed or trained in a program that meets standards specified by the Secretary of DHHS, include some requirements for the content of the training, and require that the agency include each patient's plan of care in the clinical record.

The new law also sets up a process of "standard" and "extended" surveys for home health agencies; it requires annual surveys to be conducted without prior notice and scheduled in such a way as to minimize the ability of the provider to predict the timing of the survey. The standard survey, to which each agency is to be subject, calls for visits to the homes of clients, selected on the basis of a "case-mix stratified" sample of the agency's clients, to evaluate the quality of care provided by the agency. The home visits appear to be directed at gathering outcome-based measures of quality, particularly in the areas of physical functioning. In addition, the plan of care and clinical record must be in accord with a "standardized assessment instrument." Finally, the standard survey must be based on a protocol that was to be developed, tested, and validated by the Secretary of DHHS no later than October 1, 1989.

Extended surveys would be triggered by negative findings on the standard survey, but they can also occur for other reasons. They will include a more extensive review of policies and procedures.

New standards require state surveyors to make in-home visits and interview patients. Abt Associates (with support from HCFA) is developing a patient-oriented approach to surveying home health agencies for the home visit portion of the revised Conditions of Participation. Their proposed instrument will query patients about their understanding of their medical condition and plan of care, elicit patient and family expectations for outcomes, and ascertain whether self-care techniques have been taught. Another section deals with the perceptions of patients and their families about the dependability and continuity of care and caregiver sensitivity.

OBRA 1986: Uniform Needs Assessment

Section 9305(h) of OBRA 1986 (P.L. 99-509) mandated the development (but not the implementation) of a uniform needs assessment instrument by the Secretary of DHHS. The instrument is intended to be used to evaluate the needs of patients for post-hospital extended care services, home health services, and long-term-care services of a health-related or supportive nature. It is to be used by hospital discharge planners, home health agencies, other health care providers, and fiscal intermediaries to evaluate post-discharge needs for continuing care. Content will include measures of functional capacities, nursing care requirements, and social and family supports available (DHHS, 1989c) (see also Chapter 8 in this volume). It may also be used to determine whether payment for long term care should be approved.

An advisory panel appointed by the Secretary developed a draft instrument that was reviewed by interested organizations, associations, and providers. As of November 1989, a final instrument had been prepared but not yet transmitted to Congress by the Secretary of DHHS.

Licensure

Licensure generally gives authority to organize and operate. According to a recent survey by the Intergovernmental Health Policy Project (IHPP, 1989), 36 states currently have home health agency licensure requirements in place, and 2 others (Washington and Minnesota) were to have joined them by July 1989. Three other states have licensure laws but face delays in implementing them. Some states license only proprietary agencies (ABA, 1986; Leader, 1986). In states that do license agencies, a large number of entities providing home care escape licensure altogether. Many agencies— estimates range from 15 percent of the total to a number equal to the number of licensed agencies—operate as nurse "pools" or employment agencies and thus are not required to be licensed (Harrington, 1988).

The licensure laws vary widely but generally mirror Medicare Conditions of Participation (Riley, 1988). In a survey conducted by the American Association of Retired Persons, only 9 of 25 responding states reported having licensure laws more stringent than Medicare. Twelve states mandate specific consumer rights, and 13 require specific training of personnel; a large number of states in the survey indicate a standard requiring care plans (Riley, 1988). A care plan is a written plan included in the medical record of a home health client. It includes: a listing of the patient-client problems and needs, goals that are measurable, objective outcomes, and specific activities or interventions that are planned to achieve the goals (adapted from Joint Commission, 1988).

According to the National Association for Home Care, such standards fail to ensure financial stability in agencies; adequate staffing, training, and supervision; and adequate internal quality assurance (Hawes and Powers, 1987). State efforts at quality assurance are similarly inadequate in terms of assuring home health quality.

A review of state quality assurance programs for home care conducted by Macro Systems (1988) illustrates the underdeveloped nature of standards, inspections, and enforcement mechanisms. For instance:

• Of the 19 states studied, only 3 had objective outcome criteria (Minnesota and South Carolina for Title XX and Wyoming for Title III case management programs).

• State efforts were mainly structural: worker training, training requirements for aides, licensure of home health agencies based on Medicare Conditions of Participation. Some states had additional standards involving bills of client rights and codes of ethics.

• Agency monitoring of home care was usually required, but requirements for supervision varied widely.

• Supervisory home visits were required for home health care, but the nature and frequency varied.

• Client assessment and evaluation and case management varied in model and frequency.

• Provider surveys were primarily tied to Medicare certification, state licensure, and accreditation review activities.

A few states mandate criminal record checks of job applicants, but such reviews are required more frequently for independent providers than for agency providers (Hawes and Kane, 1989).

Voluntary Accreditation (NLN, NHCC, Joint Commission)

Three voluntary accreditation programs are now in place for home health agencies. Since 1961, the National League for Nursing (NLN) in conjunction with the American Public Health Association has offered accreditation to home health care providers under a program called CHAP (Community Health Accreditation Program). The NLN has been working recently to develop improved structural and process quality standards for home health; these structural standards cover staffing, strategic planning, marketing, organization and management, and internal evaluation. The process standards include more extensive process quality measures (e.g., evaluations and discussions of patient assessment and the adequacy of the individual care plan). Other new features include adding client home visits to the accreditation surveys and shortening the period of accreditation (from 5 to 3 years).

The National HomeCaring Council (NHCC), which is now part of the Foundation for Hospice and Home Care, has accredited both home health aide and homemaker services since 1972. NHCC's standards address training, qualifications, and supervision of aide and homemaker services. The agencies accredited by NHCC are surveyed every 5 years. In addition, both the foundation and the NAHC, a trade association representing most of the Medicare-certified agencies, are working on the development of voluntary quality-of-care standards for home health agencies.

The Joint Commission now accredits community-based home health agencies in addition to existing accreditation for hospital-based agencies (Joint Commission, 1988). Standards require staff who provide home health or support services to participate in orientation, in-service training, and continuing education programs. Standards have been expanded to include quality-of-care activities for both health and support services. The Joint Commission standards address process of care (such as patients' receiving care in a timely manner), the adequacy of instruction and supervision of staff on equipment use, patients' rights, care planning and provision, and internal quality assurance.

By June 1989, the Joint Commission had completed 350 surveys and had scheduled over 700 surveys for completion in 1990 and 1991, or about 8 percent of some 13,000 home health organizations by 1991 (O'Leary, 1989).

HCFA has proposed that deemed status be accorded to agencies accredited by the NLN or the Joint Commission (*Federal Register*, December 31, 1987). Such a move awaits a decision by the HCFA Administrator and implementation of the new home health care Conditions of Participation. A Final Interim Rule on the Conditions was published in the *Federal Register* on August 14, 1989. Unless deemed status is granted, agencies have little reason to seek—and now rarely do—what is considered an expensive and added administrative burden.

From the perspective of consumers, accreditation is of limited utility because records regarding the agency's performance are not public. The Joint Commission has no mechanisms for receiving or responding to consumer complaints, and it does not have the power to sanction agencies that fail to meet accreditation standards or that, although in minimal compliance, nevertheless provide deficient care in some areas.

Case Management

Several states (e.g., Oregon, Washington, Wisconsin, and Maine) have implemented "case management" models in which professionals work with consumers to assess their needs, develop comprehensive plans of care, arrange for services, monitor service delivery, and reassess needs and revise plans regularly (Riley, 1988). States view case management (often administered through area agencies on aging) as an important quality assurance tool, for developing client advocacy and providing services based on the needs of the client (Riley, 1988). The success of these techniques for quality assurance remains unproven.

Internal Methods of Preventing Problems in Home Health Care

Methods used frequently by home health care agencies for ensuring the capacity of the organization to provide high quality in-home care include staff selection, continuing training requirements, and standards of work performance.

Staff Selection, Supervision, and Continuing Education

Staff selection begins by ensuring that those health professionals who must be licensed are, in fact, so licensed and by ensuring that those who are not required to be licensed (such as home health aides) have at least minimal training (Riley, 1988). Home health agencies may also require continuing training and allow time off from work for continuing education, provide additional in-service training as necessary for unfamiliar procedures, and make consultation arrangements for difficult cases.

During IOM site visits, staff at one visiting nurse service described their staff selection and training process as follows. Most nurses have baccalaureate degrees. Applicants must be interviewed by two different staff members and provide two references. The agency provides an extensive orientation program lasting 2 months, and evaluations occur at 2 and 6 months. Orientation includes review of necessary skills such as ostomy care, aseptic dressing, changing a tracheal tube, ventilator management, and teaching skills such as wound care and diabetic self-care to patients and caretakers.

All professional staff are required to attend 10 educational programs each year. Team meetings and conferences are held on roughly a biweekly basis to address NLN standards as well as interdisciplinary topics such as rehabilitation. A nurse accompanies the home health aide on the first visit to the home and every 2 weeks thereafter.

Backup Systems

Home health agencies have developed backup systems to assure patient safety. These may include keeping copies of patient prescriptions in the home office, requiring countersignatures of all care plans by a physician, maintaining a 24-hour hotline for emergencies, and having a tie-in to equipment recall notification (AHA, 1987). Other home health agencies require that the aide call in from the patient's home on arrival.

Patient Bill of Rights

Patients may be provided with a list of their rights: to be given information about their treatment, to refuse treatment, to be assured that caregivers are qualified, and to know that treatment is thorough. They may also be given instructions in case of emergency (such as power or equipment failure) and a pamphlet describing the duties of the health care worker (Daniels, 1986).

External Methods of Detecting Problems in Home Health Care

Assessing Care Provided in the Home

Quality assessment has typically been built on the techniques or approaches developed in the acute care sector, including admission and continuing stay reviews and medical care evaluations (Kane et al., 1979; Kane, 1981). However, these approaches must be adapted and supplemented for post-acute care because of the different goals and situations involved. Home health care often shares the objectives of acute care—in terms of patient recovery and rehabilitation—but it can be more complicated. In home health care, the determinants of need for service include not only the patient's medical condition but also cognitive and functional status. In addition, home health service episodes are typically longer and more difficult to define, and the location of service is the patient's home where many needs must be met by a combination of formal and informal care providers. The use of personnel is quite different from the acute care sector: physician participation is limited, and the number of unlicensed personnel who deliver home care services is large (Bauman et al., 1988).

Thus, quality in home health care must be defined in multidimensional terms covering health, functional, and social needs of patients. These fundamental differences have implications for how to define and measure home health quality as well as how to assure it. Issues in measuring quality in the home care setting are more fully discussed in Chapter 8 of Volume I.

Historical Efforts and Research Applicable to Internal Programs

An evaluation of the process of care looks at, first, whether care meets commonly accepted professional norms regarding the types of procedures a patient requires and, second, whether the manner in which care is provided meets professional standards. Both NLN and the Joint Commission have developed detailed process criteria for home health care (McCann and Hill, 1986; NLN, 1986). In addition, substantial work in the field of community health nursing has been done to develop process-of-care criteria in home health care (e.g., Januska et al., 1976; Daubert, 1977; Sorgen, 1986; Rinke and Wilson, 1987a, 1987b; Hawes and Kane, 1989). Further, several of the federal certification standards, such as "conformance with physician's orders," represent process criteria.

Abt Associates has developed a survey form (HomePACs) and protocol designed to measure some process aspects of home health care. The form focuses on the completeness of the initial patient assessment, content of the plan of care, evidence in the clinical record that the patient's needs have been reevaluated, and indications in the record that prescribed or ordered services have been provided.

The Abt form also involves surveyor observation of the home health caregiver. For example, it asks the surveyor to determine whether care is appropriate relative to the patient's condition, to say whether care delivered corresponds to the plan of treatment, and to assess the caregiver's capabilities based on these observations. The 1987 draft of the instrument does not distinguish between "undelivered" services and "unrecorded but delivered" services (Hawes and Kane, 1989).

Woodson et al. (1981) developed a detailed manual on quality assessment using process measures for nursing home patients. It specifies the care required for a variety of patient conditions, with appropriate exceptions for particular medical complications.

Research in outcomes measurement. Recently, outcome-based measures of patient status have commanded great attention. Whether using outcomes is desirable, much less feasible, has not been adequately addressed in home health. The strictest definition of outcomes refers to changes in patient status over time that are directly attributable to the care received, but some "intermediate" outcomes are also considered useful in evaluating acute and long term care (Kane et al., 1982; Hawes, 1983). For example, positive outcomes include improved function and discharge from care, participation in enjoyable activities, and patient satisfaction. Negative outcomes might be bedsores, urinary tract infections, and death.

As in other health care settings, selecting appropriate indicators of outcome is a challenging task. Classic measures are "the five Ds": death, disease, disability, discomfort, and dissatisfaction (Lohr, 1988). Although it is possible to conceive of indicators in more positive aspects such as survival, states of physiologic, physical, and emotional health, and satisfaction, at some level it is easier to define what is clearly a "bad" outcome than to presume that some alternative set constitutes or is a proxy for the whole of good quality. This is the rationale in nursing home regulation in New York, for example, in which "sentinel health events" represent negative outcomes (decubitus ulcers, urinary tract infections) that should have been avoided if appropriate care had been provided (Schneider et al., 1980; 1983). Outcome measures traditionally used to investigate quality in long term care are discussed below.

Strengths and limitations of the use of *mortality rates* as quality screens were discussed in Chapter 9 of Volume I and in the "Hospital" section of this chapter. To use mortality statistics as a quality measure for home health care would necessitate a sufficiently long time period as well as information about preceding and subsequent hospital care to identify any home health component that might have contributed to a patient death.

Discharge from home health care (e.g., differences in the timing of, location of, or status at discharge) is a potential indicator of quality that has been used in a number of studies (Linn et al., 1977; Lewis et al., 1985). Like mortality rates, however, this measure is heavily compromised by factors other than the quality of home health services. According to LaLonde (1988), home health agency discharge records are notably inaccurate, with "discharge to patient's home" connoting everything from full recovery to imminent death. Moreover, variations in eligibility and coverage decisions among patients may affect observed discharge and use rates more than differences in an agency's performance (Benjamin, 1986). Discharge data may also be difficult to interpret. For example, in an era of "sicker and quicker" hospital discharges to the community, the movement of an individual with part-time or intermittent home health care from the community to a nursing home may signify an accurate assessment and referral on the part of the agency rather than poor quality of care. LaLonde (1988) argues, therefore, that the type of discharge might be a trigger to generate further review if an agency's pattern makes it an "outlier." She suggests that four types of discharge are potentially troublesome; these are discharge to a hospital, discharge to a nursing home; discharge home with no referral; and death at home.

Many Medicare home health patients can be expected to improve and regain lost functioning. Both general measures of rehabilitation, such as functioning in Activities of Daily Living (ADLs) and Instrumental Activities of Daily Living (IADLs) (Rowland et al., 1988), and problem-specific measures, such as recovery from aphasia for stroke patients, have been widely used in health services research. They are also features of current home health studies and post-acute care studies, including, for instance, well-developed measures used in the University of Minnesota Study of Post Acute Care (Kane, 1987). In another HCFA-funded study, Spector et al. (1988) have developed statistical norms for expected rates of decline or improvement in areas such as physical functioning.

Discomfort, particularly in terms of alleviation of pain, is often recommended as a measure of home health quality. LaLonde (1988) developed a "general symptom distress" scale that includes the following: pain, bowel problems, nausea/vomiting, urinary/bladder problems, cough, respiratory difficulties, skin problems, swelling/fluid retention, speech problems, mood, and activity level.

The Aftercare study conducted by Mathematica Policy Research (B.R. Phillips et al., 1989) was a pilot study of almost 300 elderly patients. The study was designed to look at the adequacy of home health care under Medicare in the 2 weeks immediately after hospital discharge. It made extensive use of specific (process) guidelines designed to link services to client problems or conditions. This same condition-specific approach was then used to develop outcomes (generally adverse) for these conditions. These were complemented by more general outcomes such as functioning, rehospitalization, and death.

The data were collected primarily by telephone interviews with clients or their proxies. The method used computer-assisted interviewing techniques and a sophisticated branching approach to identify candidate conditions for the appropriate guidelines. Data from the interviews were supplemented by abstracts of the patients' hospital charts to ascertain their condition on discharge.

Dissatisfaction or satisfaction with home health services is a somewhat controversial indicator of quality, as no consensus exists about the role that satisfaction should play in the assessment of quality (Cleary and McNeil, 1988). Practitioners fear that patients who are ill will be unfairly negative in their assessments, influenced not so much by the actual quality of services as by their pre-existing health status or other sociodemographic characteristics (Lebow, 1974; Cleary and McNeil, 1988). Further, researchers recognize that satisfaction may not be an adequate indicator of quality if patients lack the knowledge to evaluate the technical aspects of care, if they feel intimidated in expressing their opinion, or if they have become habituated to lowered expectations (Kane and Kane, 1988). Some research suggests that satisfaction can be a valid indicator of the characteristics and performance of providers and their services (Lebow, 1974; Ware et al., 1978; Pascoe, 1983). Measures of patient and family or caregiver satisfaction have been developed by a variety of providers and researchers (Mumma, 1987; Reif, 1987; Hawes and Kane, 1989). After reviewing the literature and conducting her own research, Levit (1988, p. 28) strongly endorsed the structured interview that "incorporates the values upheld for the delivery service itself—the enhancement of autonomy, respect for individual differences, concern for quality of life and opportunity for remediation." These she contrasts with the more typical yes/no checklist that defines and constrains clients' responses and consequently the value of the exercise.

Client knowledge and self-care ability. As aspects of patient education, client knowledge and self-care ability are a critical dimension of home health care (Rinke and Wilson, 1987a, 1987b). Considerable work has been done on developing measures of client knowledge about warning signs and symptoms, monitoring their status, taking prescribed medications, and following prescribed care processes (Kane, 1987, Reif, 1987; Hawes and Kane, 1989; B.R. Phillips et al., 1989).

Caregiver burden. Home care is not delivered solely, or even primarily, by paid workers. Part of its goal is to relieve at least some of the burden borne by family and others who form the bulwark of the client-support system. Measures of caregiver burden are important aspects of the assessment of the overall quality of home care services. Many of these measures have been developed in the area of dementia (Gilhooly et al., 1986; Zarit et al., 1986). Others are more generic and can be applied to a range of health conditions.

Research in Case-Mix Measures

In the late 1970s state Medicaid agencies in Illinois, West Virginia, and Ohio began basing payment for certain costs on patient characteristics, but these early "case-mix" systems evolved clinically without the methodological rigor that arose with the development of classifications of patients into resource utilization groups (RUGs) (Schneider et al., 1983). The RUGs system, developed for the New York Medicaid program, sorts nursing home residents into 1 of 16 categories based on dependencies in ADLs; on the need for skilled, clinically complex, or rehabilitative care; and on the presence of severe behavior problems. These groupings, and others developed for other states (e.g., Texas and Minnesota), are associated with different levels of resource use. Case-mix measures can predict between 45 and 58 percent of the variance in use of nursing resources (Schlenker, 1984; Fries and Cooney, 1985; Hawes and Kane, 1989). Research on patient case-mix, that is, the characteristics of home health patients associated with variations in resource use (e.g., duration and intensity of services), is also under way. This work stems from the growing interest in prospective payment systems for home health and in capitated payment systems (Foley, 1987; Manton and Hausner, 1987).

Understanding patient case-mix is critical to evaluation of quality in long term care. The inherent challenge in approaching quality of home care has been to abstract the problem sufficiently to make it manageable without distorting it altogether. The challenge is to capture the dynamic character of care (both the process of care and changes in patient status) in what can only be a series of snapshots.

PRO Review

Under the Third Scope of Work, Medicare PROs must review the care of a sample of patients who receive home health care between discharge and readmission to a hospital within 31 days of discharge (so called "intervening care"). In addition, PROs are required to investigate any complaints they receive about quality of care in skilled nursing facilities, home health agencies, and hospital outpatient departments.

Complaints

Complaints about home health care may be filed with the state department of health in which the client lives. Medicare Conditions of Participation require a state or local public agency to maintain a toll-free hotline and an investigative unit to "collect, maintain, and continually update" information on agencies that are certified, as well as to receive complaints and answer questions; the unit must be empowered to investigate complaints received in this way. Information maintained must include any significant deficiencies identified through the most recent certification survey, whether corrective actions have been taken or are planned, and any sanctions imposed.

State departments of health may have their own complaint mechanisms. For example, complaints lodged with an area office of the New York State Department of Health (NYSDOH) are divided for investigation into two categories: (1) "patient care" complaints, such as patient abuse or neglect, failure to deliver services, and negligent patient care; (2) "administrative" complaints, such as billing discrepancies and personnel issues. The investigation of patient care complaints is initiated within 24 hours. In investigating complaints, NYSDOH staff may interview complainants, patients, and agency staff and may make unannounced visits to the home care agency. A letter summarizing the results of the investigation is sent to the agency administrator, the complainant, and the patient.

Long-Term-Care Ombudsman

The Older Americans Act requires state-based nursing home ombudsmen, and a few states have also developed home health care ombudsman programs. This requirement has now been consolidated in some states with current requirements for home health care hotlines. For example, the Virginia Department of Aging, through the Office of the State Long-Term Care Ombudsman, is developing a model consumer protection program for home care users that will focus on trained volunteer mediators and self-advocacy training for consumers and their families. It will train five regional ombudsmen as well as develop brochures, consumer guides, and a complaint procedure package.

Internal Methods of Detecting Problems in Home Health Care

The National Long Term Care Channeling Demonstration provided descriptive information about quality-of-care issues in the home care industry. These include caregivers' absenteeism and lateness, their failure to complete assigned tasks, their failure to follow medical instructions, rough care, theft, and inappropriate matching of home care personnel to clients' needs (ABA, 1986; DHHS, 1989a; P.D. Phillips et al., 1989). These issues remain problems that quality assurance programs must be able to detect.

Patient and Physician Assessment

Home health agencies may conduct patient satisfaction or other outcome assessments at periodic intervals or after discharge. For example, the West Georgia Medical Center uses the satisfaction survey shown in Exhibit 6.HH1. The questionnaires must be specific enough to provide information that can be used by the home health agency for appropriate action. However, home health agencies have not typically had the skills or resources to field or analyze extensive satisfaction questionnaires.

Complaints

Home care agencies that receive complaints from clients, family, or (less likely) referring providers tend to deal with them on a case-by-case basis. Some home health agencies, however, have developed systems to summarize these data to look for patterns of problems. For example, the collaborative Ohio Quality Assurance Project developed innovative quality assurance strategies that are still in use (P.D. Phillips et al., 1989). These include a problem-recording form for feedback from clients and supervisors. Logs are aggregated weekly to identify patterns of problems or excellence.

Retrospective Record Review

The Ohio Project home health agencies use their complaint recording form in conjunction with a Client Service Report, which (1) documents the client's condition, (2) assesses adherence to the care plan, and (3) evaluates the delivered service by observing and talking with the client and the client's informal caregiver and service worker. Supervisors complete a report on each client every 30 days. Homemaker supervisors must complete the reports every 90 days, and reports are then reviewed by the case manager and quality assurance coordinator.

EXHIBIT 6.HH1 Example of Home Health Care Agency Satisfaction Survey

Dear Home Health Patient:

Our Home Health Department would like to know how you feel about the care you are receiving from our staff. Please take a moment and complete the following questions by checking the appropriate box.

HOME HEALTH EVALUATION

	Yes	No	Undecided
1. Does the nurse/aide usually come on the day you expect her to come?			
2. Does the nurse/aide usually notify you of changes in her schedule?			
3. Is your nurse/aide dependable?			
4. Does the nurse/aide act as if she wants to help you?			
5. Does the nurse/aide help you feel good about yourself?			
6. Does the nurse/aide treat you in a caring way?			
7. Does the nurse/aide give you good care?			
8. Does the nurse/aide teach you things you did not know about caring for yourself?			
9. Is your nurse/aide kind to you?			
10. Does the nurse/aide make you feel safe?			
11. Do you feel you can trust your nurse/aide.			

Comments:

_____

_____

SOURCE: West Georgia Medical Center, used with permission.

In-home audits are also described in the Ohio Project for a sample of about 10 cases per month (about 2 to 4 percent of the agency's caseload). Agencies are not aware of the schedule or the cases selected for review.

Home health agencies may hold case conferences and conduct concurrent and retrospective record review for appropriateness of care from the viewpoint of overuse as well as unmet needs. For example, the Visiting Nurse Service in Rochester, New York, includes in "utilization review" the appropriateness and effectiveness of care, and the West Georgia Medical Center considers the possible need for additional services (Exhibits 6.HH2 and 6.HH3). Another home health agency described biweekly interdisciplinary conferences with the visiting nurse and occupational, physical, and speech therapists.

Retrospective chart review may be conducted on each case after discharge or by sampling according to service (e.g., transfusion therapy), and it may be coordinated with a request for the patient to evaluate services received. The reviewer seeks evidence that the appropriate services were provided and documented. For instance, a professional services committee in the Instructional Visiting Nurse Association in Richmond, Virginia, reviews 20 percent of their charts quarterly. Every staff member rotates through this committee. In another example, the Hospital Home Health Care Agency of California reviews 10 percent of patient records at discharge for compliance with the plan of care.

EXHIBIT 6.HH2 Example of Guide for Retrospective Record Review of Home Care Patients

---

1. Evaluation of appropriateness includes:
     (a) establishment of appropriate therapeutic goals and care plans
     (b) effective execution of care plans
     (c) use of appropriate levels of personnel
     (d) effective use of other community resources
     (e) timely admission and discharge
2. Assessing utilization and coordination includes:
     (a) appropriate and economical use of therapeutic services
     (b) effectiveness of communication among the disciplines
     (c) coordination of services, including MDs and other agencies
     (d) continuity from one facility to another
3. Identifying gaps in service
     need to expand or better utilize the agency services, other community services, or need for consultation services
4. Providing information necessary for program evaluation, planning, and staff development

---

SOURCE: Adapted from Rochester Visiting Nurses Service, used with permission.

These audits generally do not include health status measures. However, LaLonde (1988), in conjunction with the Home Care Association of Washington, has developed and validated seven outcome-based quality measures for use in home health settings. These include taking prescribed medications as prescribed, general symptom distress, discharge status, caregiver strain, functional status, physiological indicators, and knowledge of diagnosis and prognosis. One of these scales, The General Symptom Distress Scale, is shown in Exhibit 6.HH4.

Performance evaluation. The Visiting Nurse Service of Seattle described a performance evaluation, skills assessment, and monitoring program in which both managerial and clinical team members provide in-service training by circulating with field staff and participating in patient visits.

Incident Reporting Systems

An incident report is a written report of an actual or potential patient injury, adverse outcome, or event, or a perception of the patient or family that an injury has occurred (AHA, 1987). Incident reports are intended to provide early notification of compensable events and establish the basis for early investigation. From a quality assurance as well as risk management viewpoint they could provide a data base for problem detection, analysis, and correction. For these purposes a coding and reporting system would have to be developed so that patterns of problems can be identified. Exhibit 6.HH5 lists incidents that the American Hospital Association recommends be reported by clients, family, or caregivers.

External Methods of Correcting Problems in Home Health Care

HCFA (Medicare- and Medicaid-Certified Home Health Agencies)

For 20 years the predominant method of improving quality in long term care has been persuasion through feedback (Hawes and Kane, 1989). Home health certification surveyors make periodic visits to evaluate the agency for compliance and report back to the agency about its performance relative to these standards. The Joint Commission and NLN surveys are much the same. Although state and federal agencies can use the threat of license revocation or termination of the provider agreement ("decertification"), and agencies accredited by the Joint Commission and the NLN can lose their accreditation, these remedies have been so seldom used that even providers acknowledge that such a threat is viewed as largely symbolic (IOM, 1986). Decertification and loss of accreditation are so severe that they are not used for minor problems and, in fact, are seldom used even for major problems or deficiencies. This failure of the enforcement remedies, documented most

EXHIBIT 6.HH3 Example of Audits Using Record Review.

PART II. . NURSING AUDIT CHART REVIEW SCHEDULE

All Entries To Be Completed By A Member Of the Nursing Audit Committee
(Please check in box of choice; DO NOT obscure number in box.)

Name of patient: _____
                 (LAST)   (FIRST)

		YES	NO	UNCERTAIN	TOTALS
I.	APPLICATION AND EXECUTION OF PHYSICIAN'S LEGAL ORDERS				
1.	Medical diagnosis complete	7	0	3	
2.	Orders complete	7	0	3	
3.	Orders current	7	0	3	
4.	Orders promptly executed	7	0	3	
5.	Evidence that nurse understood cause and effect	7	0	3	
6.	Evidence that nurse took health history into account	7	0	3	
	(42) TOTALS		0		□
II.	OBSERVATION OF SYMPTOMS AND REACTIONS				
7.	Related to course of above disease(s) in general	7	0	3	
8.	Related to course of above disease(s) in patient	7	0	3	
9.	Related to complications due to therapy (each medication and each procedure)	7	0	3	
10.	Vital signs	7	0	3	
11.	Patient to his condition	7	0	3	
12.	Patient to his course of disease(s)	5	0	2	
	(40) TOTALS		0		□
III.	SUPERVISION OF THE PATIENT				
13.	Evidence that initial nursing diagnosis was made	4	0	1	
14.	Safety of patient	4	0	1	
15.	Security of patient	4	0	1	
16.	Adaptation (support of patient in reaction to condition and care)	4	0	1	
17.	Continuing assessment of patient's condition and capacity	4	0	1	
18.	Nursing plans changed in accordance with assessment	4	0	1	
19.	Interaction with family and with others considered	4	0	1	
	(28) TOTALS		0		□
IV.	SUPERVISION OF THOSE PARTICIPATING IN CARE (EXCEPT THE PHYSICIAN)				
20.	Care taught to patient, family, or others, nursing personnel	5	0	2	
21.	Physical, emotional, mental capacity to learn considered	5	0	2	
22.	Continuity of supervision to those taught	5	0	2	
23.	Support of those giving care	5	0	2	
	(20) TOTALS		0		□
V.	REPORTING AND RECORDING				
24.	Facts on which further care depended were recorded	4	0	1	
25.	Essential facts reported to physician	4	0	1	
26.	Reporting of facts included evaluation thereof	4	0	1	
27.	Patient or family alerted as to what to report to physician	4	0	1	
28.	Record permitted continuity of intramural and extramural care	4	0	1	
	(20) TOTALS		0		□

effectively in the nursing home sector (IOM, 1986), has meant that regulatory personnel have had to rely on various forms of persuasion in attempting to ensure compliance with standards.

In effect, then, feedback and, to some degree, consultation have been the major methods used by survey agencies to assure quality in nursing homes and Medicare-certified home health agencies in this country for some time. Surveyors report problems to the providers (retrospective feedback) and

EXHIBIT 6.HH3 Continued

VI. APPLICATION AND EXECUTION OF NURSING
PROCEDURES AND TECHNIQUES

		YES	NO	UNCERTAIN	TOTALS	DOES NOT APPLY
29.	Administration and/or supervision of medications	2	0	0.5		2
30.	Personal care (bathing, oral hygiene, skin, nail care, shampoo)	2	0	0.5		2
31.	Nutrition (including special diets)	2	0	0.5		2
32.	Fluid balance plus electrolytes	2	0	0.5		2
33.	Elimination	2	0	0.5		2
34.	Rest and sleep	2	0	0.5		2
35.	Physical activity	2	0	0.5		2
36.	Irrigations (including enemas)	2	0	0.5		2
37.	Dressings and bandages	2	0	0.5		2
38.	Formal exercise program	2	0	0.5		2
39.	Rehabilitation (other than formal exercise)	2	0	0.5		2
40.	Prevention of complications and infections	2	0	0.5		2
41.	Recreation, diversion	2	0	0.5		2
42.	Clinical procedures - urinalysis, B/P	2	0	0.5		2
43.	Special treatments (e.g., care of tracheotomy, use of oxygen, colostomy or catheter care, etc.)	2	0	0.5		2
44.	Procedures and techniques taught to patient	2	0	0.5		2
	(32) TOTALS		0			

VII. PROMOTION OF PHYSICAL AND EMOTIONAL
HEALTH BY DIRECTION AND TEACHING

		YES	NO	UNCERTAIN	TOTALS	DOES NOT APPLY
45.	Plans for medical emergency evident	3	0	1		3
46.	Emotional support to patient	3	0	1		3
47.	Emotional support to family	3	0	1		3
48.	Teaching promotion and maintenance of health	3	0	1		3
49.	Evaluation of need for additional resources (e.g., spiritual, social service, homemaker service, physical or occupational therapy)	3	0	1		3
50.	Action taken in regard to needs identified	3	0	1		3
	(18) TOTALS		0			

TOTAL SCORE

FINAL SCORE

SOURCE: West Georgia Medical Center, used with permission.

hope for improvement. As might be expected, this approach has had only limited success. Hawes and Kane (1989) advocate three ways in which survey findings could be better used by agencies. First, the agency's performance should be compared to that of its peers and, as appropriate, the measures adjusted to account for differences in patient case-mix and variables other than the quality of care the agency provides. Second, the feedback should include information on how the agency can improve its self-monitoring capacity. This is in line with substantial work in the health care field that argues for a regulatory process that intervenes by creating expectations for the process of internal quality assurance (Vladeck, 1988). Third, the feedback should be precise. Long-term-care providers frequently complain that the survey and certification standards and criteria are unclear and

EXHIBIT 6.HH4 Example of Outcome-Based Quality Measures for Home Health Settings

Client's Name or Number _____

Primary Diagnosis_____

GENERAL SYMPTOM DISTRESS

(Suggested Introduction To Client: May Be Paraphrased)

"BEFORE WE GO ANY FURTHER WITH TODAY'S VISIT, I WOULD LIKE TO ASK YOU ABOUT SOME SYMPTOMS YOU MAY BE EXPERIENCING. (Client's Name). **I AM GOING TO READ YOU A LIST OF SYMPTOMS. PLEASE STOP ME WHEN I READ A SYMPTOM YOU HAVE HAD A PROBLEM WITH IN THE LAST MONTH. DO YOU UNDERSTAND?"** (Allow Client to respond.) **"IN THE PAST MONTH HAVE YOU HAD A PROBLEM WITH . . ."** (Read symptoms below verbatim including the examples. Circle each symptom identified by the client as being a problem in the last month. Underline the particular subsymptom identified by the client from the examples given. If more than one subsymptom under a particular symptom is identified, ask the client which one is most distressing. Underline and interview for that particular subsymptom).

Pain	Nausea/Vomiting	Bowel Problems (e.g., diarrhea, constipation, incontinence)	Urinary/Bladder Problems (e.g., retention, incontinence)	Cough	Respiratory Difficulties (e.g., shortness of breath, congestion)
Swelling/Fluid Retention	Skin Problems (e.g., raw areas, rashes, sores, open wounds, itches)	Speech Problems (e.g., difficulty speaking, swallowing, making yourself understood)	Mood (e.g., anxiety depression)	Activity Level (e.g., weakness, coordination, endurance)	

(Enter each circled symptom in the column headings below: one symptom per column. If more than eight symptoms are circled, use a second form. Ask the client verbatim the questions on the left of the scale. Ask all applicable questions for the symptom in column 1 before going to column 2. In the appropriate boxes, enter Yes or No to each applicable question. Enter the client's final score for each symptom at the bottom of each column.)

	COL 1	COL 2	COL 3	COL 4	COL 5	COL 6	COL 7	COL 8
(WRITE IN CIRCLED SYMPTOMS) ►►								
"Are you currently taking a medication for your (name of symptom) or taking any actions for it?"								
"In the past 3 days, has your (name of symptom) been a problem for you?" (IF YES) (IF NO►►STOP. FINAL SCORE=1. ▼ GO TO NEXT SYMPTOM)								
"Can your (name of symptom) be easily ignored?" (IF NO) (IF YES►►STOP. FINAL SCORE=2. ▼ GO TO NEXT SYMPTOM)								
"In a 24 hour period, does your (name of symptom) bother you less ☐ than ½ the time or more ☐ than ½ the time?" (If exactly ½ the time, consider as more than ½ the time.) (IF LESS THAN ½ THE TIME, FINAL SCORE=3. IF ½ THE TIME OR MORE THAN ½ THE TIME, FINAL SCORE=4 GO TO NEXT SYMPTOM.)								
FINAL SCORE EACH COLUMN								

Signature _____   Date _____

(M/D/Y)

SOURCE: LaLonde, 1988, used with permission.

EXHIBIT 6.HH5 Medically Related Incidents Relevant to Quality
Assurance Activities

Falls
Burns
Medication status needing review
Medication errors
Patient refusing treatment
Failure of family member to perform procedure as taught
Mishaps due to faulty equipment
Mishaps due to misuse of equipment
Unplanned return to an inpatient setting
Adverse or allergic drug reactions
Failure to respond to patient or family request for assistance, information or
treatment

Other reportable events listed include:

Home care staff/patient disagreements
Caregiver barred from home
Unplanned absence of caregiver
Abuse of patients
Child abuse
Failure of home care staff to report accident-causing hazard in home
Patient complaints of alleged theft
Breakage or damage to personal property of patient or family

SOURCE: Adapted from AHA, 1987.

that the survey report does not convey sufficient information to explain the
deficiency or to suggest how performance might be improved (IOM, 1986;
Hawes and Kane, 1989).

OBRA 1987

In OBRA 1987 enforcement remedies were expanded to include intermediate sanctions, such as civil fines and suspension of payments. The enforcement steps can also require what is, in effect, temporary "health care
receivership" for agencies with serious violations.

State Departments of Health

Complaints made to a state department of health or hotline about home
health services are investigated by the department as described above. The
department may then take various actions, such as freezing new cases or
prohibiting the home health agency from taking new cases until the problem

has been corrected. Cases may also be reassigned to another agency. Loss of Medicare certification and monetary penalties as well as loss of state licensure are possible disciplinary actions.

NYSDOH, for instance, conducts an investigation of all complaints it receives. After the department determines whether the complaint is substantiated, it may conduct a full review of the home health agency. Penalties may include a fine, or a limitation or revocation of the certificate of approval or license. When the department receives an inquiry from the news media that involves information pertaining to a specific agency or group of agencies, it is obligated to provide information under the Public Freedom of Information Law.

Home health agencies found to provide substandard care are subject to termination of certification or intermediate sanctions, such as civil money penalties, suspension of payment, or appointment of temporary management.

Internal Methods of Correcting Problems in Home Health Care

Home health agencies use a variety of methods to correct identified problems, which can be thought of as generally similar to those available for office-based physician care. For example, the Visiting Nurse Service in Seattle uses both counseling and education, which may include a written plan of correction and supervisor-accompanied home visits.

CONCLUDING REMARKS

This chapter has described the range of methods available to prevent, detect, and correct quality problems in the three sites of care emphasized in this study—the hospital, ambulatory settings, and the home. Although this sampler includes external quality review, such as that conducted by the Medicare PROs as well as by state departments of health, data commissions, and hospital associations, it has also delineated the great variety of internal, organization-based efforts at quality assessment and assurance. It reviews some of the considerable research experience that has accumulated for developing instruments for quality review as well as numerous examples of methods shared with the committee during its site visits.

Quality assurance may legitimately be seen as spanning a very broad range of activity from seeking to prevent unwanted events that may harm a patient to the development of major data bases or controlled trials to investigate the effectiveness of medical interventions. In all such activities, the participation of professional organizations, practitioners, health care managers, and patients may vary from none to initiating and playing a central role. How such groups and their differing perspectives and approaches can be incorporated into a strategy for Medicare quality assurance merits continued attention as that strategy evolves.

NOTES

1. Much of the discussion of anti-dumping legislation is based on a paper, "Medicare Quality Assurance Mechanisms and the Law," prepared for the study by A.H. Smith and M.J. Mehlman at Case Western Reserve University School of Law, hereafter referred to as Smith and Mehlman (1989).

2. Risk management also includes legal losses arising from institutional negligence, product liability, environmental damage, breach of contract, battery, and breach of confidentiality. Nonlegal losses that can be minimized by comprehensive risk management include: machine or plant failures; interruption of sole supplier; explosion, water, and fire damage; data or record tampering; theft; embezzlement; loss of key personnel; vehicular accidents; work actions; employee benefit and workers' compensation costs; absenteeism; and injury to patients, visitors, or employees.

3. Much of this discussion is based on a paper by L.L. Roos, N.P. Roos, E.S. Fisher, and T.A. Bubolz commissioned for this study. Some of the material appears in Roos (1989) and Roos et al. (1989). The commissioned paper will hereafter be referred to as Roos et al. (1990).

4. Medical directors may be salaried or not and may be full-time or not, depending on the organization. The terms medical director, chief of staff, physician in chief, director of medical affairs, and vice president for medical affairs are all used to describe the individual responsible for managing the hospital's medical staff and the quality of care provided by the medical staff (Fisher, 1986).

5. An adverse patient occurrence was defined as any "untoward patient event which, under optimal conditions, is not the natural consequence of the patient's illness or management."

6. Much of the discussion of the rationale for the Health Care Quality Improvement Act and of the Patrick case is based on Smith and Mehlman, 1989.

7. In the Patrick case, the AMA and others supporting the defendants had argued that physicians seeking to discipline other physicians should not be liable for such large damage awards, for which insurance is unavailable, when a jury can be persuaded that the review committee members' motives are less than pure (Holthaus, 1988).

8. The ISD-A review system includes intensity of service, severity of illness, discharge screens, and ancillary service appropriateness screening criteria.

9. The hospitals of the County of Los Angeles, Department of Health Services, which is self-insured, have taken traditional risk management a step further to place a "perinatal analyst" on site in the obstetrics, delivery, and intensive care nursery to reviews records and consult with staff.

10. Much of the discussion of licensure and of specialty board certification is based on Smith and Mehlman, 1989.

11. Volume I, Chapter 10 provides a more extended discussion of appropriateness (practice) guidelines, patient management criteria sets, and algorithms.

12. An example of a statement in the PHRED criteria set is "A CBC [complete blood count] should be performed within 30 days of a diagnosis of infectious mono-

nucleosis" (Leighton, 1981, p. 92). This statement requires information about a laboratory procedure, a diagnosis, a date, and patient-specific identifier. If an additional statement is used, such as "Ampicillin should not be prescribed to patients with a diagnosis of infectious mononucleosis," then information about pharmaceuticals must also be collected.

13. Because Medicaid contracting HMOs are not paid on a fee-for-service basis and thus do not submit claims, encounter data completed at each patient visit and used internally serve as a comparable data source.

14. State legislation concerning fraud and abuse, although related to quality of care, is beyond the scope of this chapter.

15. Sabatino (1989) has summarized a remarkable list of provider, service, and funding mechanism descriptors for home care. They include the following providers: nonprofit, proprietary, free-standing, hospital-based, health department, Veterans Administration, HMO, subsidiary, independent contractor, individual, and referral agency. He listed services as "low-tech" (e.g., homemaker, personal care, supportive services, companion, chore service), skilled nursing, physical therapy, speech therapy, occupational therapy, medical social services, home health aides, and "high-tech" (e.g., infusion therapies, respiratory therapy, dialysis, enteral and parenteral nutrition, interactive monitoring systems). Funding sources include Medicare, Medicare HMOs, Medicaid, Medicaid waiver, social services, Older Americans Act, Veterans Administration benefits, state and local appropriation, private insurance, charitable giving, and out-of-pocket. He further notes all the possible hybrid combinations available and the complexity of regulating such a myriad of service arrangements.

Study site visits occurred almost exclusively at Medicare-certified home health care agencies. Thus, the quality assurance mechanisms discussed in this section are related primarily to home health services (skilled nursing and home health aide care) provided by home health agencies.

16. Much of this section is based on a paper, "Issues Related to Quality Review and Assurance in Home Care," prepared for the study by C. Hawes of Research Triangle Institute, N.C., and R.L. Kane at the University of Minnesota School of Public Health, hereafter referred to as Hawes and Kane (1989).

REFERENCES

ABA (American Bar Association). *The Black Box of Home Care Quality.* A Report Presented by the Chairman of the Select Committee on Aging: House of Representatives. Ninety-Ninth Congress. Second Session. Com. Publ. No. 99-573. Washington, D.C.: U.S. Government Printing Office, August 1986.

AHA (American Hospital Association. The Hospital Research and Educational Trust). *Managing Risk and Quality in Hospital-Sponsored Home Care.* Chicago, Ill.: HRET, 1987.

AMA (American Medical Association). Status on Medical Disciplinary Boards. *State Health Legislation Report* 14:14–25, 1986.

Aronow, D.B. Severity-of-Illness Measurement: Applications in Quality Assurance and Utilization Review. *Medical Care Review* 45:339–366, 1988.

Avorn, J. and Soumerai, S.B. Improving Drug-therapy Decisions Through Educational Outreach: A Randomized Controlled Trial of Academically Based "Detailing." *New England Journal of Medicine* 308:1457–1463, 1983.

Bader, B.S., Veatch, R., and Childress, A. Hospital Quality Data Enter the Public Domain. *The Quality Letter* 1:2–8, 1989.

Barnett, G.O. Quality Assurance Through Computer Surveillance and Feedback. *American Journal of Public Health* 67:230–231, 1977.

Barnett, G.O., Winickoff, R.N., Dorsey, J.L., et al. Quality Assurance Through Automated Monitoring and Concurrent Feedback Using a Computer-Based Medical Information System. *Medical Care* 16:962–970, 1978.

Barnett, G.O., Winickoff, R.N., Morgan, M.M., et al. A Computer-Based Monitoring System for Follow-up of Elevated Blood Pressure. *Medical Care* 21:400–409, 1983.

Batalden, P.B. and Buchanan, E.D. Industrial Models of Quality Improvement. Pp. 133–159 in *Providing Quality Care: The Challenge to Clinicians*. Goldfield, N. and Nash, D.B., eds. Philadelphia, Pa.: American College of Physicians, 1989.

Bauman, M.K., Kramer, A.M., Shaughnessy, P.W., et al. *Development of Outcome-Based Quality Measures in Home Health Services, Study Paper 1: Literature and Program Review of Quality Assurance Systems Related to Home Health Care.* HCFA Contract No. 500-88-0054. Denver, Colo.: Center for Health Policy Research, 1988.

Benjamin, T. State Variations in Home Health Expenditures and Utilization Under Medicare and Medicaid. *Home Health Care Services Quarterly* 7:5–28, 1986.

Benson, D.S., Gartner, C., Anderson, J., et al. The Ambulatory Care Parameter: A Structured Approach to Quality Assurance in the Ambulatory Care Setting. *Quality Review Bulletin* 13:51–55, 1987.

Berman, S. Quality Assurance in Ambulatory Health Care. *Quality Review Bulletin* 14:18–21, 1988.

Boland, P. Trends In Second-Generation PPOs. *Health Affairs* 6:75–81, 1987.

Bolt v. Halifax Hospital Medical Center, 851 F2d 1273 (11th Cir. 1988).

Borgiel, A.E. Assessing the Quality of Care in Family Physicians' Practices by the College of Family Physicians of Canada. Pp. 63–72 in *Quality of Care and Technology Assessment*. Lohr, K.N. and Rettig, R.A., eds. Washington, D.C.: National Academy Press, 1988.

Borgiel, A.E., Williams, J.I., Anderson, G.M., et al. Assessing the Quality of Care in Family Physicians' Practices. *Canadian Family Physician* 31:853–862, 1985.

Brook, R.H., Ware, J.E., Jr., Rogers, W.H., et al. *The Effect of Coinsurance on the Health of Adults. Results from the RAND Health Insurance Experiment.* R-3055-HHS. Santa Monica, Calif.: The RAND Corporation, 1984.

Card, W.F. and Lehmann, R. An Overview of the Methodology Used by The Joint Commission to Evaluate Medicare-Certified HMOs. *Quality Review Bulletin* 13:415–417, 1987.

Chassin, M.R., Kosecoff, J., and Dubois, R. *Value-Managed Health Care Purchasing: An Employers' Guidebook Series. Volume II: Health Quality Assessment.* Chicago, Ill.: Midwest Business Group on Health, 1989a.

Chassin, M.R., Park, R.W., Lohr, K.N., et al. Differences Among Hospitals in Medicare Patient Mortality. *Health Services Research* 24:1–31, 1989b.

Cleary, P.D. and McNeil, B.J. Patient Satisfaction as an Indicator of Quality Care. *Inquiry* 25:25–36, 1988.

Couch, J.B. The Joint Commission on Accreditation of Healthcare Organizations. Pp. 201–224 in *Providing Quality Care: The Challenge to Clinicians.* Goldfield, N. and Nash, D.B., eds. Philadelphia, Pa.: American College of Physicians, 1989.

Craddick, J.W. and Bader, B.S. *Medical Management Analysis: A Systematic Approach to Quality Assurance and Risk Management.* Vol. I. Auburn, Calif.: J.W. Craddick, 1983.

Cross, J.M. and Berman, J.A. In Search of Immunity: Hospital Peer Review and the State Action Doctrine after Patrick. *Antitrust* 3:14–18, 1988.

Daley, J.M., Gertman, P.M., and Delbanco, T.L. Looking for Quality in Primary Care Physicians. *Health Affairs* 107–113, 1988a.

Daley, J., Jencks, S., Draper, D., et al. Predicting Hospital-Associated Mortality for Medicare Patients. *Journal of the American Medical Association* 260:3617–3624, 1988b.

Daniels, K. Planning for Quality in the Home Care Systems. *Quality Review Bulletin* 12:247–251, 1986.

Daubert, E.A. A System to Evaluate Home Health Care Services. *Nursing Outlook* 25:261–268, 1977.

Davies, A.R. and Ware, J.E. Involving Consumers in Quality of Care Assessment. *Health Affairs* 7:33–48, 1988.

Dettmann, F.G. and Simmons, G.E. Remedial CME: One Physician Group's Positive Alternative to Medicare Sanctions. Presented at the Medical Directors' Section Meeting of the American Medical Peer Review Association, July 1989.

DHHS (Department of Health and Human Services). *Report of the National Conference on Home Care Quality: Issue and Accountability. Washington, D.C. June 1–2, 1988. Volume I: Proceedings.* Washington, D.C.: U.S. Government Printing Office, 1989a.

DHHS (Bureau of Data Management and Strategy). *1989 Data Users Conference. Proceedings. June 13–15, 1989. Baltimore, Md.* Baltimore, Md.: DHHS/HCFA/BDMS Publication No. 03293, 1989b.

DHHS. Background Regarding the Uniform Needs Assessment Initiative. Enclosed with a letter to Andrew Webber from Wayne Smith (Office of Survey and Certification, Health Standards and Quality Bureau), April 13, 1989c.

DiBlase, D. *Business Insurance,* October 17, 1988.

Donabedian, A. Quality and Cost: Choices and Responsibilities. *Inquiry* 25:90–99, 1988.

Dubois, R.W. Hospital Mortality as an Indicator of Quality. Pp. 107–132 in *Providing Quality Care: The Challenge to Clinicians.* Goldfield, N. and Nash, D.B., eds. Philadelphia, Pa.: American College of Physicians, 1989.

Dubois, R.W., Brook, R.H., and Rogers, W.H. Adjusted Hospital Death Rates: A Potential Screen for Quality of Medical Care. *American Journal of Public Health* 77:1162–1166, 1987a.

Dubois, R.W., Moxley, J.H., Draper D., et al. Interpreting Hospital Mortality: Is it a Predictor of Quality? *New England Journal of Medicine* 317:1674–1680, 1987b.

Ente, B.H. and Lloyd, J.S. Taking Stock of Mortality Data: A Joint Commission Conference. *Quality Review Bulletin* 15:54–57, 1989.

Federal Register, Vol. 52, pp. 49510–49517, December 31, 1987.

Federal Register, Vol. 54, pp. 33354–33373, August 14, 1989.

Fintor, L. Cost and Quality in HMOs, Conflict of Interest? *HMO Practice* 2:215–219, 1988.

Fisher, H.M. *QA Basics. Quality Assurance Issues for Hospital Trustees, Physicians and Administrators.* New York, N.Y.: Greater New York Hospital Association, 1986.

Flanagan, E. Indicators of Quality in Ambulatory Care. *Quality Review Bulletin* 11:136–137, 1985.

Foley, W. Developing a Patient Classification System for Home Health Care. *Pride Institute Journal* 6:22–24, 1987.

Fries, B.E. and Cooney, L.M., Jr. Resource Utilization Groups: A Patient Classification System for Long-Term Care. *Medical Care* 23:110–112, 1985.

GAO (General Accounting Office). *Medical Malpractice: Characteristics of Claims Closed in 1984.* HRD-87-55. Washington, D.C.: General Accounting Office, April 1987.

GAO. *Initiatives in Hospital Risk Management.* GAO/HRD-89-79. Washington, D.C.: General Accounting Office, 1989.

Geller, S. Autopsy. *Scientific American* 248:124–135, 1983.

Gertman, P.M. and Restuccia, J. The Appropriateness Evaluation Protocol: A Technique for Assessing Unnecessary Days of Hospital Care. *Medical Care* 19:855–871, 1981.

Gilhooly, M.L., Zarit, S.H., and Birren, J.E., eds. *The Dementias: Policy and Management.* Englewood Cliffs, N.J.: Prentice Hall, 1986.

Gonnella, J.S., Louis, D.Z., and McCord, J.J. The Staging Concept—An Approach to the Assessment of Outcome of Ambulatory Care. *Medical Care* 14:13–21, 1976.

Goodspeed, R.B. and Goldfield, N. Quality Assurance in a Preferred Provider Organization. *Journal of Ambulatory Care Management* 10:8–16, 1987.

Grad, F.P. and Marti, N. *Physician Licensure and Discipline: the Legal and Professional Regulation of Medical Practice.* Dobbs Ferry, N.Y.: Oceana, 1979.

Greenfield, S.F. Flaws in Mortality Data: The Hazards of Ignoring Comorbid Disease. *Journal of the American Medical Association* 260:2253–2255, 1988.

Greenfield, S.F. Measuring the Quality of Office Practice. Pp. 183–198 in *Providing Quality Care: The Challenge to Clinicians.* Goldfield, N. and Nash, D., eds. Philadelphia, Pa.: American College of Physicians, 1989.

Greenfield, S.F., Cretin, S., Worthman, L.G., et al. Comparison of a Criteria Map to a Criteria List in Quality-of-Care Assessment for Patients with Chest Pain: The Relation of Each to Outcome. *Medical Care* 19:255–272, 1981.

Haley, R.W., Whilete, J.W., Culver, D.H., et al. The Financial Incentives for Hospitals to Prevent Nosocomial Infections under the Prospective Payment System. *Journal of the American Medical Association* 257:1611–1614, 1987.

Hallowell, E. Challenging the HMO System of Incentives. *Philadelphia Inquirer,* March 28, 1989.

Hannan, E.L., Bernard, H.R., O'Donnell, J.F., et al. A Methodology for Targeting Hospital Cases for Quality of Care Record Reviews. *American Journal of Public Health* 79:430–436, 1989a.

Hannan, E.L., O'Donnell, J.F., Kilburn, H., et al. Investigation of the Relationship Between Volume and Mortality for Surgical Procedures Performed in New York State Hospitals. *Journal of the American Medical Association* 262:503–510, 1989b.

Harrington, C. *Quality, Access, and Costs: Public Policy Issues of Home Health Care Services*. San Francisco, Calif.: Institute for Health and Aging, University of California, 1988.

Hartman, S.E. Voluntary Reimbursement Successfully Controls Cost Increases. *Michigan Hospitals* (no vol.):40–44, 1988.

Hattwick, M.A., Hart, R.J., and Weiss, S. Using the Information Tool To Improve Preventive Medical Care. Pp. 182–186 in *Proceedings of the Fifth Annual Symposium on Computer Applications in Medical Care*. New York: Institute of Electrical and Electronic Engineers. November 1981.

Havighurst, C.C. *Public Law and Policy: Readings, Notes, and Questions*. Westbury, N.Y.: Foundation Press, 1988.

Havighurst, C.C. and King, N.M. Private Credentialing in the Health Care Field. *American Journal of Law & Medicine* 9:131–201, 1983.

Hawes, C. *Public Policy and Long-Term Care: Defining, Measuring and Assuring Quality*. Final report for the Robert Wood Johnson Foundation, Princeton, New Jersey, 1983.

Hawes, C. and Kane, R.L. Issues Related to Quality Review and Assurance in Home Care. Paper prepared for the Institute of Medicine Study to Design a Strategy for Quality Review and Assurance in Medicare, 1989.

Hawes, C. and Powers, L. Quality Assurance in Long-Term Care: Special Issues for Patients with Dementia. Pp. 369–412 in *Losing a Million Minds*. Cook-Deegan, R., ed. Washington, D.C.: Office of Technology Assessment, 1987.

Holthaus, D. Peer Review After Patrick Case is Alive and Well. *Hospitals* 62:34, 1988.

IHPP (Intergovernmental Health Policy Project). Regulation of In-Home Care: An Overview of State Activity. *State Health Notes* 92:1–4, 1989.

InterQual. *The ISD-A Review System with Adult Criteria*. Chicago, Ill.: InterQual, 1987.

IOM (Institute of Medicine, Committee on Nursing Home Regulation). *Improving Quality of Care in Nursing Homes*. Washington, D.C.: National Academy Press, 1986.

Januska, C., Engle, J., and Wood, J. Status of Quality Assurance in Public Health Nursing. Presented at the Annual Meeting of the American Public Health Association, Public Health Section, Miami Beach, Fla., October 1976.

Jencks, S.F., Daley, J., and Draper, D. Interpreting Hospital Mortality Data: The Role of Clinical Risk Adjustment. *Journal of the American Medical Association* 260:3611–3616, 1988.

Johnsson, J. Kaiser Plans' HMOs Test Quality Management System. *Contract Healthcare* (no vol.):30–31, 1988.

Joint Commission (Joint Commission on Accreditation of Healthcare Organizations). *Agenda for Change Update* 1:1, September, 1987.

Joint Commission. *1988 Home Care Standards for Accreditation*. Chicago, Ill.: Joint Commission, 1988.

Joint Commission. *Agenda for Change Update* 3:1,5, October, 1989a.

Joint Commission. *1990 AMH Accreditation Manual for Hospitals.* Chicago, Ill.: Joint Commission, 1989b.

Joint Commission. *1990 AHC Ambulatory Health Care Standards Manual.* Chicago, Ill.: Joint Commission, 1989c.

Joint Commission. Characteristics of Clinical Indicators. *Quality Review Bulletin* 15:330–339, 1989d.

Joint Commission. Monitoring and Evaluating the Quality and Appropriateness of Care. Background paper for the National Invitational Forum on Clinical Indicator Development, Chicago, Ill., March, 1989e.

Kahn, K.L., Brook, R.H., Draper, D., et al. Interpreting Hospital Mortality Data. How Can We Proceed? *Journal of the American Medical Association* 260:3625–3628, 1988.

Kane, R.A. and Kane, R.L. Long-Term Care: Variations on a Quality Assurance Theme. *Inquiry* 25:132–146, 1988.

Kane, R.L. Assuring Quality of Care and Quality of Life in Long-Term Care. *Quality Review Bulletin* 7:3–10, 1981.

Kane, R.L. A National Study of Post Acute Care. HCFA Contract No. 17-C-98891/5-01. Washington, D.C.: Assistant Secretary for Planning and Evaluation, DHHS, 1987.

Kane, R.L., Kane, R.A., Kleffel, D., et al. *The PSRO and the Nursing Home. Volume I, An Assessment of PSRO Long-Term Care Review.* R-2459/1-HCFA. Santa Monica, Calif.: The RAND Corporation, 1979.

Kane, R.L., Riegler, S., Bell, R., et al. *Predicting the Course of Nursing Home Patients.* A RAND Note. Santa Monica, Calif.: The RAND Corporation, 1982.

Kessner, D.M., Kalk, C.E., and Singer, J. Assessing Health Quality: The Case for Tracers. *New England Journal of Medicine* 288:189–194, 1973.

Knaus, W.A., Draper, E.A., Wagner, D.P., et al. An Evaluation of Outcome from Intensive Care in Major Medical Centers. *Annals of Internal Medicine* 104:410–418, 1986.

Koizumi, L. and Sorian, R., eds. PPOs: Insurers, Employers Get More Involved. *Medicine and Health (Perspectives),* December 5, 1988.

LaLonde, B. *Quality Assurance Manual of the Home Care Association of Washington, 2nd Edition.* Edmonds, Wash.: The Home Care Association of Washington, 1988.

Landefeld, C.S. and Goldman, L. The Autopsy in Quality Assurance: History, Current Status, and Future Directions. *Quality Review Bulletin* 15:42–48, 1989.

Leader, S. *Home Health Benefits Under Medicare.* Washington, D.C.: American Association of Retired Persons, September 1986.

Leape, L.L., Park, R.E., Solomon, D.H., et al. Relation Between Surgeons' Practice Volume and Geographic Variation in the Rate of Carotid Endarterectomy. *New England Journal of Medicine* 321:653–657, 1989.

Lebow, J.L. Consumer Assessments of the Quality of Medical Care. *Medical Care* 12:328–337, 1974.

Lehmann, R. Forum on Clinical Indicator Development: A Discussion of the Use and Development of Indicators. *Quality Review Bulletin* 15:223–227, 1989.

Leighton, R. *Synthesis and Documentation of the PHRED Quality Assurance Demonstration.* Sacramento, Calif.: Department of Health Services, Organized Health Systems Division, 1981.

Levit, G.E.   Assuring the Quality of Quality Assurance.   Improving Service to Homebound Elderly Through their Engagement in Evaluation.   Unpublished study for the Suburban Area Agency on Aging (Illinois), October, 1988.

Lewis, M.A., Kane, R.L., Cretin, S., et al.   The Immediate and Subsequent Outcomes of Nursing Home Care. *American Journal of Public Health* 75: 758–762, 1985.

Linn, M.W., Gurel, L., and Linn, B.S.   Patient Outcome as a Measure of Quality of Nursing Home Care. *American Journal of Public Health* 67:337–344, 1977.

Logsdon, D.N.   A Selected Bibliography of Literature on Ambulatory Health Care. *Quality Review Bulletin* 5:22–27, 1979.

Lohr, K.N.   *Quality of Care for Respiratory Illness in Disadvantaged Populations.* P-6570.   Santa Monica, Calif.: The RAND Corporation, 1980a.

Lohr, K.N.   Quality of Care in the New Mexico Medicaid Program (1971–1975). *Medical Care* 18:1–129 (January Supplement), 1980b.

Lohr, K.N.   Outcome Measurement: Concepts and Questions. *Inquiry* 25:37–50, 1988.

Longo, D.R., Ciccone, K.R., and Lord, J.T.   *Integrated Quality Assessment: A Model for Concurrent Review.*   Chicago, Ill.: American Hospital Association Publishing Co., 1989.

Luft, H.S.   HMOs and the Quality of Care. *Inquiry* 25:147–156, 1988.

Macro Systems.   *Review of State Quality Assurance Programs for Home Care.*   Submitted to U.S. DHHS Office of the Assistant Secretary for Planning and Evaluation.   Washington, D.C.: DHHS, 1988.

Manton, K.G. and Hausner, T.   A Multidimensional Approach to Case Mix for Home Health Services. *Health Care Financing Review* 8:37–54, 1987.

McAllister, J.C., III, Black, B.L., Griffin, R.E., et al.   Controversial Issues in Home Health Care: A Roundtable Discussion. *American Journal of Hospital Pharmacy* 43:933–946, 1986.

McCann, B.A. and Hill, K.L.   The JCAH Home Care Project. *Quality Review Bulletin* 12:191–193, 1986.

McDonald, C.J.   Protocol-Based Computer Reminders, the Quality of Care and the Non-Perfectability of Man. *New England Journal of Medicine* 295:1351–1355, 1976.

McDonald, C.J., Hui, S.L., Smith, D.M., et al.   Reminders to Physician From an Introspective Computer Medical Record: A Two-Year Randomized Trial. *Annals of Internal Medicine* 100:130–138, 1984.

MediQual.   *MedisGroups Software for Medical Care Quality Control.*   Westborough, Mass.: MediQual Systems, Inc., 1986.

Merlis, M.   *Medicare: Risk Contracts With Health Maintenance Organizations and Competitive Medical Plans.*   Washington, D.C.: The Library of Congress, 1988.

Meyer, H.   Peer Review's Limits Visible Once Again. *American Medical News,* May 5, 1989.

Meyer, W., Clinton, J.J., and Newhall, D.   A First Report of the Department of Defense External Civilian Peer Review of Medical Care. *Journal of the American Medical Association* 260:2690–2693, 1988.

Mitchell v. Howard Memorial Hospital, 853 F.2d 762 (9th cir. 1988).

MMAF (Maine Medical Assessment Foundation). *Confronting the Healthcare Challenge*. (Pamphlet.) Manchester, Maine: MMAF, 1989.

MMWR. *Morbidity and Mortality Weekly Report*. Autopsy frequency - United States (1980–1985). *MMWR* 37:191–194, 1988.

Morlock, L., Lindgren, O., and Mills, D. Malpractice, Clinical Risk Assessment, and Quality Assessment. Pp. 225–259 in *Providing Quality Care: The Challenge to Clinicians*. Goldfield, N. and Nash, D., eds. Philadelphia, Pa.: American College of Physicians, 1989.

Mumma, N. Quality and Cost of Home Care Services: Coordinated Funding. Pp. 105–112 in *Quality and Home Health Care: Redefining the Tradition*. Fisher, K. and Gardner, K., eds. Chicago, Ill.: Joint Commission on Accreditation of Healthcare Organizations, 1987.

NAHC (National Association for Home Care). *Quality Assurance Survey*. Unpublished report from NAHC. Washington, D.C., 1986.

NAHDO (National Association of Health Data Organizations). *Resource Manual*. Volume I & II. Washington, D.C.: NAHDO, 1988.

NCHSR (National Center for Health Services Research). *Research Activities*. No. 124, December 1989.

Nelson, A.R. Orphan Data and the Unclosed Loop: A Dilemma in PSRO and Medical Audit. *New England Journal of Medicine* 295:617–619, 1976.

Nelson, E.C. and Berwick, D.M. The Measurement of Health Status in Clinical Practice. *Medical Care* 27:S77-S90, (March Supplement) 1989.

Nelson, E.C., Wasson, J.H., Kirk, J.W., et al. Assessment of Function in Routine Clinical Practice: Description of the COOP Chart Method and Preliminary Findings. *Journal of Clinical Diseases* 40:55S-63S, (Supplement) 1987.

Nelson, E.C., Hays, R.D., Larson, C., et al. The Patient Judgment System: Reliability and Validity. *Quality Review Bulletin* 15:185–191, 1989.

NLN (National League for Nursing, Accreditation Program for Home Care and Community Health). *Policies and Procedures for the NLN Accreditation Program*. New York, N.Y.: NLN, 1986.

O'Leary, D. *Future Trends in Evaluating Quality Care*. Lecture delivered at the McCormick Center Hotel, Chicago, Ill., May 13, 1988.

O'Leary, D. Keeping an Eye on Health Care Quality. *The Internist* (no vol.) 17–20, 1989.

Oswald, E.M. and Winer, I.K. A Simple Approach to Quality Assurance in a Complex Ambulatory Care Setting. *Quality Review Bulletin* 13:56–60, 1987.

OTA (Office of Technology Assessment). *The Quality of Medical Care. Information for Consumers*. OTA-H-386. Washington, D.C.: U.S. Government Printing Office, June 1988.

Palmer, R.H., Strain, R., Maurer, J.V.W., et al. Quality Assurance in Eight Adult Medicine Group Practices. *Medical Care* 22:632–643, 1984.

Palmer, R.H., Louis, T.A., Hsu, L.N., et al. A Randomized Controlled Trial of Quality Assurance in Sixteen Ambulatory Care Practices. *Medical Care* 23:751–768, 1985.

Pascoe, G.C. Patient Satisfaction in Primary Health Care: A Literature Review and Analysis. *Evaluation and Program Planning* 6:185–210, 1983.

Patrick v. Burget, 108 S. Ct. 1658 (1988), rev'g 800 F2d 1498 (9th Cir. 1986).

Payne, S.M. Identifying and Managing Inappropriate Hospital Utilization: A Policy Synthesis. *Health Services Research* 22:710–769, 1987.

PCA Today. Reporting to the Medical Board. *PCA Today. Technical Advice Bulletin of the Patient Care Assessment Unit of the Massachusetts Board of Registration in Medicine* 1:4, April 1987.

Perry, B.C. and Kirz, H.L. Quality Management in a Staff-Model HMO. *HMO Practice* 3:164–168, 1989.

PHCCCC (Pennsylvania Health Care Cost Containment Council). *Hospital Effectiveness Report . . . A Model Report.* HE 5—Volume I. Harrisburg, Pa.: PHCCCC, 1989.

Phillips, B.R., Schneider, B.W., Steele, K., et al. *A Pilot Study of the Adequacy of Post-Hospital Community Care of the Elderly: Final Report.* MPR No. 7886-100. Princeton, N.J.: Mathematica Policy Research (September), 1989.

Phillips, P.D., Applebaum, R.A., Atchley, S.J., et al. Quality Assurance Strategies for Home-Delivered Long-Term Care. *Quality Review Bulletin* 15:156–162, 1989.

Ray, W.A., Fink, R., and Federspiel, W. Improving Antibiotic Prescribing in Outpatient Practice: Non-association of Outcome With Prescriber Characteristics and Measures of Receptivity. *Medical Care* 23:1307–1313, 1985.

Reerink, E. Report on International Aspects of Quality Assurance. Paper prepared for the Institute of Medicine Study to Design a Strategy for Quality Review and Assurance in Medicare, 1989.

Reif, L. Measuring the Quality of Home Care: Assessing Providers' Performance from a Consumer's Perspective. Paper presented at Nursing Leadership in Home Care Research, an invitational conference sponsored by the National League for Nursing and the National Center for Homecare Education and Research, Chicago, Ill., November 9–10, 1987.

Retchin, S., Brown, B., Wooldridge, J., et al. National Medicare Competition Evaluation. An Evaluation of the Quality of the Process of Care. Final Analysis Report. RFP No. HCFA-83-ORD-29/CP. Richmond, Va.: Williamson Institute for Health Studies at the Medical College of Virginia, Virginia Commonwealth University, 1988.

Riley, P.A. *Quality Assurance in Home Care.* Report prepared for the National Academy for State Health Policy, an affiliate of the Center for Health Policy Development. Washington, D.C., December 1988.

Rinke, L.T. and Wilson, A.A. *Outcomes Measures in Home Care: Volume I Research.* New York, N.Y.: National League for Nursing, 1987a.

Rinke, L.T. and Wilson, A.A. *Outcomes Measures in Home Care: Volume II Service.* New York, N.Y.: National League for Nursing, 1987b.

Roos, L.L. Nonexperimental Data Systems in Surgery. *International Journal of Technology Assessment in Health Care* 5:341–386, 1989.

Roos, L.L., Sharp, S.M., Cohen, M.M., et al. Risk Adjustment in Claims-Based Research: The Search for Efficient Approaches. *Journal of Clinical Epidemiology* 42:1193–1206, 1989.

Roos, L. L., Roos, N.P., Fisher, E.S., et al. Strengths and Weaknesses of Health Insurance Data Systems for Assessing Outcomes. Paper prepared for the Institute of Medicine Study to Design a Strategy for Quality Review and Assurance in Medicare, 1989. Also published in Gelijns, A.C., ed., *Medical Innovation at the Crossroads. Volume I. Modern Methods of Clinical Investigation.* Washington, D.C.: National Academy Press, (in press).

Rowland, D., Lyons, B., Neuman, P., et al. Defining the Functionally Impaired Elderly Populations. Center for Hospital Finance. Baltimore, Md.: The Department of Health Policy and Management, School of Hygiene and Public Health, The Johns Hopkins University. Report prepared under a grant from the American Association of Retired Persons, 1988.

RTI (Research Triangle Institute). *Nationwide Evaluation of Medicaid Competition Demonstrations.* Final Report. NTIS # PB-89-209688/AS. Research Triangle Park, N.C.: RTI, 1988.

Rubin, L. *Comprehensive Quality Assurance System. The Kaiser-Permanente Approach.* Alexandria, Va.: American Group Practice Association, 1975.

Rutstein, D.D., Berenberg, W.B., Chalmers, T.C., et al. Measuring the Quality of Medical Care (Tables Revised, 9/1/77) A Clinical Method. *New England Journal of Medicine* 294:582–588, 1976.

Sabatino, C. Putting Public Accountability to the Test. Homecare Quality. *Generations* 13:12–16, Winter, 1989.

Sanazaro, P.J. Determining Physicians' Performance: Continuing Medical Education and Other Interacting Variables. *Evaluation and the Health Professions* 6:197–210, 1983.

Sanazaro, P.J. and Worth, R.M. Measuring Clinical Performance of Individual Internists in Office and Hospital Practice. *Medical Care* 23:1097–1114, 1985.

Schlackman, N. Integrating Quality Assessment and Physician Incentive Payment. *Quality Review Bulletin* 15:234–237, 1989.

Schlenker, R.E. Nursing Home Reimbursement, Quality, and Access—A Synthesis of Research. Paper prepared for the Institute of Medicine Conference on Reimbursement, Anaheim, Calif., 1984.

Schneider, D., Hatcher, G., and O'Sullivan, A. Quality Assurance for Long Term Care: The Sentinel Health Event System. Final Report to New York State Health Planning Commission, Albany, New York. Troy, N.Y.: Rensselaer Polytechnic Institute, 1980.

Schneider, D., Fries, B. and Desmond, M. *Incentives and Basic Principles for Long-Term Care Patient Classification Development. Report 1.* New York State Case Mix Prospective Reimbursement System for Long-Term Care. Troy, N.Y.: Rensselaer Polytechnic Institute, 1983.

Schroeder, S.A. and Donaldson, M.S. The Feasibility of an Outcome Approach to Quality Assurance: A Report from One HMO. *Medical Care* 14:49–55, 1976.

Schwartz, W.B. and Mendelson, D.N. The Role of Physician-Owned Insurance Companies in the Detection and Deterrence of Negligence. *Journal of the American Medical Association* 262:1342–1346, 1989.

Smith, A.H. and Mehlman, M.J. Medicare Quality Assurance Mechanisms and the Law. Paper prepared for the Institute of Medicine Study to Design a Strategy for Quality Review and Assurance in Medicare, 1989.

Solberg, L.I., Peterson, K.E., Ellis, R.W., et al. *The Minnesota Project: A Focused Approach to Ambulatory Quality Assurance.* St. Paul, Minn.: Group Health, Inc., 1987.

Sorgen, L.M. The Development of a Home Care Quality Assurance Program in Alberta. *Home Health Care Services Quarterly* 7:13–28, 1986.

Spector, W., Kapp, M., Eichorn, A., et al. *Longitudinal Study of Case Mix, Outcomes, and Resource Use in Nursing Homes.* Providence, R.I.: Center for Gerontology and Health Care Research, Brown University, 1988.

SRI (SRI International). *Evaluation of the Arizona Health Care Cost Containment System. Quality of Care Report.* Washington, D.C.: NTIS No. PB-89-156210/AS, January 1989.

Steinwachs, D.M., Weiner, J.P., and Shapiro, S. Management Information Systems and Quality. Pp. 160–182 in *Providing Quality Care: The Challenge to Clinicians.* Goldfield, N. and Nash, D.B., eds. Philadelphia, Pa.: American College of Physicians, 1989.

Stewart, A.L., Hays, R.D., and Ware, J.E. The MOS Short-Form General Health Survey: Reliability and Validity in a Patient Population. *Medical Care* 26:724–732, 1988.

Stewart, A.L., Greenfield, S., Hays, R.D., et al. Functional Status and Well-Being of Patients with Chronic Conditions: Results from the Medical Outcomes Study. *Journal of the American Medical Association* 262:907–943, 1989.

Stocker, M.A. Quality Assurance in an IPA. *HMO Practice* 3:183–187, 1989.

Summer, S.J. Maryland's Experiment with Quality Measures. *Business and Health* (no vol.):14–16, November 1987.

Tarlov, A.R., Ware, J.E., Greenfield, S., et al. The Medical Outcomes Study: An Application of Methods for Monitoring the Results of Medical Care. *Journal of the American Medical Association* 262:925–930, 1989.

Tierney, W.M., Hui, S.L., and McDonald, C.J. Delayed Feedback of Physician Performance Versus Immediate Reminders to Perform Preventive Care: Effects on Physician Compliance. *Medical Care* 24:659–666, 1986.

Tierney, W.M., McDonald, C.J., Hui, S.L., et al. Computer Predictions of Abnormal Test Results: Effects On Outpatient Testing. *Journal of the American Medical Association* 259:1194–1198, 1988.

Vladeck, B.C. Quality Assurance Through External Controls. *Inquiry* 25:100–107, 1988.

Ware, J.E., Davies-Avery, A., and Stewart, A.L. The Measurement and Meaning of Patient Satisfaction. A Review of the Recent Literature. *Health and Medical Care Services Review,* 1:1–15, January/February 1978.

Warner, C.K. Peer Review in Quality Assurance. *HMO Practice* 3:178–182, 1989.

Weiner, J., Powe, N., Steinwachs, D., et al. Quality of Care Indicators for Potential Application to Insurance Claims/Encounter Data. Report to the CIGNA Foundation. Baltimore, Md.: Johns Hopkins University Research and Development Center, 1989a.

Weiner, J., Steinwachs, D., and Powe, N. Applying Insurance Claims to Quality Measurement: Perspectives and Challenges. Paper presented at a special session of the Committee of Health Services Research of the Medical Care Section, Annual Meeting of the American Public Health Association, Chicago, Ill., 1989b.

Williams, K.N. and Brook, R.H. A Review of the Recent Literature. Quality Measurement and Assurance. *Health and Medical Care Services Review* 1:1–15, May/June 1978.

Williamson, J.W. Evaluating Quality of Patient Care: A Strategy Relating Outcome and Process Assessment. *Journal of the American Medical Association* 218:564–568, 1971.

Williamson, J.W. *Improving Medical Practice and Health Care: A Bibliographic Guide to Information Management In Quality Assurance and Continuing Education.* Cambridge, Mass.: Ballinger Publishing Co., 1977.

Williamson, J.W. Formulating Priorities For Quality Assurance Activity: Description of a Method and its Application. *Journal of the American Medical Association* 239:631–637, 1978.

Williamson, J.W., Aronovitch, S., Kelly, D., et al. Health Accounting: An Outcome-Based System of Quality Assurance: Illustrative Application to Hypertension. *Bulletin of the New York Academy of Medicine* 51:727–738, 1975.

Wilner, S., Coltin, K., and Winickoff, R. Classifying Problems and Selecting Intervention Strategies. Medical Care Roundtable Session, Annual Meeting of the American Public Health Association, Los Angeles, Calif., October 1978.

Woodson, A.S., Foley, S.M., Daniels, P.J., et al. *Long-Term Care Guidelines for Quality.* Denver, Colo.: Center for Health Services Research, University of Colorado Health Sciences Center, 1981.

Zarit, S.H., Todd, P., and Zarit, J. Subjective Burden of Husbands and Wives as Caregivers: A Longitudinal Study. *The Gerontologist* 26:260–266, 1986.

APPENDIX

MERCY HEALTH SERVICES SURVEY OF QUALITY MANAGEMENT PROGRAMS, STAFF, AND RESOURCES

During the spring of 1989, Mercy Health Services in Farmington, Michigan, conducted a survey of hospital systems and their member hospitals.[1] The purpose of the survey was to gather information on the resources allocated to quality management[2] at both the corporate level and by individual member hospitals. The Institute of Medicine (IOM) study commissioned an analysis of some of the data collected for the survey. The purpose was to obtain empirical information on the resources devoted to quality measurement and assurance, because such data are very difficult to amass on a systematic basis.

Methods

Survey Methodology

The investigators at Mercy Health Services (MHS) identified hospital systems willing to participate. The various corporate offices distributed surveys to individuals in their hospital who had appropriate responsibility and knowledge. For instance, information on quality management in a given hospital was provided by the director of the department with responsibility for the quality assurance program.

Participation in this project by individual hospitals belonging to various systems was voluntary, and it depended to some extent on encouragement and facilitation by the corporate office. Methods of distribution of the surveys by corporate offices varied considerably. In one system the chief executive officer had the survey mailed to all the hospitals without further endorsement. At another it was distributed at the end of a meeting of hospital representatives. In other systems, interested corporate staff wrote personal distribution letters and held meetings with quality managers to explain the survey and urge participation. Because methods of distribution varied, neither an exact count nor a response rate can be calculated. Five systems with three or four member hospitals had 100 percent return rates. In contrast, only 4 of a possible 10 surveys were received from one system.

Survey Responses

The survey analysis is based on responses from 11 corporate offices and 58 hospitals. The hospital responses represent 13 multihospital systems and 2 unaffiliated hospitals in 21 states. Eleven of the 13 systems are sponsored by the Catholic Church; all of the hospitals are nonprofit. The hospitals range from sole community rural providers to major urban medical centers, but it is not known how many of the hospitals have major teaching responsibilities. The number of beds for medical-surgical services in responding hospitals ranged from 19 to 747.

Survey Analysis

Data collection and analysis was commissioned by the IOM study on quality assurance in Medicare. Data verification, coding, and analysis were done in three phases by the MHS principal investigators with participation by the IOM study staff. This Appendix discusses only data that were designated as pertinent to quality management functions conducted at corporate or individual hospitals. It does not include the considerable data also collected on utilization management, risk management, and other topics. Where joint activities are carried out in departments, the MHS investigators apportioned time and resources as described below.

Content Validation and Decision Rules. One MHS investigator reviewed surveys and coding before data entry to ensure consistency in interpretations. This included checks on the internal consistency of the information, such as the consistency between the time allotted to various functions and the number of full-time–equivalent staffing positions reported. Similarly, percentages of time devoted to various functions corresponded to 100 percent.

Many hospitals have combinations of programs (e.g., quality and risk management, quality and utilization management, risk management and medical staff office). Among the integrated programs were many instances in which budget information and staffing information were provided in only one of the seven programmatic survey sections, but the survey notes or organizational charts indicated that the information supported two or more programs. In these instances, the reported budget or staffing data were divided equally between the programs.

The numbers of responses for each survey variable are shown in the tables. In some cases data were missing or the category was not applicable. For example, budget information may not have been known or the respondent may have preferred not to answer. In other cases a quality management function may not be performed at the hospital.

Results

Corporate Resources and Assessment

Table A.1a shows the number of corporate offices, among the 11 responding, that had formal programs at the corporate level supporting the areas of quality management, risk management, and utilization management. Only about half had programs designated, even partly, to quality management. Table A.1b shows the functional areas supported at the corporate level. Six of 11 hospital systems reported that quality management is supported at the corporate level; 4 with distinct program responsibility, 1 combined with utilization management, and 1 combined with risk management.

Table A.2 shows the percentage of time spent by the responsible individuals at the corporate level in the three core functions and constituent

TABLE A.1a Number and Percentage of Respondents that Identify Program Responsibility at the Corporate Level, by Type of Core Area

Core Area	Number	Percentage
Quality management	6	56
Risk management	3	27
Utilization management	1	9

NOTE: Number of respondents was 11.

TABLE A.1b Number and Percentage of Respondents with Formal Programs at the Corporate Level, by Type of Functional Area

Functional Area	Number	Percentage
Nursing	7	64
Medical staff	6	54
Quality management	4	36
Risk management	2	18
Quality and risk management	1	9
Quality and utilization management	1	9
Medical records	2	18
Pharmacy	2	18
Medical education	1	9
Ethics	1	9

NOTE: Number of respondents was 11.

tasks now and 3 years ago. The bulk of time is devoted to reporting to the hospitals' governing boards, preparing comparative reports, and making consultation visits to hospitals. In comparison with risk management and utilization management tasks, which have remained fairly stable, many quality-related tasks are reported to have increased during this period. Increases evidently occurred in time spent providing comparative reports, developing clinical guidelines, and reviewing institutional quality reports.

Table A.3 shows corporate responses to questions about the strengths of their program (aspects that others might emulate), needs of their program, and the challenges foreseen during the next 5 years. Five systems singled out systemwide quality indicators as sources of pride, and four systems identified their insurance and claims management systems. The greatest need identified was for better data systems. Challenges included the "commitment of senior leadership" and the "development of effective, integrated quality, utilization, and risk management programs." These were followed in decreasing frequency of mention by the "proliferation of external demands" and the need to find a way to document improvements in quality.

Hospital Characteristics

Location, size, type of patients served, average length of stay, and severity. Fifty-eight hospitals in 21 states responded to the MHS survey, and they were located in all geographic regions of the United States. Hospitals were divided into three groups for the IOM analysis according to the number of medical and surgical beds they reported staffing—11 had less than

100 beds (19 percent), 23 had 100 to 250 beds (40 percent), and 24 had more than 250 beds (41 percent). Further information about the hospital services is shown in Table A.4. Volume of services, as predictable, rose with increasing hospital size. In this group of hospitals, average length of stay and Medicare Case Mix Index also rose with size, but percentage of patients on Medicaid decreased.

The percentage of Medicare patients among the entire patient census for these hospitals ranged from a low of 24 percent to a high of 68 percent; overall, these hospitals averaged 41 percent Medicare patients. Reported average length of stay ranged from 3.3 days to 10.6 days, with 6.6 days being the overall average. The Medicare Case Mix Index, a measure of the severity of illness of the hospital's patient population, averaged 1.28 and ranged from 0.94 to 1.67. A Case Mix Index of 1.0 is defined as the national average.

Hospital committees and services. The average number of hospital staff departments and services and medical staff departments rose with the number of hospital beds (Table A.5). The number of hospital departments was markedly different between the smallest hospitals and the other two categories (17 as compared with about 51); the overall average was 45 with a range of 4 to 174. The average number of medical staff departments per hospital was just under 10, with a range of 1 to 27. The average number of medical staff committees doubled between the smallest hospital (9) and the two larger groups (about 19). The overall average was almost 18 with a range of 3 to 46.

Just over one-half of the 54 hospitals responding to these items (56 percent) reported that medical staff are paid for their participation in utilization management. By contrast, only 24 percent of medical staff are paid for quality management, and only 19 percent for participation in infection control programs. Forty-nine percent of hospitals (26 of 53) have a paid medical director; of those, 60 percent are part-time and 40 percent full-time.

Quality Management Programs

Table A.6 shows the types of quality management programs reported by each hospital. Combined programs are the most prevalent type in the small hospitals (4 of 11 hospitals); 3 hospitals reported that quality management was combined with the Medical Staff Office. The 23 medium-size hospitals (100 to 250 medical and surgical beds) also reported combined programs of quality, utilization, and risk management in 9 hospitals and quality and utilization management in 7 hospitals. The 24 larger hospitals were most likely to have combined quality and utilization management programs (10 of 24 hospitals).

TABLE A.2 Percentage of Time Allocated to Corporate Quality Management Tasks now and 3 Years Ago, by Type of Function

Tasks	Now			Three Years Ago		
	No. of Respondents	Mean Time (%)	Range (%)	No. of Respondents	Mean Time (%)	Range (%)
Quality management						
Provide comparative reports for analyses of clinical practices patterns using national, corporate, and regional data	10	11	0–25	10	2	0–10
Consultation visits to hospitals	8	10	0–20	10	10	0–50
Assist in preparation for Joint Commission on Accreditation for Healthcare Organizations	10	8	0–25	10	8	0–40
Periodic systemwide meetings with hospitals' quality management staffs	10	6	0–20	10	4	0–20
Provide assistance with peer review programs	9	4	0–10	9	1	0–10
Develop clinical guidelines, protocols, and standards with interdisciplinary groups	9	5	0–20	9	1	0–5
Conduct research projects on emerging quality-of-care issues	9	5	0–10	9	9	0–3
Miscellaneous department administration	7	5	0–10	7	3	0–10

Board-Governance quality reporting interface[a]	2	12	5–20	2	12	5–20
Review of institution quality reports[a]	2	9	8–10	2	2	0–5
Task force[a]	1	20		1	2	
Strategic planning[a]	1	19		1	24	
Risk management interface[a]	1	25		1	30	
External requirements and requests[a]	1	10		1	5	
Unspecified interface[a]	1	62		0	0	
Utilization management						
Consultation visits to hospitals	5	27	0–76	4	21	0–85
Contacts with state peer review organizations	5	5	1–15	4	0	
Contacts with managed care contracts (HMO's[b] payor request)	5	7	0–10	4	0	
Miscellaneous department administration	5	4	0–15	4	4	0–15
Risk management consultation						
Program management	9	5	1–10	9	4	0–10
Financial management	9	4	0–20	9	3	0–20
Insurance management	10	5	0–10	10	5	0–20
Employee benefits	8	3	0–25	8	3	0–13
Claims management	9	12	0–40	10	10	0–55
Loss control and prevention	10	10	0–50	10	7	0–50

[a]Additions by respondents
[b]HMO is Health Maintenance Organization

TABLE A.3 Number and Percentage of Responses Citing Strengths, Needs, and Challenges of Respondents' Quality Management Programs

Response Category	Number of Responses[a]	Percentage
Strengths		
Systemwide quality indicators	5	26
Insurance and claims management	4	21
Coordination with the Joint Commission	3	16
Governance focus on quality	2	11
Staff in facilities serve as systems	2	11
Same studies in hospitals	1	5
Integration of quality, utilization, and risk management	1	5
Consultation	1	5
Needs		
Data systems and capabilities	7	35
Financial impact and implications of quality	3	15
Increased integration of quality, utilization, and risk activities	3	15
Governance-level quality reporting	2	10
Applications	1	5
Joint studies	1	5
Relationship with PROs[b]	1	5
Medical staff issues	1	5
Standardization among facilities	1	5
Challenges		
Senior leadership commitment to quality	4	19
Develop effective, integrated quality/ utilization risk processes	4	19
Proliferation of external demands	3	14
Document improvements in quality	3	14
Increase in the system's reputation for quality	2	10
Software and hardware updates	2	10
Sources and uses of valid data	1	5
Communication with organizations in the system	1	5
Fiscal issues	1	5

[a]Number of respondents was 11. Some respondents gave multiple answers. Number of responses for the Strengths, Needs, and Challenges categories were 19, 20, and 21, respectively.

[b]PRO is Utilization and Quality Control Peer Review Organization.

TABLE A.4 Volume, Payment Source, and Case Mix Index of Responding Hospitals, by Hospital Size (Number of Beds)

Characteristics of Hospitals	<100 Beds			100–250 Beds			>250 Beds		
	N	Mean	SD[a]	N	Mean	SD	N	Mean	SD
Inpatient admissions	10	3,575	5,332	23	8,572	3,553	23	17,338	7,234
Outpatient visits	10	16,895	15,969	23	45,737	27,984	23	148,680	164,990
Emergency room visits	10	11,937	14,694	23	22,043	6,723	23	32,032	11,053
Average length of stay (days)	10	5.2	1.7	23	6.6	1.3	24	7.1	1.4
Medicare patients (%)	10	41.5	12.5	23	44.2	10.5	24	38.0	7.0
Medicaid patients (%)	10	12.4	15.0	22	10.3	6.2	23	8.8	6.0
Capitated patients per diem (%)	6	5.6	6.4	13	6.2	6.7	18	3.9	5.9
Medicare Case Mix Index	9	1.17	0.16	22	1.32	0.18	23	1.36	0.16

[a]Standard deviation

TABLE A.5 Average Number of Hospital Departments and
Services, Medical Staff Departments, and Medical Staff Committees,
by Hospital Size

	Hospital Size (No. of Beds)		
Organizational Components	<100	100-250	>250
Hospital departments and services	17	49	51
Medical staff departments	5	9	12
Number of medical staff committees	9	20	18

TABLE A.6 Types of Quality Assurance Programs in Hospitals, by
Hospital Size

	Hospital Size (No. of Beds)			
Type of Program	<100	100-250	>250	All Hospitals
QM/UM[a]	1	7	10	18
Combined QM/UM/RM[a]	4	9	4	17
Combination with medical staff office	3	3	3	9
Separate QM	1	2	4	7
Information systems	1	2	2	5
QM/RM	0	0	1	1
Combination with focus on nursing	1	0	0	1
Total	11	23	24	58

[a]QM is quality management, UM is utilization management, RM is risk management.

Staff time spent on quality management functions. Tables A.7 to A.11
show the amounts of time in hours per quarter estimated by respondents to
be spent on various functions. The tables are divided by type of program
and hospital size; for instance, hospitals with 100 to 250 beds and combined
quality and utilization management programs. The hours, however, refer
only to quality management functions. Despite this attempt at homogene-
ous grouping, there are enormous ranges reported in the amount of time
spent for many functions. For instance, Table A.10 shows that for combined quality, utilization, and risk management programs, the time spent on
concurrent record review ranges from 72 to 1,040 hours per quarter in
midsize hospitals.

TABLE A.7 Hours Per Quarter (Hrs/Q) for Quality Management Functions in Quality Management Departments, by Hospital Size (Number of Beds)

Activity	<100 Beds		100–250 Beds			>250 Beds		
	N	Mean (Hrs/Q)	N	Mean (Hrs/Q)	Range	N	Mean (Hrs/Q)	Range
Hospitalwide functions								
Indicator development	1		3	5	2–8	2	3	3–6
Committee time	1	38	3	42	9–102	4	45	8–98
Concurrent record review			1	12		1	400	
Retrospective record review			1	72		3	56	45–78
Adverse patient occurrence	1	24	1	51		2	68	30–105
Data collection/analysis	1	120	2	112	18–207	3	64	42–105
Medical staff								
Indicator development	1	72	3	5	2–8	1	6	
Committee time	1	21	2	96	15–177	2	110	26–195
Concurrent record review	1	80	1	6				
Retrospective record review	1	120	2	168	120–216	2	240	216–264
Adverse patient occurrence	1	153	2	30	30–24	1	78	
Data collection/analysis	1	160	3	69	12–180	2	238	54–423
Reappointment/privileging			1	10		2	36	24–48
Medical staff functions								
Blood usage	1	16	1	20		2	142	24–260
Surgical case review	1	24	2	46	20–72	2	202	144–260
Medical records	1	40				1	138	
Pharmacy and therapeutics	1	32						

TABLE A.8 Hours Per Quarter (Hrs/Q) for Quality Management Functions in Quality/Risk Management Departments, by Hospital Size (Number of Beds)

| Activity | <100 Beds[a] | | >250 Beds | | |
	N	Mean (Hrs/Q)	N	Mean (Hrs/Q)	Range
Hospitalwide functions					
Indicator development	1	150	1	5	
Committee time	1	750	2	23	21– 25
Concurrent record review					
Retrospective record review	1	54	1	256	
Adverse patient occurrence	1	21	2	92	64–120
Data collection/analysis	1	90	1	9	
Medical staff					
Indicator development			1	5	
Committee time	1	420	2	372	9–735
Concurrent record review					
Retrospective record review			1	1,500	
Adverse patient occurrence			2	78	27–130
Data collection/analysis			2	170	144–195
Reappointment/privileging			1	30	
Medical staff functions					
Blood usage			1	36	
Surgical case review			1	108	
Medical records					
Pharmacy and therapeutics					

[a]Table A.6 shows no respondent in this category.

Total resources for quality management functions. Tables A.12 to A.15 show the resources—total budget, personnel budget, and full-time equivalent staff (FTEs)—now and 3 years ago. Resources are also grouped by program type and hospital size. Again, reported budgets for quality management in large hospitals ranged from $13,000 to $127,000.

Patient surveys. Table A.16 shows the frequency of patient surveys as reported by hospitals. Ninety-four percent of hospitals reported using inpatient surveys, generally at the time of discharge, but they also report conducting surveys monthly, quarterly, and according to special sampling frames.

About half of the hospitals (52.9 percent) reported surveying outpatients. It is likely that the hospitals that survey patients "constantly" were referring to readily available patient comment forms.

285

TABLE A.9 Hours Per Quarter (Hrs/Q) for Quality Management Functions in Quality/Utilization Management Departments, by Hospital Size (Number of Beds)

Activity	<100 Beds N	<100 Beds Mean (Hrs/Q)	100–250 Beds N	100–250 Beds Mean (Hrs/Q)	100–250 Beds Range	>250 Beds N	>250 Beds Mean (Hrs/Q)	>250 Beds Range
Hospitalwide functions								
Indicator development			2	2	2–3	3	2	1–3
Committee time			6	42	14–96	7	63	20–126
Concurrent record review			4	237	7–492			
Retrospective record review			4	311	153–432	1	5,700	
Adverse patient occurrence			4	97	2–336	2	5	2–8
Data collection/analysis			3	42	11–78	3	65	18–104
Medical staff								
Indicator development	0	0	0	0	0	5	18	1–30
Committee time	1	93	3	78	39–98	7	118	7–288
Concurrent record review	1	9	4	154	4–420	3	92	6–260
Retrospective record review	1	12	4	171	30–360	4	491	63–1560
Adverse patient occurrence	1	4	2	18	3–33	2	114	3–225
Data collection/analysis	1	288	5	100	15–312	4	139	48–394
Reappointment/privileging	1	96	3	22	12–40	5	9	1–24
Medical staff functions								
Blood usage	1	4	5	23	3–72	2	108	30–186
Surgical case review	1	10	3	68	6–180	3	110	6–180
Medical records	1	3	3	13	2–30	1	30	
Pharmacy and therapeutics	0	0	1	12		1	12	
Drug utilization	0	0	1	132		1	12	

TABLE A.10 Hours Per Quarter (Hrs/Q) for Quality Management Functions in Quality/Utilization/Risk Management Departments, by Hospital Size (Number of Beds)

Activity	<100 Beds			100–250 Beds			>250 Beds		
	N	Mean (Hrs/Q)	Range	N	Mean (Hrs/Q)	Range	N	Mean (Hrs/Q)	Range
Hospitalwide functions									
Indicator development	2	2	2–3	3	16	2–40	2	20	4–35
Committee time	4	23	4–53	5	81	19–294	4	45	20–105
Concurrent record review	1	120		3	82	2–240	1	120	
Retrospective record review	3	17	1–31	2	121	2–240	2	42	12–72
Adverse patient occurrence				4	31	10–60	1	20	
Data collection/analysis				5	10	6–18	3	96	39–96
Medical staff									
Indicator development	2	7	6–8	5	12	4–24	3	15	10–22
Committee time	2	68	12–123	6	196	9–506	4	72	55–115
Concurrent record review	2	250	60–440	6	397	72–1040	4	239	120–472
Retrospective record review	1	72		7	156	30–600	5	86	6–195
Adverse patient occurrence	2	36	6–65	5	80	8–162	3	212	24–484
Data collection/analysis	2	12	12	7	97	9–264	4	163	36–321
Reappointment/privileging	1	9		4	9	6–12	3	16	3–38
Medical staff functions									
Blood usage	1	32		5	20	2–48	4	45	3–99
Surgical case review	2	14	4–24	6	27	4–120	4	46	6–99
Medical records	1	32		4	155	4–570	2	38	14–64
Pharmacy and therapeutics	1	32		1	4		2	16	14–18
Drug utilization				1	4		1	14	

TABLE A.11 Hours Per Quarter (Hrs/Q) for Quality Management Functions in Information Systems Departments, by Hospital Size (Number of Beds)

Activity	<100 Beds		100–250 Beds			>250 Beds		
	N	Mean (Hrs/Q)	N	Mean (Hrs/Q)	Range	N	Mean (Hrs/Q)	Range
Hospitalwide functions								
Indicator development	1	2	1	30		2	9	
Committee time	1	69	2	122	76–168	2	28	22–33
Concurrent record review	1	180	1	483		1	9	
Retrospective record review	1	60	1	483		2	31	21–40
Adverse patient occurrence	1	1						
Data collection/analysis	1	11						
Medical staff								
Indicator development	1	52				2	8	6–10
Committee time	1	60	1	314		1	34	
Concurrent record review	1	60				1	360	
Retrospective record review	1	1				1	120	
Adverse patient occurrence			1	15		1	186	
Data collection/analysis	1	6	1	33		2	66	33–99
Reappointment/privileging	1	15	2	24	9–40	1	15	
Medical staff functions								
Blood usage	1	6	2	38	16–60	2	129	48–210
Surgical case review	1	15	2	62	12–112	2	192	24–360
Medical records	1	12	2	17	3–30	2	78	60–96
Pharmacy and therapeutics	1	2						
Drug utilization	1	2						

TABLE A.12 Quality Assurance Resources by Hospital Size. Program Type: Quality Management

Variable	<100 Beds			100–250 Beds			>250 Beds		
	N	Mean	Range	N	Mean	Range	N	Mean	Range
Total budget ($)	3	30,358	15,632–85,667	9	68,000	6,673[a]–100,000	3	77,336	13,349–126,990
Personnel budget ($)	3	33,395	1,583–83,852	9	61,334	29,287– 80,000	3	65,779	11,870–108,80
Consulting ($)	0			3	644	0–1,933	1	4,233	
Travel & education ($)	3	471	432–500	8	1,729	166–3,400	3	344	67–666
Total FTEs[b]	1	1		9	2.8	1.5–6.2	3	4.8	4.0–6.2
Change in FTEs in 3 years	1	–4.0		9	0	–4.4– to +3.4	3	+0.9	0 to +2.1

[a]Figure given but appears to be out of range.
[b]FTE is full-time-equivalent staff.

TABLE A.13 Quality Assurance Resources by Hospital Size. Program Type: Quality/Risk Management

Variable	<100 Beds			100–250 Beds			>250 Beds		
	N	Mean	Range	N	Mean	Range	N	Mean	Range
Total budget ($)	1	19,823		2	239,830	238,270–241,380	2	66,543	2,000–113,090
Personnel budget ($)	1	16,834		2	185,580	166,380–204,770	1	83,195	
Consulting ($)	1	2,358		2	1,125	500–1,750	1	6,393	
Travel & education ($)	2	167	134–200	2	4,759	1,500–8,018	1	2,594	
Total FTEs[a]	3	1.7	1–3	3	2.2	1–3	2	2.5	1.5–3.5
Change in FTEs in 3 years	3	+0.5	0 to +1.7	3	+0.7	0 to +1.0	2	+1.0	+1.0 to +1.1

[a]FTE is full-time-equivalent staff.

TABLE A.14 Quality Assurance Resources By Hospital Size. Program Type: Quality/Utilization Management

Variable	<100 Beds		100–250 Beds			>250 Beds		
	N	Mean	N	Mean	Range	N	Mean	Range
Total budget ($)			1	292,670		2	23,620	72,255–400,270
Personnel budget ($)			1	2,743		2	240,600	69,496–411,710
Consulting ($)			1	0				
Travel & education ($)			1	4,175		2	757	240–1275
Total FTEs[a]	1	1.8	2	6.7	3.6–9.7	2	3.2	2.0–4.5
Change in FTEs in 3 years	1		2	+4.4	0 to +8.7	2	+1.5	+1.0 to +2.0

[a]FTE is full-time-equivalent staff.

TABLE A.15 Quality Assurance Resources by Bed Type. Program Type: Quality/Utilization/Risk Management

Variable	<100 Beds		100–250 Beds			>250 Beds		
	N	Mean	N	Mean	Range	N	Mean	Range
Total budget ($)	1	58,506	7	117,530	50,552–175,000	9	193,610	2,400[a]–550,000
Personnel budget ($)	1	43,447	7	104,880	48,141–137,500	9	189,440	104,000–400,000
Consulting ($)	1	745	4	2,312	0–6,000	1	0	
Travel & education ($)	1	1,640	7	3,468	675–15,540	9	1,767	200–3,000
Total FTEs[b]	1	1.8	7	4.1	0.6–11.0	9	5.6	1.7–10.0
Change in FTEs in 3 years	1	+0.5	7	−0.3	−3.4 to +1.2	8	+2.3	−1.8 to +6.5

[a]Figure given but appears to be out of range.
[b]FTE is full-time-equivalent staff.

TABLE 6A.16 Type and Frequency of Patient Surveys

| Setting | Any Surveys? | | How Often? | | | | | | | |
	N	Percentage Yes	Constantly	Sample	Monthly	Quarterly	Annual	Semi-annual	Irregular
Inpatient	51	94.1	23	5	7	6	1	3	0
Outpatient	51	52.9	14	4	2	1	1	0	1
Emergency room	49	59.2	14	6	2	2	1	0	0
Short stay	44	47.7	18	1	0	1	0	0	0

Discussion

The survey was not conducted with a random sample of hospitals, and response rate could not be determined. Nor is it possible, except very crudely, to determine the understanding of respondents, the accuracy of their responses, or any systematic bias in response. However, the survey includes a wide range of hospital sizes, geographic regions, organizational arrangements, and resources allocated to quality management. The numbers of departments, committees, functions, staff, and approaches are probably representative of many U.S. hospitals and demonstrate patterns in program organization and resources by hospital size. The smaller hospitals have simpler organizational arrangements and fewer staff and resources, and the two larger groupings are more comparable and tend to divide departments and personnel among their dozens of functions.

Although corporate offices, by and large, do not yet have separate quality management functions, it appears that they have begun to move in the last few years to greater integration of activities (e.g., systemwide quality indicators) between hospitals and to see this as a desired task. Very little specifically designed computer support, other than spreadsheet applications and word processing, was reported in the survey. The need for data system support was widely voiced.

Notes

1. For follow-up, contact Joann Richards, R.N., M.S.N., Principal Investigator, whose current address is Visiting Assistant Professor, 434 O'Dowd Hall, School of Nursing, Oakland University, Rochester, Michigan 48309. Telephone: (313) 370-4070.

2. The term quality management used in this survey instrument broadly encompasses the monitoring and evaluation resources, management, and reporting related to quality management and assurance, utilization management, and risk management activities, regardless of the hospital department in which the function might be located.

7

Medicare Conditions of Participation and Accreditation for Hospitals

Michael G. H. McGeary

Since the passage of Medicare legislation in 1965, Section 1861 of the Social Security Act has stated that hospitals participating in Medicare must meet certain requirements specified in the act and that the Secretary of the Department of Health, Education and Welfare (HEW) [now the Department of Health and Human Services (DHHS)] may impose additional requirements found necessary to ensure the health and safety of Medicare beneficiaries receiving services in hospitals. On this basis, the Conditions of Participation, a set of regulations setting minimum health and safety standards for hospitals participating in Medicare, were promulgated in 1966 and substantially revised in 1986.

Also since 1965, under authority of Section 1865 of the Social Security Act, hospitals accredited by the Joint Commission on Accreditation of Healthcare Organizations (JCAHO or the Joint Commission) or the American Osteopathic Association (AOA) have been automatically "deemed" to meet all the health and safety requirements for participation except the utilization review requirement, the psychiatric hospital special conditions, and the special requirements for hospital providers of long-term-care services. As a result of this deemed status provision, most hospitals participating in Medicare do so by meeting the standards of a private body governed by representatives of the health providers themselves. Currently, about 5,400 (77.1 percent) of the 7,000 or so hospitals participating in Medicare are accredited. The 1,600 or so participating hospitals that are unaccredited[1] tend to be small and located in nonurbanized areas. A 1980 study found that about 70 percent of the unaccredited hospitals had fewer than 50 beds, compared with only 13 percent of the accredited hospitals (see Table 7.1).

The current federal standards for hospitals participating in Medicare are presented in the Code of Federal Regulations (CFR) as 24 "Conditions of

TABLE 7.1 Medicare Participating Hospitals, 1980

Number of Beds	Total Participating Hospitals	JCAHO/AOA[a] Accredited Hospitals[b]	Unaccredited Hospitals
<50	1,772	679	1,093
50–99	1,607	1,253	354
100–199	1,444	1,366	78
200–299	786	761	25
300–399	444	433	11
400–499	293	288	5
500–999	343	338	5
1,000+	56	54	2
Total	6,745	5,172	1,573

[a]JCAHO is the Joint Commission on Accreditation of Healthcare Organizations; AOA is the American Osteopathic Association.
[b]115 are accredited by AOA.

SOURCE: DHHS, 1980.

Participation," containing 75 specific standards (see Table 7.2).[2] The responsibility for revising the Conditions of Participation lies with the Bureau of Eligibility, Reimbursement and Coverage of the Health Care Financing Administration (HCFA). A separate HCFA unit, the Bureau of Health Standards and Quality (HSQB), is responsible for administering and enforcing the Conditions of Participation. In addition to overseeing about 1,600 certified and 5,400 accredited hospitals, HSQB enforces separate sets of Conditions of Participation for over 25,000 other Medicare providers, including approximately 10,000 skilled nursing facilities, 5,700 home health agencies, and 4,775 laboratories. The actual compliance of hospitals with the Conditions of Participation is monitored for the federal government by each state through periodic on-site surveys by personnel of the state agency that licenses hospitals and other health facilities (or, in a few cases, by an equivalent agency).

The Joint Commission on Accreditation of Hospitals (JCAH) was created in 1951 to accredit hospitals that met its minimum health and safety standards. In 1987, JCAH changed its name to the Joint Commission on Accreditation of Healthcare Organizations in recognition that since 1970 it had developed accreditation programs for additional health services organizations delivering long term care, ambulatory health care, home care, hospice care, mental health care, and "managed" care [for example, health maintenance organizations (HMOs) and preferred provider organizations (PPOs)].

TABLE 7.2 Current Medicare Conditions of Participation and Standards for Hospitals

Conditions of Participation	Standards
1. Provision of emergency services by nonparticipating hospitals	
2. Compliance with federal, state, and local laws	(a) Federal laws (b) State licensure (c) Personnel licensure
3. Governing body	(a) Medical staff (b) Chief executive officer (c) Care of patients (d) Institutional plan and budget (e) Contracted services (f) Emergency services
4. Quality assurance	(a) Clinical plan (b) Medically related patient care services (c) Implementation
5. Medical staff	(a) Composition of the medical staff (b) Medical staff organization and accountability (c) Medical staff bylaws (d) Autopsies
6. Nursing services	(a) Organization (b) Staffing and delivery of care (c) Preparation and administration of drugs
7. Medical record services	(a) Organization and staffing (b) Form and retention of record (c) Content of record
8. Pharmaceutical services	(a) Pharmacy management and administration (b) Delivery of services
9. Radiologic services	(a) Radiologic services (b) Safety for patients and personnel (c) Personnel (d) Records
10. Laboratory services	(a) Adequacy of laboratory services (b) Laboratory management (c) Personnel (d) Blood and blood products (e) Proficiency testing (f) Quality control
11. Food and dietetic services	(a) Organization (b) Diets
12. Utilization review	(a) Applicability (b) Composition of utilization review committee (c) Scope and frequency of review (d) Determination regarding admissions or continued stays (e) Extended stay review (f) Review of professional services

Conditions of Participation	Standards
13. Physical environment	(a) Buildings (b) Life safety from fire (c) Facilities
14. Infection control	(a) Organization and policies (b) Responsibilities of chief executive officer, medical staff, and director of nursing services
15. Surgical services	(a) Organization and staffing (b) Delivery of service
16. Anesthesia services	(a) Organization and staffing (b) Delivery of services
17. Nuclear medicine services	(a) Organization and staffing (b) Delivery of service (c) Facilities (d) Records
18. Outpatient services	(a) Organization (b) Personnel
19. Emergency services	(a) Organization and direction (b) Personnel
20. Rehabilitation services	(a) Organization and staffing (b) Delivery of services
21. Special provisions applying to psychiatric hospitals	
22. Special medical record requirements for psychiatric hospitals	(a) Development of assessment and diagnostic data (b) Psychiatric evaluation (c) Treatment plan (d) Recording progress (e) Discharge planning and discharge summary
23. Special staff requirements for psychiatric hospitals	(a) Personnel (b) Director of inpatient psychiatric services; medical staff (c) Availability of medical personnel (d) Nursing services (e) Psychological services (f) Social services (g) Therapeutic activities
24. Special requirements for hospital providers of long-term-care services ("swing-beds")	(a) Eligibility (b) Skilled nursing facility services

SOURCE: 42 CFR Part 482, effective September 15, 1986

The Joint Commission's standards for the 5,400 hospitals it accredits currently are contained in the Accreditation Manual for Hospitals, some sections of which are revised each year through an elaborate process of professional consensus coordinated by its department of standards (see Table 7.3 for the outline of the Joint Commission's hospital standards). The Joint Commission currently is governed by a board of 24 commissioners, 7 each appointed by the American Medical Association (AMA) and the American Hospital Association (AHA), 3 each by the American College of Surgeons (ACS) and the American College of Physicians, 1 by the American Dental Association, and 3 private citizens appointed by the board to add the consumer perspective (JCAHO, 1988a).[3] As of late 1988, the Joint Commission had a staff of 320 at its headquarters in Chicago and 310 surveyors located around the country.

Both governmental regulation by HCFA and professional self-regulation by the Joint Commission are aimed at assuring the quality of care provided in hospitals.[4] Both sets of standards have evolved from efforts to assure a minimum capacity to provide adequate care to more ambitious efforts to make hospitals assess and improve their organizational and clinical performance in a comprehensive and continuous manner.

HOSPITAL STANDARDS: ORIGIN AND DEVELOPMENT

Private, voluntary efforts to improve the quality of care in hospitals by setting minimum, and later, optimum standards date from 1918. However, federal facility standards have inevitably accompanied any significant federal expenditures on hospital services or construction, beginning with the first grant-in-aid program for maternal and child health services, the Sheppard-Towner Act of 1921. The two approaches were formally joined in 1965, when the Social Security Act amendments creating Medicare specified that accreditation by JCAH meant that a participating hospital was automatically deemed to meet the federal Conditions of Participation in the Medicare program. Initially, about 60 percent of participating hospitals qualified through accreditation; today about four-fifths of the participating hospitals are accredited by the Joint Commission or, in some cases, the AOA.

Development of Early Voluntary Standards by the ACS and JCAH

The first standards for the organization and operation of hospitals were set forth by the ACS in 1918 (Davis, 1973; Stephenson, 1981; Roberts et al., 1987). The founders of the ACS considered conditions in many hospitals to be deplorable for patients and physicians alike, and hospital standardization was a stated purpose of the organization at its founding in 1912.

TABLE 7.3 Joint Commission on Accreditation of Healthcare Organizations' Hospital Standards, 1990

Chapter	Standard
Alcoholism and Other Drug Dependence Services (AL)	AL.1 Objectives and scope AL.2 Assessment AL.3 Treatment planning AL.4 Monitoring and evaluation AL.5 Discharge planning
Diagnostic Radiology Services (DR)	DR.1 Direction and staffing DR.2 Policies and procedures DR.3 Diagnostic studies and therapeutic procedures DR.4 Monitoring and evaluation
Dietetic Services (DT)	DT.1 Organization, direction, staffing, and integration DT.2 Orientation, education, and training DT.3 Policies and procedures DT.4 Facility design and equipment DT.5 Medical record DT.6 Quality control mechanisms DT.7 Monitoring and evaluation
Emergency Services (ER)	ER.1 Plan ER.2 Organization, direction, and staffing ER.3 Integration ER.4 Training and education ER.5 Policies and procedures ER.6 Facility design and equipment ER.7 Medical record ER.8 Quality control mechanisms ER.9 Monitoring and evaluation
Governing Body (GB)	GB.1 Responsibilities GB.2 Conflict of interest GB.3 Fulfillment of responsibilities
Hospital-Sponsored Ambulatory Care Services (HO)	HO.1 Availability HO.2 Education and training HO.3 Policies and procedures HO.4 Safety, equipment, and utilities management and life safety HO.5 Medical record HO.6 Quality control mechanisms HO.7 Monitoring and evaluation
Infection Control (IC)	IC.1 Program IC.2 Committee IC.3 Management IC.4 Policies and procedures IC.5 Support services/ departments

TABLE 7.3 continues

TABLE 7.3 Continued

Chapter	Standard
Management and Administration (MA)	MA.1 Responsibilities
Medical Record Services (MR)	MR.1 Purposes MR.2 Content MR.3 Confidentiality and completeness MR.4 Direction, staffing, and facilities MR.5 Staff role in committee functions
Medical Staff (MS)	MS.1 Membership MS.2 Bylaws and rules and regulations MS.3 Organization MS.4 Privilege delineation MS.5 Reappointment and reappraisal MS.6 Monitoring and evaluation MS.7 Continuing education
Nuclear Medicine Services (NM)	NM.1 Direction and staffing NM.2 Policies and procedures NM.3 Diagnostic studies and therapeutic procedures NM.4 Monitoring and evaluation
Nursing Services (NR)	NR.1 Responsibilities NR.2 Direction and integration NR.3 Organization NR.4 Assignments NR.5 Care NR.6 Education and training NR.7 Policies and procedures NR.8 Monitoring and evaluation
Pathology and Medical Laboratory Services (PA)	PA.1 Availability PA.2 Facility design and equipment PA.3 Communication PA.4 Records and reports PA.5 Quality control systems PA.6 Additional specific requirements PA.7 Monitoring and evaluation
Pharmaceutical Services (PH)	PH.1 Direction and staffing PH.2 Facility design and equipment PH.3 Scope of service PH.4 Intrahospital drug distribution system PH.5 Administration of drugs PH.6 Monitoring and evaluation
Physical Rehabilitation Services (RH)	RH.1 Availability RH.2 Services

Chapter	Standard
	RH.3 Comprehensive physical rehabilitation services
	RH.4 Monitoring and evaluation
Plant, Technology, and Safety Management (PL)	PL.1 Safety management program
	PL.2 Life safety management program
	PL.3 Equipment management program
	PL.4 Utilities management program
Professional Library Services (PR)	PR.1 Availability
	PR.2 Policies and procedures
Quality Assurance (QA)	QA.1 Program
	QA.2 Scope
	QA.3 Monitoring and evaluation
	QA.4 Administration and coordination
Radiation Oncology Services (RA)	RA.1 Direction and staffing
	RA.2 Policies and procedures
	RA.3 Consultations and procedures
	RA.4 Monitoring and evaluation
Respiratory Care Services (RP)	RP.1 Availability
	RP.2 Training and education
	RP.3 Policies and procedures
	RP.4 Facility design and equipment
	RP.5 Documentation
	RP.6 Monitoring and evaluation
Social Work Services (SO)	SO.1 Availability
	SO.2 Training and education
	SO.3 Policies and procedures
	SO.4 Documentation
	SO.5 Monitoring and evaluation
Special Care Units (SP)	SP.1 Availability
	SP.2 Direction and staffing
	SP.3 Training and education
	SP.4 Policies and procedures
	SP.5 Facility design and equipment
	SP.6 Monitoring and evaluation
	SP.7 Specific-purpose units
Surgical and Anesthesia Services (SA)	SA.1 Availability
	SA.2 Comparable quality
	SA.3 Policies and procedures
	SA.4 Monitoring and evaluation
Utilization Review (UR)	UR.1 Program

SOURCE: JCAHO, 1989

Sixty percent of the applicants for fellowship in the first 3 years of the ACS were rejected because the information in their medical case records was inadequate to judge clinical competence. Thus, the ACS formally established the Hospital Standardization Program, which existed until it was superseded by the JCAH in 1951.

Although the ACS initially only promulgated five requirements, called the "Minimum Standard," only 89 of the 692 hospitals inspected in 1919 met these requirements. The number of accredited hospitals increased steadily, however; by 1950 nearly 3,300 hospitals met the Minimum Standard, which accounted for more than half the hospitals in the United States.[5]

The Minimum Standard emphasized basic structural characteristics considered to be essential to "safeguard the care of every patient within a hospital" (Roberts et al., 1987, p. 937). It required an organized medical staff of licensed medical school graduates who were competent, worthy in character, and ethical. The medical staff had to develop policies and rules approved by the governing body that governed the professional work of the hospital. The rules had to require medical staff meetings at least monthly and periodic reviews of patient care in each department, based on patient records. The specifications for complete patient medical records were detailed, including condition on discharge, follow-up, and autopsy findings in the case of death. Finally, diagnostic and therapeutic facilities had to include at least a clinical laboratory and X-ray department (the entire minimum standard is reproduced in Roberts et al., 1987).

The Minimum Standard had dramatic results (Jost, 1983). By 1935, for example, the proportion of hospitals with organized medical staffs increased from 20 percent to 90 percent. The ACS standards were revised and expanded a number of times over the years. By 1941 an additional 16 standards addressing physical plant, equipment, and administrative organization supplemented the Minimum Standard. Eventually, however, the burden of accrediting several thousand hospitals became too great for the ACS to carry alone. In 1951 it joined with the American College of Physicians, the AHA, and the AMA to form the JCAH (Jost, 1983).[6]

JCAH carried on the ACS principles for improving health care in hospitals—voluntary private accreditation, minimum health and safety standards based on the consensus of health professionals, and confidential on-site surveys that involved education and consultation as well as evaluation (Roberts et al., 1987). In 1961 JCAH began to hire its own surveyors rather than use ACS and AMA staff and in 1964 it began to charge a fee for inspections (Jost, 1983). By 1965, when the legislation creating Medicare and Medicaid was passed, JCAH was already accrediting 60 percent of the hospitals (4,308 of 7,123) with 66 percent of the beds (1.13 million of 1.7 million) (AHA, 1966).

Early Government Standards

State licensing programs for hospitals were not common until the early 1950s. Most were stimulated by federal requirements (the link in timing between federal requirements and state regulatory activity is evident from inspecting the tables in Fry, 1965). Fewer than a dozen states had hospital regulations before World War II (Worthington and Silver, 1970). Federal hospital standards were imposed in 1935 for maternity and children's services, under regulatory authority contained in Title V of the Social Security Act (Somers, 1969). In 1946 the Hospital Survey and Construction (Hill-Burton) Act required the states to establish minimum standards for maintaining and operating hospital buildings aided by the act. At that time the AHA, the Public Health Service (PHS), the Council of State Governments, and other organizations sponsored a model hospital licensing law. This model law was adopted in many states, especially after 1950 amendments to the Social Security Act required states using federal matching funds for the payment of health care for welfare recipients to designate an agency to establish and maintain standards for facilities providing the care (Somers, 1969).

In 1964 the Hill-Harris amendments to the Hill-Burton Act required state licensure programs that went beyond building conditions to the administration of services. Nevertheless, in 1965 one state (Delaware) still did not license hospitals and Ohio and Wisconsin only licensed maternity hospitals and maternity units in general hospitals. Connecticut, on the other hand, had an extensive program for inspecting and licensing hospitals (Foster, 1965). New York and Michigan had just passed the first comprehensive hospital codes that addressed the quality of medical service organization and delivery (Worthington and Silver, 1970).

A series of studies and surveys in the late 1950s and early 1960s also found that the hospital survey programs of the states varied greatly in focus, intensity, and composition of the inspection team (Taylor and Donald, 1957; McNerney, 1962; Foster, 1965; Fry, 1965). Nearly all emphasized fire safety and sanitation, but fewer than 40 looked at nurse staffing and practices and fewer than 30 looked at medical staffing and practices. Just 37 states inspected hospitals annually. Nurses were on inspection teams in only 27 states and the use of physicians in state licensure programs was rare (Foster, 1965).

Development of the Medicare Conditions of Participation, 1965–1966

The drafters of the Medicare legislation were aware of the variability in the extent and application of state licensure standards. They knew that several thousand, primarily small rural or proprietary hospitals, with a third of the nation's bed supply, were not in JCAH's voluntary accreditation program. In order to maximize access of beneficiaries to services, they did not want to exclude unaccredited hospitals from participating in the Medicare program. They could not rely, therefore, on licensure or accreditation to ensure minimum health and safety conditions in all hospitals. At the same time, federal policymakers did not want to create a national licensure program with federal inspectors. Accordingly, the Medicare legislation outlined a program in which hospitals and other providers could participate voluntarily if employees of a state health facility inspection agency certified that the providers met certain federal statutory and regulatory requirements or if they were accredited by JCAH or another nationally recognized accreditation organization.

The 1965 amendments to the Social Security Act that established Medicare contained certain minimum requirements for hospitals, including the maintenance of clinical records, medical staff bylaws, a 24-hour nursing service supervised by a registered nurse, utilization review planning, institutional planning and capital budgeting, and state licensure. Hospitals also had to meet any other requirements as the Secretary of HEW found necessary that were in the interest of the health and safety of individuals furnished services in the institution, provided that such other requirements were not higher than the comparable requirements prescribed for the accreditation of hospitals by JCAH. In addition, institutions accredited as hospitals by JCAH were "deemed" by the law to meet federal requirements without additional inspection or documentation (except the legislative requirements for utilization review, psychiatric hospital special conditions, and special requirements for hospitals providing long-term-care services).

The Bureau of Health Insurance (BHI) of the Social Security Administration's Medicare Bureau was responsible for drafting the Conditions of Participation. Staff of the Division of Medical Care Administration in the PHS served as technical advisors, and a task force made up of representatives of major hospitals and health care and consumer organizations participated in the drafting of the conditions (HCFA, personal communication, 1989). Although the opportunity existed to develop model national standards, the efforts were severely constrained by the wording of the law, political and time pressures, the need to rely on state agency surveyors to inspect unaccredited hospitals, and the lack of knowledge about how to measure and achieve quality of medical care (Cashman and Myers, 1967). Except for utilization review, Congress prohibited standards higher than those of JCAH, even though JCAH itself described its 1965 accreditation standards as the minimum ones necessary to assure an acceptable level of quality. Congressmen and administration officials had assured the hospital community since 1961 that JCAH-accredited hospitals would automatically be eligible for participation in Medicare.[7] There was tremendous political pressure to deliver Medicare benefits quickly and universally and therefore to involve as many hospitals as possible in order that every Social Security recipient would have access to hospital care (Feder, 1977a, 1977b).[8] The conditions and procedures for applying them had to be developed in a few months; the law passed on July 30, 1965, and the conditions were mailed to hospitals at the end of January, 1966. The standards could not be too complicated because they had to be applied by state surveyors with widely varying experience and training, who, in most cases, were new to their jobs. Finally, even the best standards of the time were considered to be, at best, merely indicators of the structural and organizational capacity to deliver quality care. In the words of the PHS advisors on the conditions (Cashman and Myers, 1967, p. 1108), ". . . when a provider complies with the standards, it has demonstrated a capacity to furnish a stated level of quality of care. The key element here is that standards define a certain capacity for quality and not quality itself. We assume that, given this capacity, a level of quality will result. And experience informs us that without this capacity, achievement of quality is difficult, if not impossible."

BHI proceeded to draft Conditions of Participation that would be equivalent to those of JCAH. Except for utilization review, the 16 standards corresponded to the areas covered in JCAH's 1965 hospital accreditation standards. The standards were mostly qualitative and subjective rather than quantitative. For example, they did not specify staffing ratios but referred to "adequate" staffing, "qualified" personnel, and an "effective" staff organization.

Next, procedures had to be worked out by which a number of hospitals that could not meet the standards, at least initially, could participate in Medicare while, hopefully, bringing themselves into compliance (Cashman and Myers, 1967). The solution was the concept of substantial compliance, which meant that a hospital could be certified for participation even if it had significant deficiencies in meeting one or more standards, as long as the significant deficiencies did not interfere with adequate care or represent a hazard to patient health and safety. Meanwhile, the hospital had to develop and make an adequate effort to complete a plan of correction. However, as the starting date of July 1, 1966, approached, the pressure to make the program universal was overwhelming, and there was notable resistance to denying certification to any hospital that could meet the basic statutory requirements, which were embodied in 8 of the 100 standards (Cashman and Myers, 1967). Also, provisions were made for special certification of hospitals in geographically remote areas where denial would have a major impact on the access of beneficiaries to services.[9]

The federal standard-setters expected and found widely varying state-to-state interpretations of the conditions (Cashman and Myers, 1967). Of the 2,700 unaccredited hospitals applying by September 30, 1966, less than 8 percent could not meet the conditions according to state surveyors, but the rate of denial recommendations varied from 0 in 18 states to 20 percent or more in 7 states. In all, just 15 percent of the 2,400 unaccredited hospitals that were certified were in compliance without any significant deficiencies. Nearly a third (1,556) were certified with correctable deficiencies, and more than a fifth (545) were not in compliance but were certified in the special categories to ensure access. Some states did not recommend special certification for any hospitals; others recommended special certification for half their hospitals. In all, some 700 hospitals had significant deficiencies in at least 6 of the conditions.[10]

Given that the federal requirements were minimum standards, the authors of the original Conditions of Participation concluded that future progress would have to take place through innovative leadership by professionals through the accreditation process. They called on professional standard-setters to establish optimal rather than minimum standards for medical care (Cashman and Myers, 1967).

JCAH and Medicare

In 1966, with its standards forming the basis for the hospital Conditions of Participation in the Medicare program, JCAH found that the federal government was "usurping" its traditional role of guaranteeing minimum hospital standards (Roberts et al., 1987). Already, in December 1965, the JCAH board of commissioners had adopted a utilization review standard.[11] In August 1966, JCAH's board of commissioners decided to issue optimum achievable standards rather than minimum essential standards for hospital accreditation. The resulting *1970 Accreditation Manual for Hospitals* contained 152 pages of standards, compared with just 10 pages of standards in 1965 (JCAH, 1965, 1971). Meanwhile, however, JCAH went through a period of negative publicity that culminated in legislative changes in 1972 that imposed federal oversight of the accreditation process. In 1969 the Health Insurance Benefits Advisory Council, the advisory group to the Social Security Administration on the implementation of Medicare, criticized JCAH's standards and inspection process in its first report. According to the report, some JCAH standards were too low, the inspection cycle (2 years at that time) was too infrequent, and the surveyors (then just physicians) were too narrowly focused on medical staff and medical record issues. The council recommended that the Secretary of HEW be given authority to set standards higher than those of JCAH and that state agencies be given the authority to inspect accredited hospitals (Health Insurance Benefits Advisory Council, 1969).

In 1969 and 1970, JCAH accredited (but with 1-year provisional certificates) Boston City Hospital, D.C. General Hospital, San Francisco General Hospital, St. Louis City Hospital, and other major urban hospitals despite extensive publicity about serious problems in patient care (Worthington and Silver, 1970). Consumer groups presented JCAH with demands for patient rights and consumer participation in the accreditation process (Silver, 1974). Some groups sued HEW, arguing that the delegation of Medicare certification to the private JCAH was unconstitutional, and legislation was even introduced to establish a federal accreditation commission (Jost, 1983).

In 1972 Congress responded with amendments to the Social Security Act that gave the HEW Secretary the authority to promulgate standards higher than those of JCAH, to conduct inspections of a random sample of accredited hospitals each year, to investigate allegations of substantial deficiencies in accredited hospitals, and, finally, to decertify hospitals that failed to meet federal requirements even though they were accredited. As a result of the first year of validation surveys, 107 of the 163 hospitals inspected by state agencies for HEW lost deemed status for being out of compliance with the Conditions of Participation. The state inspectors found 4,300 deficiencies where JCAH had only found 2,993 contingencies; moreover, only 7 percent of the deficiencies cited by both groups were similar. JCAH and the AHA responded that the discrepancies had more to do with differences in the size and composition of the survey teams and duration of the inspection visit than real differences in hospital conditions (Phillips and Kessler, 1975). For example, more than half of the deficiencies found by state inspectors (2,305) related to the Life Safety Code (LSC), which, JCAH argued, were not significantly related to quality of patient care or safety. In contrast, JCAH surveyors found more deficiencies than state inspectors concerning patient care; that is, in such areas as medical staff, medical records, and radiology. The first annual validation report strongly recommended that JCAH strengthen its capacity to evaluate and enforce fire safety requirements. As a result, JCAH introduced revised fire safety standards and procedures in October 1976.

A study of the situation by the General Accounting Office (GAO, 1979) was more critical of HEW and its loose oversight of state agency operations than of JCAH. The GAO found that JCAH was finding more violations of requirements identified as essential by HEW and obtaining faster compliance, although state agency surveyors often found some deficiencies that JCAH did not. The GAO report concluded that state survey results were less reliable and had less impact than those of JCAH because HEW guidelines for compliance were inadequate and federal specifications for survey team composition and training and survey duration were too weak to ensure consistency. Among alternatives for improving the certification process, GAO gave its highest recommendation to contracting with JCAH for the

conduct of all certification surveys, subject to validation by federal surveyors, because "this arrangement would provide a better, more consistent evaluation of hospitals and eliminate the problems associated with having more
than 50 independent decision makers" (GAO, 1979, p. 31).

The discrepancies between JCAH and state agency surveys were much
reduced with the introduction of the Fire Safety Evaluation System (FSES),
a system for evaluating alternative ways of meeting the intent of the LSC.
The FSES was developed for HEW by the National Bureau of Standards.
Although more recent annual reports on validation surveys continued to
recommend improvements in JCAH surveying of the LSC, they concluded
that JCAH's surveying of accredited hospitals is "equivalent" to state agency
surveying of unaccredited hospitals (DHHS, 1988). For example, the proportion of JCAH-accredited hospitals subject to validation surveys that was
found out of compliance with one or more conditions was 20 percent in
fiscal year (FY) 1982, 15 percent in FY 1983, 20 percent in FY 1984, and
29 percent in FY 1985, compared with an average of 25 percent among
unaccredited hospitals (Table 7.4). Also, the proportion of noncompliance
with each condition is similar for accredited and unaccredited hospitals
(Table 7.5).

In other words, HCFA has concluded that compliance with the Conditions of Participation is about the same in accredited and unaccredited hospitals.[12] This does not, however, preclude the possibility that Joint Commission accreditation has a greater positive impact on quality of patient
care than the federal-state survey and certification program, because in recent years, as will be seen below, the former's standards have been higher

TABLE 7.4 Noncompliance of Joint Commission on Accreditation of
Hospitals (JCAH)–Accredited and Unaccredited Hospitals with One or
More Medicare Conditions of Participation, Fiscal Year 1985

Medicare-Certified Hospitals Surveyed by State Agencies	JCAH-Accredited Hospitals		Unaccredited Hospitals	
	Number	Percentage	Number	Percentage
In compliance	328	70.7	1,168	75.6
Out of compliance	136	29.3	377	24.4
Total	464	100.0	1,545	100.0

NOTE: The JCAH-accredited, Medicare-certified hospitals surveyed by state
agencies included 66 randomly selected for validation purposes and 398 hospitals
surveyed on the basis of allegations of serious deficiencies that could affect the
health and safety of patients.

SOURCE: DHHS, 1988.

TABLE 7.5 Noncompliance of Joint Commission on Accreditation of Hospitals (JCAH)–Accredited and Unaccredited Hospitals by Medicare Condition of Participation, Fiscal Year 1985

Condition of Participation	Noncompliant, JCAH-Accredited, Certified Hospitals		Noncompliant, Unaccredited, Certified Hospitals	
	Frequency	Percentage[a]	Frequency	Percentage[b]
State and local law	2	3.0	64	4.0
Governing body	2	3.0	58	4.0
Physical environment	2	3.0	81	5.0
Medical staff	4	6.0	69	4.0
Nursing	2	3.0	92	6.0
Dietary	0	0.0	32	2.0
Medical record	3	5.0	56	3.0
Pharmacy	3	5.0	77	5.0
Laboratories	3	5.0	89	6.0
Radiology	0	0.0	18	1.0
Complementary	2	3.0	21	1.0
Outpatient	0	0.0	23	1.0
Emergency	3	5.0	88	6.0
Social work	0	0.0	15	1.0

[a]Of the total of 66 JCAH-accredited, Medicare-certified hospitals that were randomly selected to be surveyed by state agencies for compliance with the Medicare Conditions of Participation in fiscal year 1985.

[b]Of the total of 1,545 unaccredited, Medicare-certified hospitals that were surveyed by state agencies for compliance with the Medicare Conditions of Participation in fiscal year 1985.

SOURCE: DHHS, 1988.

and much more detailed with regard to quality assurance processes than the conditions.

Despite the drastic revision and expansion of the accreditation standards in 1970, the JCAH standards still emphasized the structure and process features of hospital organization and administration that were believed to create the capacity to deliver quality patient care rather than evaluating the hospital's actual performance (JCAHO, 1987). In the early 1970s, aware of criticism of the emphasis on organizational and clinical capacity rather than actual performance (Somers, 1969), and stimulated by the advent of the Professional Standards Review Organizations (PSROs) with their mandate to review quality of care, JCAH began to emphasize the medical audit as the mechanism for assuring quality of care and to specify the use of explicit criteria and formal procedures in place of the informal and subjective review processes already presumed to take place at the monthly medical staff and department meetings required since 1918 (Roberts and Walczak, 1984). For example, JCAH sponsored the development of PEP, the Performance Evaluation Procedure for Auditing and Improving Patient Care, an elaborate medical audit system that was taught in workshops for accredited hospitals (JCAH, 1975; Jacobs et al., 1976). The PEP methodology was based on several decades of efforts to develop objective methods of appraising clinical performance through retrospective auditing of medical charts using explicit criteria (Sanazaro, 1980).

In 1976 a new section of the accreditation manual for hospitals on quality of professional services called for a certain number of medical audits depending on hospital size, but it soon became apparent that the methodology was being applied mechanistically with little impact on medical practice. Meanwhile, JCAH survey results indicated that surgical case review, drug and blood utilization review, and review of appointments and reappointments by the medical staff were subjective and informal and often ineffective in finding or resolving patient care and clinical performance problems (Affeldt et al., 1983).

In 1979, JCAH dropped numerical medical audit requirements and introduced a new quality assurance standard in a separate chapter of the accreditation manual. The new standard required the development of a hospitalwide program that not only identified specific problems in patient care and clinical performance but documented attempts to resolve them. Since 1979 the accreditation manual for hospitals has undergone substantial change in an effort to incorporate quality assurance activities in each clinical activity of a hospital. The revised standards are analyzed and recent efforts to develop explicit indicators of clinical and organizational performance are described in later sections of this chapter.

Evolution of the Hospital Conditions of Participation, 1966–1986

The final regulations on the original Conditions of Participation that were promulgated in late 1966 were basically the same as those issued earlier in the year, except they accorded deemed status to hospitals accredited by the AOA. Those regulations included 16 conditions, broken down into about 100 standards and several hundred explanatory factors (Table 7.6). The conditions were criticized from the beginning for only looking at the capacity of a hospital to provide adequate quality of care rather than its actual performance or effect on patient well-being. Nevertheless, the conditions were not revised in a significant way for 20 years.

Generally, the conditions in effect from 1966 until 1986 emphasized structure over process measures of organizational and clinical capacity, such

TABLE 7.6 Medicare Conditions of Participation for Hospitals, 1965

1. Compliance with state and local laws
2. Governing body
3. Physical environment
4. Medical staff
5. Nursing department
6. Dietary department
7. Medical record department
8. Pharmacy or drug room
9. Laboratories
10. Radiology department
11. Medical library
12. Complementary departments (surgery; anesthesia; dentistry and dental staff; rehabilitation, physical therapy, and occupational therapy)
13. Outpatient department
14. Emergency service or department
15. Social work department
16. Utilization review plan

as staff qualifications, written policies and procedures, and committee structure, which were usually specified at the standard level. The process aspects of quality-of-care standards were usually suggested as explanatory factors that could be used to evaluate compliance with the standard. For example, there was no quality-of-care or quality assurance condition or standard. Instead, the medical staff condition had a meetings standard, calling for regular meetings of the medical staff to review, analyze, and evaluate the clinical work of its members, using an adequate evaluation method. The explanatory factors that surveyors were supposed to use to determine compliance with the standard included attendance records at staff or departmental meetings and minutes that showed reviews of clinical practice at least monthly. The reviews were supposed to consider selected deaths, unimproved cases, infections, complications, errors in diagnosis, results of treatment, and review of transfusions, based on the hospital statistical report on admissions, discharges, clinical classifications of patients, autopsy rates, hospital infections, and other pertinent hospital statistics. The minutes were also supposed to contain short synopses of the cases discussed, the names of the discussants, and the duration of the meeting.

In the 1970s there were several unsuccessful efforts by the government to revise the conditions. In 1977, HCFA developed specifications for revising the Conditions of Participation and invited comments from interested parties in the Federal Register. After considering more than 2,000 comments, HCFA published draft revised conditions in the Federal Register in

1980 (*Federal Register,* 1980, p. 41794). Generally, the new conditions proposed in 1980 would have eliminated a number of prescriptive requirements, especially those specifying personnel credentials and certain committees of the governing board and medical staff, replacing them with statements of the functions to be performed. The new conditions also recognized changes in medical practice by adopting JCAH definitions and standards in new conditions for nuclear medicine; for rehabilitative, respiratory, and psychiatric services; and for special care units.

The proposed 1980 regulations also included a new standard, Quality Assurance, in the governing body condition. The new standard would have required a hospitalwide quality assurance program involving the medical staff in peer review and requiring performance evaluations by each organized service.

Although the Reagan administration withdrew the proposed new Conditions of Participation for hospitals when it took office in January 1981, they were among the top five sets of regulations addressed by the Vice President's task force on deregulation. A committee of top political appointees and career staff in HCFA reviewed the Conditions of Participation line by line, developing detailed worksheets analyzing each condition and standard in terms of its statutory basis, pertinent public comments on the proposed 1980 regulations, and, in the several cases where they existed, research findings.[13]

The revised conditions that were proposed in 1983 (*Federal Register,* 1983, p. 299) and finalized in 1986 (*Federal Register,* 1986, p. 22010) were based in part on those proposed in 1980, although, in line with the Reagan administration's emphasis on deregulation, the resulting regulations carried further the process of eliminating prescriptive requirements specifying credentials or committees, departments, and other organizational arrangements. They were replaced with more general statements of desired performance or outcome in order to increase administrative flexibility (see statements on the proposed and final regulations in the Federal Registers cited above). On the other hand, the activities proposed for elevation to the condition level in 1980 to give them more emphasis in the certification process were retained as new conditions, including infection control and surgical and anesthesia services. In addition, quality assurance was made a separate condition. The possible impact of the new condition on quality of care is analyzed in a later section of this chapter, along with the JCAH quality assurance standards.

The new Conditions of Participation took effect on September 15, 1986. They were accompanied by interpretive guidelines and detailed survey procedures developed by HCFA to increase consistency of interpretation and application by the state agency surveyors (HCFA, 1986). Use of the new quality assurance condition as a basis for decertification was delayed for a year. The state inspectors did survey the condition, however. After the first 2 years, 128 (9 percent) of the 1,420 hospitals surveyed were found to be out of compliance with the new quality assurance condition (data supplied by HSQB). The states with the most hospitals failing this condition were Texas, with 23 (15 percent) of its 150 unaccredited hospitals, and Montana, with 10 (23 percent) of its 43 unaccredited hospitals. Other states with smaller numbers of unaccredited hospitals had higher rates of noncompliance: 6 of 10 in South Carolina; 2 of 4 in Virginia, and 1 of 3 in New Jersey.

MEDICARE CERTIFICATION AND JOINT COMMISSION ACCREDITATION STANDARDS AND PROCEDURES FOR ASSURING QUALITY OF PATIENT CARE IN HOSPITALS

Although one is governmental and the other private, both HCFA and the Joint Commission are regulatory in their approach. They each attempt to assure quality of care by influencing individual and institutional behavior. As in any regulatory system, quality assurance in health delivery organizations has three components (IOM, 1986). First, standards have to be set that relate to quality of care. Second, the extent of compliance of hospitals with the standards must be monitored. Third, procedures for enforcing compliance are necessary. The HCFA and Joint Commission standards and their procedures for monitoring and enforcing compliance with the standards are described, analyzed, and compared in this section.

Standards

In 1966, at the time the Conditions of Participation were first drafted, Donabedian (1966) identified three aspects of patient care that could be measured in assessing the quality of care: structure, process, and outcome. Theoretically, structure, process, and outcome are related, and, ideally, a good structure for patient care (e.g., safe and sanitary buildings, necessary equipment, qualified personnel, and properly organized staff) increases the likelihood of a good process of patient care (e.g., the right diagnosis and best treatment available), and a good process increases the likelihood of a good outcome (e.g., the highest health status possible) (Donabedian, 1988).

Structure and Process Orientation of Hospital Standards

The original conditions of 1966, and the JCAH standards they were based on, were almost exclusively based on structural aspects of patient care, because structural measures are the easiest for standard-setters to specify, for surveyors to assess, and for enforcers to use in justifying their actions.

Unfortunately, there is very little knowledge about the relations between structural characteristics and process features or outcomes of care. What knowledge exists on the relations between structure and process indicates that they are weak (Palmer and Reilly, 1979; Donabedian, 1985). At best, then, the use of structurally oriented standards ensures that care is given in an environment that is conducive to good care (Donabedian, 1988). Not meeting minimum structural standards may make it impossible to provide good care. Thus, structural standards may be necessary, but they are far from sufficient guarantors of good care.

Clinical decision making is very complex, and, despite the development of complex clinical decision-making algorithms for assessing quality (Greenfield et al., 1975, 1977, 1981), it has proved to be difficult to develop objective criteria for assessing the quality of clinical processes in particular cases. In some instances, something is known about the relations between clinical processes and clinical outcomes, for example, where properly controlled experiments have been conducted. In most instances, however, standards for best clinical practices are based on professional consensus, even though the relations between clinical practices considered by professional consensus to be best and favorable outcomes are generally weak (Schroeder, 1987).

Outcome-based standards are the most difficult to apply or justify. Consider, for example, a standard that stated that the death rate should be no more than X percent during a specified time period among patients who had a particular diagnosis or who underwent a particular procedure. Because a number of factors influence death rates besides the clinical setting and processes used, death rates would have to be carefully adjusted for initial severity of illness and other case-mix differences before they could be used in setting regulatory standards. In any case, for compliance and enforcement purposes, outcome measures such as death rates, however adjusted, would have to be followed by assessment and documentation of the processes used in particular cases that caused the adverse outcomes.

Both HCFA and the Joint Commission are severely constrained in their efforts to assure quality of care in hospitals or other health care organizations by this fundamental lack of knowledge about relations between the aspects of care that can be most easily regulated (such as building specifications, staff credentials, regular committee meetings, complete medical records, written quality assurance plans, and number of medical care audits) and those aspects of patient care that pertain more directly to quality (such as how well each patient is treated, how each patient's health status is affected by the care provided, or how the health status of the population served is being affected by a hospital's services).

Traditionally, given these limitations, HCFA and the Joint Commission standard-setters did not try to assess the quality of care actually given.

Instead, they adopted standards that, if met, would indicate that a hospital had the capacity to provide a minimum level of quality of care. Both sets of standards have always included standards for the construction, maintenance, and safe operation of hospital buildings. Currently, for example, compliance with the 1981 LSC and infection control standards (elevated to a Medicare Condition of Participation in 1986) are required. Both sets of standards require an organized medical staff and appointment of a hospital administrator, although the requirements have become less prescriptive over the years. For example, rather than require certain committees or credentials, the standards specify the functions that must be carried out.

By and large, these capacity-oriented standards are based on professional consensus, although some are based on research. The LSC is a set of consensus-based standards for fire safety developed by the National Fire Protection Association. Infection control was raised to a condition in 1986, in part because of research by the Centers for Disease Control showing that 5 percent of patients in acute care hospitals contracted nosocomial infections, necessitating several days of additional hospitalization at a cost of $1 billion a year (*Federal Register*, 1983, p. 303). The requirements that the medical staff be organized under bylaws and that the medical staff and hospital administrator be accountable to a governing body were retained in the 1986 revision of the conditions in part because of research indicating that medical care is better in well-organized and supervised hospitals (HCFA Task Force, 1982).

Shift from Capacity Standards to Performance Standards

In recent years, HCFA and the Joint Commission have tried to revise their standards in ways that would impel hospitals to examine and, hopefully, improve the quality of their organizational and clinical performance. Thus, for example, both organizations have adopted quality assurance standards that call for hospitals to set up structures and processes for monitoring patient care, identifying and resolving problems, and evaluating the impact of quality assurance activities. Under these standards, the medical staff is required to develop or adopt indicators of quality of care, gather information on the indicators, select criteria for deciding when an indicator is signaling a possible problem, and act on those signals.

The Joint Commission calls these quality assurance activities "outcome-oriented," although the main emphasis of the new standards is to make hospitals adopt processes for monitoring indicators of the quality of their performance. Only a few of the indicators are likely to be outcomes, and those are most likely to be intermediate outcomes. For example, a radiology department might agree that the accuracy of upper gastrointestinal (GI) contrast studies is an important indicator of quality (JCAH, 1986). Data from the records of 20 percent of the department's patients would be collected monthly and aggregated by the radiologist and physician ordering an upper GI series, to determine whether or not the criteria for upper GI series are being met. Some of the criteria might be: 100 (or 98) percent of the requisitions for upper GI series contain the pertinent history, physical findings, and suspected diagnosis, or that radiologic interpretations shall be consistent with endoscopic findings 100 (or 97) percent of the time. Other indicators (for other departments or hospitalwide) might be: hospital-acquired infections, severe adverse drug reactions, agreement of final pathology diagnoses with patients' previous diagnoses, or transfer of patients from postsurgical recovery units to operating rooms (JCAHO, 1988c).

Evolution of the Joint Commission's Quality Assurance Standards

The shift from prescriptive to performance-oriented standards began at JCAH in 1978, when the board of commissioners decided to replace the numerical medical audit requirement with a new quality assurance standard that mandated an ongoing, hospitalwide effort to monitor care, identify problems or ways to improve care, and resolve any problems (Affeldt et al., 1983). The new quality assurance program was to involve all departments and services, not just a quality assurance unit. It was to be problem-focused rather than mindlessly to collect vast quantities of data for their own sake, which the old medical audit standard had encouraged. The new standard was approved in 1979 but not implemented until 1981, to give hospitals time to develop systematic quality assurance programs. In 1981 the JCAH board voted to revise all the hospital standards by 1983 according to five principles (JCAH, 1981):

1. The standards would be essential ones that any hospital should meet.
2. The standards should be statements of objectives, leaving the means to achieve their intent to the discretion of individual hospitals.
3. The standards should focus on elements essential to high-quality patient care, including the environment in which that care is given.
4. The standards must be reasonable and surveyable.
5. The standards should reflect the current state of the art.

The standards for governing bodies, medical staffs, management and administrative services, medical records, and quality and appropriateness review for support services were revised first. Despite the intention to simplify the standards and make them less prescriptive and more goal-oriented, the revision process ended up involving substantial expansion and formalization of quality assurance activities in each chapter of the hospital accreditation manual, including an increasing specification of processes needed to achieve the objectives of JCAH's new quality assurance standard.

In 1981 the new quality assurance chapter of the hospital accreditation manual had one standard: There shall be evidence of a well-defined, organized program designed to enhance patient care through the ongoing objective assessment of important aspects of patient care and the correction of identified problems. According to a standard in the governing body chapter, the governing body was to hold the medical staff responsible for establishing quality assurance mechanisms. One of the medical staff standards required regular review, evaluation, and monitoring of the quality and appropriateness of patient care provided by each member of the medical staff as well as surgical case (tissue) review, review of pharmacy and therapeutic activities, review of medical records, blood utilization review, review of the clinical use of antibiotics, and participation in hospitalwide functions such as infection control, safety and sanitation, and utilization review.

In 1984 uniform language for the monitoring and evaluation of quality and appropriateness of care was added into each of 14 chapters on specific clinical services, e.g., anesthesia, nursing, radiology, and social work services: "As part of the hospital's quality assurance program, the quality and appropriateness of patient care provided by the X department/service are monitored and evaluated, and identified problems are resolved" (JCAH, 1983, p. 6). The required characteristics of an acceptable process for carrying out the standard included: designation of the department head as responsible for the process, routine collection of data about important aspects of the care provided, periodic assessment of the data to identify problems or opportunities to improve care, use of objective criteria that reflect current knowledge and clinical experience, taking actions to address problems and document and report problems to the hospitalwide quality assurance program, and, finally, evaluating the impact of the actions taken (JCAH, 1983).

In 1984, after four field reviews of several drafts, revised medical staff standards were included in the hospital accreditation manual but not used for accreditation decisions until 1985. The standard for medical staff monitoring and evaluation of the quality and appropriateness of patient care now included departmental review of the clinical performance of all individuals with clinical privileges and went on to specify the same required characteristics included in the other chapters on clinical services (JCAH, 1984a).

In 1985 the quality assurance chapter was revised to add three standards. The second standard codified the monitoring and evaluation functions already specified in the medical staff chapter and in each of the chapters on other services. It mandated certain hospitalwide activities (infection control, utilization control, and review of accidents, injuries, and safety hazards) and required that the relevant findings of quality assurance activities were considered in the reappraisal or reappointment of medical staff members and renewal of clinical privileges of independent practitioners. The third standard required the use of the same steps for carrying out monitoring and evaluation activities already listed as required characteristics in each of the clinical chapters in the 1984 manual. The fourth standard called for hospitalwide coordination and oversight of quality assurance activities (JCAH, 1984b) (see Table 7.7).

By 1985, then, an elaborate set of quality assurance processes had evolved as standards and required characteristics in every chapter of the hospital accreditation manual. The object of these processes is aimed at making hospitals, through their medical staff, review and assess the quality of care given by each person with clinical privileges and in each clinical department and to act on problems or opportunities that are identified. Most hospitals, however, have had significant problems complying with the standards. As already noted, the quality assurance standard adopted in 1979 was not implemented until 1981. Even then, hospitals only had to comply with the first three steps: assignment of authority and responsibility for quality assurance activities to a specific individual or group; progress in coordinating existing quality assurance mechanisms; written plan (JCAH, 1981). In 1982 more than 60 percent of the 12,000 contingencies given by JCAH to the 1,150 hospitals surveyed were for quality assurance problems. The proportion of hospitals with contingencies or recommendations for credentialing was 63 percent and for surgical case review was 45 percent (Roberts and Walczak, 1984).

Despite compliance problems, JCAH increased the level of compliance required with the quality assurance standard during 1983, requiring evidence that quality assurance information was being integrated, that patient care problems were being identified through the monitoring and evaluation activities of the medical staff and support services, and that the problems were being resolved (JCAH, 1982). Medical staff quality assurance activities still accounted for a large proportion of the contingencies and recommendations given in 1984, in areas such as the following: monthly department meetings to consider monitoring and evaluation findings (46 percent of hospitals surveyed); medical staff monitoring and evaluation actions are documented and reported (44 percent); and when important problems in patient care or opportunities to improve care are identified, problems are resolved (32 percent) (Longo et al., 1986).

In 1985, JCAH introduced implementation monitoring, by which certain standards would be surveyed and recommendations made, but lack of compliance would not affect accreditation decisions. JCAH explained that some changes in standards were taking more than 3 years for full implementation because they were difficult for hospitals to meet and required more time for learning (and for education of surveyors) (JCAH, 1985). Not surprisingly, most of the standards placed on implementation-monitoring status initially, from January 1986 through June 1987, pertained to quality assurance: some parts of medical staff departmental monitoring and evaluation, use of medical staff quality assurance findings, and quality and appropriateness review in support services.

In early 1988 the Joint Commission again eased implementation of the quality assurance standards. It no longer gave contingencies if hospitals were using only generic rather than department-specific indicators in monitoring and evaluating the quality and appropriateness of care in the various departments and services. The explanation for the change in contingency policies referred to the problems the Joint Commission itself had encountered in developing quality indicators for various types of care: "As the Agenda for Change activities have moved forward, it has become evident that the clinical literature does not provide sufficient information to permit health care organizations to select a full set of validated indicators for each area of clinical practice" (JCAHO, 1988b, p. 5).

The problems that many hospitals were having in complying with the Joint Commission standards for outcome-oriented monitoring and evaluating quality of care were part of the impetus for the Joint Commission effort, called the Agenda for Change, to develop indicators of organizational and clinical performance for the hospitals to use (JCAHO, 1988c, 1988d, 1988e). The data on such indicators would be transmitted by each hospital to the Joint Commission for use in developing empirical norms for hospitals to use in comparing their performance. Eventually, such indicator data could be used by the Joint Commission for monitoring compliance with accreditation standards.

Development of the Quality Assurance Condition of Participation

The quality assurance condition implemented in late 1986 by HCFA is similar in approach to, although less elaborate than, the Joint Commission's quality assurance standards. The task force of HCFA officials that developed the revised conditions in 1981–1982 consciously tried to make the new requirements consistent with JCAH standards. In the preface of their recommendations, HCFA noted that in 1966 the conditions were similar to JCAH standards in 1966 but no longer were. JCAH had revised and updated its standards continuously while Medicare had not. The task force stated: "Another recent consideration is the movement toward providing hospitals with greater flexibility in determining how they can best assure the health and safety of patients. The current regulations are, in many cases, overly prescriptive and not sufficiently outcome oriented. This trend toward increased internal hospital accountability has been reflected in recent revisions to JCAH standards" (HCFA Task Force, 1982).

Task force members agreed that a quality assurance program aimed at the identification and correction of patient care problems should be a condition because it was important and cut across all aspects of direct patient

TABLE 7.7 Joint Commission on Accreditation of Healthcare Organizations Quality Assurance Standards for Hospitals

---

Standard

QA.1: There is an ongoing quality assurance program designed to objectively and systematically monitor and evaluate the quality and appropriateness of patient care, pursue opportunities to improve patient care, and resolve identified problems.

Required characteristics

QA.1.1   The governing body strives to assure quality patient care by requiring and supporting the establishment and maintenance of an effective hospital wide quality assurance program.

QA.1.2   Clinical and administrative staff monitor and evaluate the quality and appropriateness of patient care and clinical performance, pursue identified problems, and report information to the governing body that the governing body needs to assist it in fulfilling its responsibility for the quality of patient care.

QA.1.3   There is a written plan for the quality assurance program that describes the program's objectives, organization, scope, and mechanisms for overseeing the effectiveness of monitoring, evaluation, and problem-solving activities.

QA.1.4   There are operational linkages between the risk management functions related to the clinical aspects of patient care and safety and quality assurance functions.

QA.1.5   Existing information from risk management activities that may be useful in identifying clinical problems and/or opportunities to improve the quality of patient care is accessible to the quality assurance function.

Standard

QA.2:   The scope of the quality assurance program includes at least the activities listed in Required Characteristics QA.2.1 through QA.2.5.3 and described in other chapters of this Manual.

Required characteristics

QA.2.1   The following medical staff functions are performed:

        QA.2.1.1   The monitoring and evaluation of the quality and appropriateness of patient care and clinical performance of all individuals with clinical privileges through

            QA.2.1.1.1 monthly meetings of clinical departments or major clinical services (or the medical staff, for a nondepartmentalized medical staff) to consider findings from the ongoing monitoring activities of the medical staff;

            QA.2.1.1.2 surgical case review;

QA.2.1.1.3 drug usage evaluation;

QA.2.1.1.4 the medical record review function;

QA.2.1.1.5 blood usage review;

QA.2.1.1.6 the pharmacy and therapeutics function.

QA.2.2 The quality and appropriateness of patient care in at least the following services are monitored and evaluated.

QA.2.2.1   Alcoholism and other drug dependence services, when provided;

QA.2.2.2   Diagnostic radiology services;

QA.2.2.3   Dietetic services;

QA.2.2.4   Emergency services;

QA.2.2.5   Hospital-sponsored ambulatory care services;

QA.2.2.6   Nuclear medicine services;

QA.2.2.7   Nursing services;

QA.2.2.8   Pathology and medical laboratory services;

QA.2.2.9   Pharmaceutical services;

QA.2.2.10 Physical rehabilitation services;

QA.2.2.11 Radiation oncology services;

QA.2.2.12 Respiratory care services;

QA.2.2.13 Social work services;

QA.2.2.14 Special care units; and

QA.2.2.15 Surgical and anesthesia services.

QA.2.3 The following hospital wide functions are performed:

QA.2.3.1   Infection control;

QA.2.3.2   Utilization review; and

QA.2.3.3   Review of accidents, injuries, patient safety, and safety hazards

QA.2.4 The quality of patient care and the clinical performance of those individuals who are not permitted by the hospital to practice independently are monitored and evaluated through the mechanisms described in Required Characteristics QA.2.1 through QA.2.3.3 or through other mechanisms implemented by the hospitals.

TABLE 7.7 continues

TABLE 7.7 Continued

QA.2.5 Relevant findings from the quality assurance activities listed in Required Characteristics QA.2.1 through QA.2.3.3 are considered as part of

> QA.2.5.1 the reappraisal/reappointment of medical staff members;
>
> QA.2.5.2 the renewal or revision of the clinical privileges of individuals who practice independently; and
>
> QA.2.5.3 the mechanisms used to appraise the competence of all those individuals not permitted by the hospital to practice independently.

Standard

QA.3: Monitoring and evaluation activities, including those described in Standard QA.2, Required Characteristics QA.2.1 through QA.2.4, reflect the activities described in this standard, Required Characteristics QA.3.1 through QA.3.4.

Required Characteristics

QA.3.1 There is ongoing collection and/or screening of, and evaluation of information about, important aspects of patient care to identify opportunities for improving care and to identify problems that have an impact on patient care and clinical performance.

> QA.3.1.1 Such information is collected and/or screened by a department/service or through the overall quality assurance program.

QA.3.2 Objective criteria that reflect current knowledge and clinical experience are used.

> QA.3.2.1 Each department/service participates in
>
> > QA.3.2.1.1 the development and/or application of criteria relating to the care or service it provides; and
> >
> > QA.3.2.1.2 the evaluation of the information collected in order to identify important problems in, or opportunities to improve, patient care and clinical performance.

QA.3.2 The quality of patient care is improved and identified problems are resolved through actions taken, as appropriate,

> QA.3.3.1 by the hospital's administrative and supervisory staffs; and
>
> QA.3.3.2 through medical staff functions, including
>
> > QA.3.3.2.1 activities of the executive committee,
> >
> > QA.3.3.2.2 activities of departments/services,
> >
> > QA.3.3.2.3 the delineation and renewal or revision of clinical privileges, and

QA.3.3.2.4 the enforcement of medical staff or department rules and regulations.

QA.3.4 The findings, conclusions, recommendations, actions taken, and results of actions taken are documented and reported through channels established by the hospital.

Standard

QA.4: The administration and coordination of the hospital's overall quality assurance programs are designed to assure that the activities described in Required Characteristics QA.4.1 through QA.4.5 are undertaken.

Required characteristics

QA.4.1 Each of the monitoring and evaluation activities outlined in Standard QA.2 and QA.3 is performed appropriately and effectively.

QA.4.2 Necessary information is communicated among departments/services when problems or opportunities to improve patient care involve more than one department/service.

QA.4.3 The status of identified problems is tracked to assure improvement or resolution.

QA.4.4 Information from department/services and the findings of discrete quality assurance activities are used to detect trends, patterns of performance, or potential problems that affect more than one department/service.

QA.4.5 The objectives, scope, organization, and effectiveness of the quality assurance program are evaluated at least annually and revised as necessary.

SOURCE: JCAH, 1984b

care. The task force suggested three minimal standards: (1) the organized, hospitalwide quality assurance program must be ongoing and have a written plan of implementation; (2) the hospital must take appropriate remedial action to address any deficiencies found; and (3) there must be evaluations of all organized services and of nosocomial infections, medicine therapy, and tissue removal.

The new quality assurance condition as finally promulgated calls for a formal, ongoing, hospitalwide program that evaluates all patient care services (Table 7.8), although the explicit references to nosocomial infections, medicine therapy, and tissue removal were dropped. The interpretive guide-

TABLE 7.8 Medicare's Quality Assurance Condition of Participation

---

Condition of Participation: Quality Assurance (QA)
The governing body must ensure that there is an effective, hospital-wide QA program to evaluate the provision of patient care.

> Interpretive guidelines: The condition requires that each hospital develop its own QA program to meet its needs. The methods used by each hospital for self-assessment (QA) are flexible. There are a wide variety of techniques used by hospitals to gather information to be monitored. These may include document-based review (e.g., review of medical records, computer profile data, continuous monitors, patient care indicators or screens, incident reports, etc.); direct observation of clinical performance and of operating systems and interviews with patients, and/or staff. The information gathered by the hospital should be based on criteria and/or measures generated by the medical and professional/technical staffs and reflect hospital practice patterns, staff performance, and patient outcomes.

(a) Standard: Clinical Plan.
The organized hospital-wide QA program must be ongoing and have a written plan of implementation.

> Interpretive guidelines: Ongoing means that there is a continuous and periodic collection and assessment of data concerning the important aspects of patient care. Assessment of such data enables areas of potential problems to be identified and indicates additional data which should be collected and assessed in order to identify whether a problem exists. The QA program must provide the hospital with findings regarding quality of care.
>
> The QA plan should include at least the following: program objectives; organization involved; hospital-wide in scope; all patient care disciplines involved; description of how the program will be administered and coordinated; methodology for monitoring and evaluating the quality of care; ongoing; setting of priorities for resolution of programs; monitoring to determine effectiveness of action; oversight responsibility—reports to governing body; documentation of the review of its own QA plan.

(1) All organized services related to patient care including services furnished by a contractor must be evaluated.

> Interpretive guidelines: "All organized services" means all services provided to patients by staff accountable to the hospital through employment or contract. All patient care services furnished under contract must be evaluated as though they were provided by hospital staff.
>
> This means that all patient services must be evaluated as part of the QA program, that is: dietetic services; medical records; medical staff care—appropriateness and quality of diagnosis and treatment; laboratory service;

nursing service; pharmaceutical service; radiology service; hospital-wide functions—infection control, utilization review (for hospitals under PRO review this requirement does not apply), discharge planning programs.

If the hospital offers these optional services, they must also be evaluated: anesthesia services; emergency services; nuclear medicine services; outpatient services; psychiatric services; rehabilitation services; respiratory services; surgical services.

Each department or service should address: patient care problems; cause of problems; documented corrective actions; monitoring or follow-up to determine effectiveness of actions taken.

(2)   Nosocomial infections and medication therapy must be evaluated.

(3)   All medical and surgical services performed in the hospital must be evaluated as they relate to appropriateness of diagnosis and treatment.

Interpretive guidelines: All services provided in the hospital must be periodically evaluated to determine whether an acceptable level of quality is provided. The services provided by each practitioner with hospital privileges must be periodically evaluated to determine whether they are of an acceptable level of quality and appropriateness.

(b) Standard: Medically-related patient care services.
The hospital must have an ongoing plan, consistent with available community and hospital resources, to provide or make available social work, psychological, and educational services to meet the medically-related needs of its patients. The hospital also must have an effective, ongoing discharge planning program that facilitates the provision of followup care.

Interpretive guidelines: To be considered effective, the discharge planning program must result in each patient's record being annotated with a note regarding the nature of post-hospital care arrangements.

(1)   Discharge planning must be initiated in a timely manner.

(2)   Patients, along with necessary medical information, must be transferred or referred to appropriate facilities, agencies, or outpatient services, as needed, for follow-up or ancillary care.

(c) Standard: Implementation
The hospital must take and document appropriate remedial action to address deficiencies found through the QA program. The hospital must document the outcome of the remedial action.

SOURCE: HCFA, 1986.

lines state that information gathered by the hospital to monitor and evaluate the provision of patient care should be based on criteria and measures generated by the medical and professional staffs and reflect hospital practice patterns, staff performance, and patient outcomes. The term outcome does not appear in the language of the conditions or standards, however, because the majority of the task force did not think that outcome measures could be used in the survey process. The discussion in the task force report of the new condition pointed out that outcomes were difficult to use because of the differences in the pre-operative condition of patients. Although outcome measures were desirable, because they promised maximum flexibility to hospitals, they were difficult to assess without undertaking longitudinal studies beyond the given episode of care, which would be too cumbersome for hospitals and surveyors and difficult to use in enforcement.

One objective of the 1986 revision of the Conditions of Participation was simplification of the regulations, and overlapping language in different conditions was usually eliminated. Accordingly, the monitoring and evaluation activities in each department and service implied by the quality assurance condition are not repeated under the other conditions, whereas the appropriate quality assurance standards are repeated in the various chapters of the Joint Commission's hospital accreditation manual and are cross-referenced with the quality assurance chapter. There are few other references to quality in the other conditions. However, the governing body condition has a standard for ensuring that the medical staff is accountable for the quality of patient care, and the medical staff condition has a parallel standard: The medical staff must be well organized and accountable to the governing body for the quality of the medical care provided to the patients. The interpretive guidelines for the medical staff condition also require that periodic appraisals of staff include information on competence from the quality assurance program. The only other reference to the quality assurance program outside the quality assurance condition itself is in the infection control condition, where a standard assigns responsibility to the chief executive officer, medical staff, and director of nursing services to assure that hospitalwide quality assurance and training programs address problems identified by the infection control officers.

The 1986 revisions of the Conditions of Participation, including the new quality assurance condition, were based in part on work done in the late 1970s and very early 1980s. They resemble the evolution of the JCAH standards in the same time period, when JCAH adopted a quality assurance standard and began to revise the other standards to make them more flexible and less prescriptive. However, the Joint Commission's standards have undergone substantial evolution since the early 1980s. The latter's quality assurance standard in particular has undergone a great deal of elaboration in the process of trying to help hospitals understand how to comply with its intent.

Survey Process

Compliance with hospital regulatory standards is monitored and enforced through a process of on-site surveying by health professionals. The resources and procedures of Medicare and the Joint Commission for surveying are described and compared in this section.

Surveyors and Survey Teams

Section 1864 of the Social Security Act directs the Secretary of DHHS to enter into agreements with any "able and willing" state, under which the state health department or other appropriate state agency surveys health facilities wishing to participate in Medicare and certifies whether they meet the federal Conditions of Participation and other requirements. In return, the secretary agrees to pay for the reasonable costs of the survey and certification activities of the state agency. With very few exceptions, the same state agencies conduct state licensure and federal certification surveys of all health providers in their states, including nursing homes, laboratories, home health agencies, and hospitals. Most of the state agency survey load consists of nursing homes, because they are much more numerous than hospitals but do not have Joint Commission deemed status.

Funding for Medicare certification activities comes from the Medicare trust funds. For FY 1990, HSQB has budgeted $91.2 million for state surveys of facilities participating in Medicare, about $10.0 million of it for surveys and follow-up visits to unaccredited hospitals. HSQB estimates average survey costs by type of facility and allocates the funds to each federal regional office by its share of each type of facility. In FY 1990, for example, the unit cost for a survey of an unaccredited hospital was $7,500. Each regional office, however, uses a different method of distributing survey funds to the states.

The states are also reimbursed for surveys of Medicaid facilities and use state funds for licensure activities. An Institute of Medicine (IOM) study of nursing home regulations in 1986 found great variation in state survey agency budgets and policies. As a result, the number of surveyors and the intensity of the surveys, as measured by average person-days at a facility, varied tremendously (IOM, 1986).

Federal regulations and HCFA's state operations manual are very general regarding survey agency staffing levels and qualifications. As a result, there are large state-to-state differences in the experience and educational backgrounds as well as numbers of the surveyors. This affects the composition of survey teams—e.g., how many nurses, generalists, sanitarians, and other specialists such as pharmacists and physicians are on the teams or available as consultants. Nationally about half are nurses, 20 percent are sanitarians, and most of the rest are engineers, administrators, and generalists (DHHS, 1983). But in 1983, eight states had only one or two licensed nurses on staff (Association of Health Facility Licensure and Certification Agency Directors, 1983). Only a few state agencies have physicians on staff.

The Joint Commission has 190 surveyors in its hospital accreditation program, 61 full-time, 74 part-time, and 55 consultants, who are based around the country (JCAHO, 1988f). Most of the consultants are physician rehabilitation and psychiatric specialists who survey rehabilitation and psychiatric hospitals and those same services in general hospitals, if provided. Joint Commission survey team composition for the typical general acute-care hospital is a physician, an administrator, a registered nurse, and a medical technologist. The survey team may be tailored for hospitals that offer psychiatric, substance abuse, or rehabilitation services by including or adding physician surveyors with the appropriate specialty to the team.

In 1988 the Joint Commission adopted a formula for determining survey costs, which are paid by the hospital desiring accreditation. The fee consists of a base fee and an additional charge that varies with the annual number of total patient encounters. A hospital with 150,000 inpatient and outpatient encounters a year would pay $8,652 for a full accreditation survey. A follow-up visit to verify correction of a problem (contingency) found in the full survey would cost $900 per surveyor. In recent years, fees have amounted to about 70 percent of the Joint Commission's revenues; most of the rest is derived from the sale of publications and educational services.

Survey Cycle

HCFA does not have a fixed survey cycle for hospitals. Beginning in FY 1991, state agencies were funded to survey 100 percent of unaccredited hospitals (currently, 75 percent). The visits are scheduled ahead of time. Once certified, a hospital stays certified until and if a subsequent survey finds it out of compliance with one or more conditions, which could be more than a year.

Until 1982, hospitals meeting JCAH standards were accredited for 2 years or, if there were problems, 1 year. Since 1982, a hospital found to be in substantial compliance with Joint Commission standards has been awarded accreditation for 3 years. The surveys are scheduled in writing at least 4 weeks ahead of time.

Survey Procedures

Both state agency and Joint Commission surveyors use survey report forms. State agency surveyors fill out survey forms provided by HCFA (Form HCFA-1537), which permit the surveyor to mark as "met" or "not met" each condition, each standard under a condition, and each element of a standard if specified in the regulations. Altogether more than 300 items are checked as met or not met.

The surveyors may refer to interpretive guidelines in the HCFA state operations manual (HCFA, 1986), which provide further guidance for evaluating compliance with the regulation (condition, standard, or element) but do not have force of law. The interpretive guidelines also specify the survey procedures to be used in verifying compliance. For example, element (3) of the quality assurance standard, Clinical Plan, states: "All medical and surgical services performed in the hospital must be evaluated as they relate to appropriateness of diagnosis and treatment" (see Table 7.8, and HCFA, 1986, p. A16). The language is further explicated in the interpretive guidelines: "All services provided in the hospital must be periodically evaluated to determine whether an acceptable level of quality is provided. The services provided by each practitioner with hospital privileges must be periodically evaluated to determine whether they are of an acceptable level of quality and appropriateness." Finally, a surveyor may refer to the survey procedures column: "Determine that the hospital is monitoring patient care including clinical performance. Determine that a review of medical records is conducted and that the records contain sufficient data to support the diagnosis and to determine that the procedures are appropriate to the diagnosis."

The Joint Commission survey report forms (one for each surveyor discipline, e.g., physician, nurse, etc.) list the hundreds of standards and associated required characteristics (350 items in the case of the physician surveyor) and provide a scale for rating compliance with most of them. The scale goes from 1 for substantial compliance to 5 for noncompliance. To help the surveyors to determine the degree of compliance with an item, the Joint Commission has developed explicit scoring guidelines for most chapters in the hospital accreditation manual as well as for the monitoring and evaluation of quality and appropriateness of care in each of the clinical services chapters. The scoring guidelines have been published and are available for sale to the hospitals.

Table 7.9 provides an example of how the first nursing services standard should be scored. If the standard or required characteristic receives a score of 3 for partial compliance, 4 for minimal compliance, or 5 for no compliance, the surveyor must document the findings on blank pages that face each page of items in the survey report form.

TABLE 7.9 Method of the Joint Commission on Accreditation of Healthcare Organizations for Scoring the First Nursing Services Standard

Defining The Standard

The following are elements of satisfactory performance for the first nursing standard, which is: "There is an organized nursing department/service":

A. The nursing department or service is organized with appropriate nursing direction;
B. The department or service provides quality care as shown by
    - use of the nursing process,
    - adequate professional nurse staffing,
    - findings of monitoring and evaluation that indicate high-quality care is provided and that actions are taken to solve identified problems, and
    - documentation of adequate participation in orientation and in-service education of nursing personnel; and
C. The department or service maintains optimal professional conduct and practice as shown by
    - policies and procedures relating to ethical conduct and professional practices,
    - monitoring and evaluation findings that identify instances of substandard practice and/or unethical conduct, and
    - actions taken according to an established disciplinary process when problems in professional conduct and practice are identified.

Scoring the Standard[a]

Score 1 if these elements have been fulfilled for at least the previous 24 months.

Score 2 if the major requirements of all elements listed are fulfilled, but have been fulfilled for only 18 to 23 months.

Score 3 if two of the three elements are fulfilled OR the elements have been fulfilled for 12 to 17 months.

Score 4 if one of the three elements is fulfilled OR the elements have been fulfilled for 6 to 11 months.

Score 5 if none of the elements are fulfilled OR the elements have been fulfilled for less than 6 months.

---

[a]All Joint Commission standards and required characteristics are scored on a scale from 1 to 5, depending on degree of compliance:

1. Substantial compliance (the organization consistently meets all major provisions of the standard or required characteristic).
2. Significant compliance (meets most provisions).
3. Partial compliance (meets some provisions).
4. Minimal compliance (meets few provisions).
5. Noncompliance (fails to meet the provisions).

SOURCE: JCAH, 1987.

State agency and Joint Commission survey teams present their findings at exit conferences, and hospitals with significant problems may begin to make corrections to head off a possible decertification or nonaccreditation action. Some state surveyors obtain plans of correction at this time, whereas others ask for them after reviewing the findings at the office.

Enforcement Procedures

Enforcement begins with a formal finding of noncompliance that necessitates correction. This is a deficiency in HCFA's lexicon, a contingency in the Joint Commission's. In both cases the facility may be and usually is certified or accredited on the basis of, or contingent on, a plan of correction that will, if carried out, bring the hospital into compliance. Depending on the nature and seriousness of the problem, the state agency or the Joint Commission may require written documentation of corrective action or may decide to schedule an on-site visit by a surveyor to verify compliance. In most cases, enforcement ends when the plan of correction is carried out, and more formal enforcement action is rarely taken.

In about 15 percent of the cases (100 of the 700 hospitals surveyed per year), problems are of a nature or degree of seriousness that an unaccredited hospital may be found out of compliance with a Condition of Participation, and decertification proceedings are begun. If it is an "immediate and serious" deficiency, a fast-track termination process is triggered that results in decertification within 23 days. In other cases, and in fast-track cases when the immediate jeopardy is removed, the process takes 90 days. In most cases, the hospitals move to make the changes necessary to have the proceedings dropped, but about 10 to 20 are terminated each year.

Traditionally, the Joint Commission has denied accreditation to between 10 and 15 hospitals a year (about 1 percent of those surveyed). When the 3-year survey cycle with the contingency system was started in 1982, about 15 percent of hospitals were accredited without contingencies and the rest, 83 to 84 percent, were accredited with contingencies that had to be removed within a certain time period, usually 6 months. More recently, 99 percent of the accredited hospitals have been receiving contingencies, several hundred of them serious enough to trigger tentative nonaccreditation procedures, but, due to serious lags in computerizing the new procedures, only four lost accreditation in 1986 and five in 1987 (Bogdanich, 1988). As a result, several hospitals with very serious problems identified in Joint Commission surveys were able to retain their accreditation status for months and even years. Meanwhile, they had lost their Medicare certification as a result of validation surveys triggered by complaints.

Enforcement Criteria

HCFA, in its state operations manual or otherwise, provides little guidance to the state agencies on how to decide whether the deficiencies found by surveyors amount to noncompliance with a Condition of Participation. For example, Hospital A may have deficiencies in four of the five standards comprising a condition but still be judged in compliance with the condition, whereas Hospital B may only have deficiencies in three standards and be ruled out of compliance with the condition. The judgment is left to the state survey agency.

In contrast, the Joint Commission has developed a complex algorithm for converting the scores on completed survey report forms for each standard and required characteristic into summary ratings on a decision grid sheet for each of the major performance-related functions that are taken into account in making accreditation decisions and decisions on whether to assign contingencies or not. In some cases, such as medical staff appointment, clinical privileges, and monitoring functions (e.g., reviews of blood utilization, medical records, and surgical cases), the score is taken directly from the survey form. In most cases, a set of scores of related items on the survey report form are aggregated according to specific written rules into a summary score. For example, the summary score for "evidence of quality assurance actions taken" is aggregated from some 21 scores on related items in 18 chapters of the accreditation manual.

The accreditation decision grid, then, aggregates the hundreds of scores given by surveyors into 43 summary scores under 10 headings (e.g., medical staff, monitoring functions, nursing services, quality assurance, medical records). Another 7 scores for standards on implementation monitoring status are listed but not used in making the accreditation decision. Another set of rules is then applied to determine whether the hospital should be accredited. This set of rules is also used to decide whether contingencies should be assigned, with what deadlines, and whether subject to a follow-up visit or just written documentation of corrective action. For example, a tentative nonaccreditation decision is forwarded to the Accreditation Committee of the Joint Commission's board of commissioners if the four elements under the medical staff heading are scored 4 or 5, or five of the seven elements under the monitoring heading are scored 4 or 5, and so forth. Similarly specific rules determine whether 1-month, 3-month, 6-month, or 9-month written progress reports are required, or 6-month, 9-month, or 12-month on-site surveys are necessary.

These three sets of decision rules (surveyor scoring of individual items on the survey report form, aggregation of the individual surveyor scores into summary scores on the accreditation grid sheet, and the rules used to make nonaccreditation and contingency decisions) are new and constantly evolving as they are used in practice. They were adopted in response to complaints about variations in surveyor judgment and in Joint Commission decision making about accreditation; the advent of computers has made it possible.

CONCLUSIONS, ISSUES, AND OPTIONS

Conclusion: Quality Assurance Through Certification and Accreditation is Limited

Federal and Joint Commission efforts to develop and apply quality assurance standards are hampered in several ways. First, despite 70 years of efforts, we still do not have adequate and valid outcome standards.[14] Because outcomes by themselves are affected by many factors besides what happens in hospitals, adverse or even improved outcomes can only be indicators of possible quality problems or opportunities that, in turn, trigger further investigation to see if some aspect of hospital care was involved (Donabedian, 1966, 1988; Lohr, 1988). Medicare and Joint Commission standard-setters therefore have tried to mandate quality assurance processes in which hospitals use indicators of quality—outcome-oriented if possible but usually process and even structural in nature—to examine quality of care. However, few clinical indicators have been adequately validated through research. Even fewer indicators of the quality of organizational performance exist. Nevertheless, to the extent there is knowledge about how to improve quality or make quality assurance more effective, it should be reflected in the Medicare and Joint Commission standards and survey processes.

The second barrier to quality assurance through certification and accreditation is the limited surveillance capacity inherent in any system of periodic inspections. A 2-day visit every year or two limits the ability of even the best surveyors to see if the process of care conforms to standards of best practice in an adequate sample of cases, let alone to see what the outcomes were. This "distance" problem is another reason why the standard-setters have tried externally to impose quality assurance standards that make the hospital itself conduct such surveillance continuously after the inspectors leave (Vladeck, 1988).

A third impediment to using regulatory, or self-regulatory, standards to assure quality is the ambivalent attitude of Medicare officials, the state agencies that actually survey the facilities, and Joint Commission leaders toward the use of sanctions. The raison d'etre of the Joint Commission is professional self-improvement. Federal and state officials are primarily motivated by the desire to make Medicare benefits widely available, and they are also subject to political pressure to keep facilities open, if at all possible. The only formal sanction is loss of formal certification or accreditation, a drastic step that officials are reluctant to take except in extreme cases. The due process protections of the legal system also discourage enforcement attempts, as do the difficulties of documenting quality problems more subtle than gross negligence or death. Thus, for a variety of reasons, officials are very reluctant to take formal enforcement actions, especially to the extent of terminating a facility, preferring instead to work with substandard or marginal facilities over time and bring them into compliance. This approach works well if the hospitals involved have the will and capacity to improve, if shown how to do it, but it is ill-equipped to deal with places that cannot or will not improve.

Fourth, while the federal government has delegated much of the standard-setting and enforcement to private accreditation bodies on the one hand, it has given away much discretion to the states on the other. The states have always varied greatly in their interpretation of federal standards, and little has been done to increase consistency. HCFA requirements for state survey programs are very loose. Federal officials recognized from the beginning that who does the surveying is critical, "since this greatly influences what the emphasis will be, regardless of what the standard-setters think the emphasis should be" (Cashman and Myers, 1967, p. 1112), but little has been done to standardize state survey capacity or process. The development of interpretive guidelines and survey procedures for the new Conditions of Participation was a step in the right direction. HCFA could develop more sophisticated decision rules for state agencies to use in determining compliance and making enforcement decisions. It also could develop a more statistically credible survey validation program to check the performance of the Joint Commission and the states.[15]

Conclusion: Certification and Accreditation Could Play a Role in Quality Assurance

Many of the obstacles to more effective quality assurance facing HCFA's survey and certification and the Joint Commission's accreditation efforts are those facing Medicare's Utilization and Quality Control Peer Review Organizations (PROs): lack of knowledge about the relations among structure, process, and outcome; distance; and political pressure. One of the advantages of the PRO program is its continuous access to information on individuals and the episodes of care they experience. Unlike the survey agencies or the Joint Commission (at least until and if its plan to develop and then collect data on clinical and organizational indicators is carried out), PROs can actively screen data using indicators of poor quality or inappropriate care. This at least allows them to identify statistically aberrant hospitals and physicians through the use of aggregate profiles. However, the PROs are not well able to make the in-depth on-site investigations of places the indicators may identify, especially small, remote hospitals in rural areas.

The survey agencies, on the other hand, can and do mandate certain minimum capacity characteristics of hospitals. In addition, they can require that hospitals have and use internal quality assurance standards and procedures. They can require those specific process characteristics that research has or will show are associated with favorable outcomes. In the meantime, the standards should be periodically revised in accord with expert consensus about best practices. Finally, survey agencies could be involved formally and systematically in investigations of hospitals where PRO-derived quality indicators signal possible quality problems and could use their legal authority to mandate changes needed.

Issues and Options

Major Issue 1: Role of Certification in Quality Assurance

The Conditions of Participation and procedures for enforcing them are a part of the federal government's quality assurance effort, and, as such, they should be the best possible, given the state of current knowledge and availability of resources, and they should be consistent with and supportive of other federal quality assurance activities.

Pros:

• A large number of hospitals (1,600) with a significant number of beds are outside the accreditation system, and they tend to be the only hospitals in their area.

• Hospitals that have lost accreditation have applied for and received certification.

• The conditions mandate some important basic structure and process standards (e.g., life safety code, sanitation and infection control, etc.) that can be enforced legally if there are related quality problems found by PROs or otherwise (e.g., through complaints).

• State health facility surveyors are useful for investigating the causes of indicators of poor quality revealed through surveillance of case statistics.

• Quality is multifaceted and multiple systems of surveillance and enforcement are useful.

Cons:

• The inherent limits on the ability of periodic facility inspections to find problems in the quality of patient care are too great (compared to, say, a peer review approach) to justify more investment in this approach.

• Quality-of-care problems in unaccredited hospitals could be effectively dealt with by the PROs or other programs based on systematic, ongoing review of cases.

• Political pressures on state health agencies and HCFA to keep hospitals open, especially in rural areas, are too great.

• The need to keep PRO data confidential precludes coordination with the certification process; potential triggering of regulatory enforcement would poison the peer review process.

Related issue: Improving the standards. If certification is considered to be an important part of the federal quality assurance effort, the standards (Conditions of Participation) should be revised to be consistent and supportive of the overall federal quality assurance effort and kept up to date.

Pros:

• The current conditions and related standards and elements were developed in the early 1980s and do not reflect recent advances in measuring and assuring quality of care.

• State licensure standards even for basic structural aspects of hospitals vary widely and certification assures conformity to a uniform set of standards.

Cons:

• It is not realistic to expect that the conditions, which must go through the formal federal rule-making process, can be updated continuously.

• Little or no relation has been shown between facility-based standards and quality of patient care.

Related issue: Improving enforcement. HCFA should take a number of steps to increase enforcement capacity (some of them already adopted in nursing home regulation), including the following: specification of survey team size and composition; use of survey procedures and instruments that focus more on patients and less on records; development of explicit decision rules for determining enforcement actions; adoption of intermediate sanctions, such as fines and bans on admissions, so the punishment can fit the crime; and more use of federal inspectors to evaluate state agency performance through validation surveys and to inspect state hospital facilities.

Pros:

• Increasing competition and price regulation (e.g., prospective payment) in the hospital sector call for more attention to quality assurance and enforcement, especially in small rural hospitals.

• Enforcement can be increased through these kinds of federal actions, as has been done with certified nursing homes.

Cons:

• These steps are not worth the cost, given the limits on their effectiveness.

Major Issue 2: Role of the Joint Commission in Assuring Quality of Care for Medicare Patients

Deemed status should continue, and the Joint Commission should be encouraged in its efforts to develop a state-of-the-art quality assurance program, but, at the same time, federal oversight of the Joint Commission should be increased to ensure accountability and there should be more disclosure of information about hospitals with quality problems discovered by the Joint Commission.

Pros:

• Joint Commission standards are higher and more up-to-date than the Conditions of Participation.
• Accreditation is a positive incentive that motivates hospitals to improve more than certification does or can (the Joint Commission is planning to reinforce this by recognizing "superior" hospitals).
• Joint Commission inspectors have better clinical credentials and make more consistent decisions.
• The Joint Commission may achieve better compliance than the state agencies because accreditation is highly valued and the state agencies are hampered procedurally and politically (e.g., due process, lack of authority to deal with repeat deficiencies, political pressure to assure access to Medicare services); in fact, HCFA might contract with the Joint Commission to conduct all certification surveys, subject to closer monitoring, rather than deal with the inconsistencies and administrative costs of dealing with more than 50 state survey agencies.
• The Joint Commission is planning voluntarily to release information to HCFA on hospitals with significant quality problems whose continued accreditation is conditional on major changes. These would be the 7 to 8 percent of hospitals surveyed each year that trigger one or more of the Joint Commission's nonaccreditation decision rules.

Cons:

• Higher standards are not meaningful if they are not enforced vigorously.
• In any case, the Joint Commission is a private organization governed by associations of the providers it is regulating; its survey findings are confidential (except in 13 states—e.g., New York, Pennsylvania, Arizona—

where the survey is a public document under state law). The Joint Commission is not publicly accountable and, therefore, responsibility for assuring the health and safety of Medicare beneficiaries should not be delegated to it.

• The Joint Commission is still relatively weak in enforcing environmental and life safety code standards.

• HCFA must maintain a certification program with adequate standards and sufficient capacity (resources and procedures) in any case, to deal with small and rural hospitals that are not accredited, and this program could and should be applied to all (hospitals would still be encouraged to seek accreditation).

• The resources for increasing federal oversight—more funding for more intensive state inspections, more federal inspectors to conduct validation surveys—would be better used elsewhere in the federal quality assurance program.

Major Issue 3: Improving Coordination of Federal Quality Assurance Efforts

HCFA should develop criteria and procedures for referring cases in which there are indications of serious quality-of-care problems from PROs to the Office of Survey and Certification and vice versa.

Pros:

• The quality-of-care screens used by PROs include only indicators of quality-of-care problems, and the actual role of a hospital in producing adverse indicators has to be investigated further before changes can be required or sanctions applied. In many cases, on-site surveys by health facility inspectors could usefully supplement central reviews of cases by PRO clinicians.

• The state inspection agencies and federal regional offices, in turn, could alert PROs when they find hospitals with possible quality-of-care problems; the PROs could then initiate focused reviews to document process-of-care or patient-outcome problems, if any.

Cons:

• Most state inspection agencies do not have physician inspectors and some do not have that many nurses, which limits their capacity to look at quality of clinical care or to justify findings in court against a facility's physician consultants.

• Any additional resources for handling quality-of-care problems should go to building up PROs or some other peer review-oriented mechanism.

CONCLUDING REMARKS

About 7,000 hospitals provide services to Medicare patients. The Secretary of DHHS has the regulatory authority to promulgate standards called Conditions of Participation in order to assure the adequate health and safety of Medicare patients in those hospitals, although the 5,400 hospitals accredited by the private Joint Commission and the AOA are deemed to meet the federal standards without further inspection by a public agency (except for a small number of accredited hospitals that are subject to validation surveys each year). In effect, then, Joint Commission standards are the Medicare standards for most Medicare beneficiaries using hospital services. At the same time, the users of 1,600 hospitals rely on the standards in the Medicare Conditions of Participation. These are mostly small, primarily rural hospitals where Medicare beneficiaries do not have the alternative of going to an accredited hospital. Both sets of standards, therefore, affect a large number of people and should be as effective as possible in achieving the goal of assuring adequate care.

This chapter has examined the evolution of Medicare and the Joint Commission hospital standards from mostly structural standards (aimed at assuring that a hospital has the minimum capacity to provide quality care) to mostly process standards (aimed at making hospitals assess in a systematic and ongoing way the actual quality of care provided on their premises). Also, certain structural standards, such as those for fire safety, that continue to be mandated and enforced through the certification and accreditation standards may not be closely related to patient care but are important factors in patient safety.

The certification and accreditation programs are inherently limited in their capacity to assure quality of care. They are hampered by the lack of knowledge about the interrelations between structure and process features of a hospital and patient outcomes. They are limited because periodic inspections cannot reveal much about how well the process of care conforms to the standards of best practice, or what the outcomes of care are. They rely on the subjective judgment of their inspectors and the enforcement attitudes of the inspection agencies.

Certification and accreditation could play a significant role in Medicare's quality assurance efforts if several issues are addressed. Pros and cons of suggested strategies are identified for consideration.

NOTES

1. Throughout this chapter, we use the terms nonaccredited and unaccredited. Nonaccredited hospitals are those that have lost accreditation from the Joint Com-

mission. Unaccredited hospitals are those hospitals that have never been accredited by the Joint Commission or who were accredited but subsequently lost accreditation and are not actively pursuing accreditation with the Joint Commission.

2. Another regulation automatically permits hospitals that meet the Medicare Conditions of Participation to participate in Medicaid.

3. One consumer representative has served on the board since 1981. In late 1989, two more public members were added to the Joint Commission board.

4. The author wishes to acknowledge the helpful comments provided by staff of the Joint Commission, HSQB, and HCFA's Office of Policy Development on earlier drafts of this chapter.

5. Most of the unaccredited hospitals had fewer than 25 beds and therefore were not eligible for accreditation under ACS rules at that time.

6. The Canadian Medical Association was also a founder of JCAH but withdrew in 1959 to develop the Canadian Council on Hospital Accreditation. The American Dental Association joined JCAH in 1980.

7. At 1961 hearings on health services for the aged, HEW Secretary Ribicoff said he would "hand down an order that any hospital that was accredited by the Joint Commission on Accreditation would be prima facie eligible" (quoted in Jost, 1983, p. 853). The report of the Senate Finance Committee accompanying the Medicare bill said that hospitals accredited by JCAH would be "conclusively presumed to meet all the conditions for participation, except for the requirement of utilization review" (quoted in Worthington and Silver, 1970, p. 314).

8. Art Hess, first head of Medicare, told the American Public Health Association at its 1965 annual meeting that the Social Security Administration did not want to pay for services that did not meet "minimal quality standards," but "the intention . . . is not to impose requirements that cannot be met." He went on to say that "the program, through its definitions, provides support to what has now been achieved, and makes continued upgrading possible as progress in standards is made in the private sector through accreditation activities" (Hess, 1966, p. 14).

9. Two special certification provisions were implemented in 1966 for certifying hospitals that did not meet the Conditions of Participation. The access provision allowed for the certifying of rural hospitals out of compliance with one or more conditions but in compliance with all statutory provisions provided the hospital was located in a rural area where access by Medicare enrollees to fully participating hospitals would be limited. The second provision, based upon the Burleson amendment, waived the statutory 24-hour registered nurse requirement for rural hospitals meeting all other requirements. Both provisions have since been terminated.

10. As of 1970, 98 hospitals that had applied in 1966 were still not in the program and 411 hospitals were participating through the special access certification provision (Worthington and Silver, 1970).

11. JCAH apparently adopted the utilization review requirement (implemented in 1967) in the hope that accredited hospitals could be deemed to meet all federal requirements without state agency inspection. The Secretary of the DHHS, however, has never agreed to let this accreditation standard be deemed to meet the federal utilization review requirement. More recently, however, hospitals have been able to meet the requirement if they are reviewed through Medicare's Utilization and Quality Control Peer Review Organization (PRO) program.

12. Even though compliance at the condition level may be similar, it is interesting to note that more detailed analyses in earlier reports found that only about 10 to 14 percent of the specific deficiencies cited were the same (DHHS, 1979, 1980; GAO, 1979).

13. These worksheets, which provide insight into the thinking that went into the revision of the Conditions of Participation for hospitals during the 1981–1983 period, are in the HCFA files (HCFA Task Force, 1982).

14. For example, comparative hospital mortality figures have no meaning without consideration of many factors such as case-mix, severity of illness, geographic differences, and patterns of care of the terminally ill among hospitals, hospices, nursing homes, and family homes.

15. As of late 1989 HCFA was considering a revision of its sampling methodology to improve the effectiveness of its validation efforts. Also, beginning in FY 1989, the number of validation surveys performed by state agency staff was increased to approximately 200 per year (HCFA, personal communication, 1989).

REFERENCES

Affeldt, J.E., Roberts, J.S., and Walczak, R.M. Quality Assurance: Its Origin, Status, and Future Direction—A JCAH Perspective. *Evaluation and the Health Professions* 6:245–255, 1983.

AHA (American Hospital Association). *Hospitals, Journal of the American Hospital Association* (Guide Issue, Part 2), 40 (August 1, 1966).

Association of Health Facility Licensure and Certification Agency Directors. Summary Report: Licensure and Certification Operations. Unpublished report submitted to Health Standards and Quality Bureau, Health Care Financing Administration, Baltimore, Md., 1983.

Bogdanich, W. Prized by Hospitals, Accreditation Hides Perils Patients Face. *Wall Street Journal* October 12, 1988, pp. A1, A12.

Cashman, J.W. and Myers, B.A. Medicare: Standards of Service in a New Program—Licensure, Certification, Accreditation. *American Journal of Public Health* 57:1107–1117, 1967.

Davis, L. *Fellowship of Surgeons: A History of the American College of Surgeons.* Chicago, Ill.: American College of Surgeons, 1973.

DHHS (Department of Health and Human Services). *Medicare Validation Surveys of Hospitals Accredited by the JCAH: Annual Report for FY 1979.* Washington, D.C.: U.S. Department of Health and Human Services, 1979.

DHHS. *Medicare Validation Surveys of Hospitals Accredited by the JCAH: Annual Report for FY 1980.* Washington, D.C.: U.S. Department of Health and Human Services, 1980.

DHHS. *Inventory of Surveyors of Medicare and Medicaid Programs, United States, 1983.* Baltimore, Md.: Health Care Financing Administration, 1983.

DHHS. Report on Medicare Validation Surveys of Hospitals Accredited by the Joint Commission on Accreditation of Hospitals (JCAH): Fiscal year 1985. In *Report of the Secretary of DHHS on Medicare.* Washington, D.C.: U.S. Government Printing Office, 1988.

Donabedian, A. Evaluating the Quality of Medical Care. *Milbank Memorial Fund Quarterly* 44:166–203, 1966.

Donabedian, A. The Epidemiology of Quality. *Inquiry* 22:282–292, 1985.

Donabedian, A. The Quality of Care: How Can It Be Assessed? *Journal of the American Medical Association* 260:1743–1748, 1988.

Feder, J. *Medicare: The Politics of Federal Hospital Insurance.* Lexington, Mass.: D.C. Heath, 1977a.

Feder, J. The Social Security Administration and Medicare: A Strategy for Implementation. Pp. 19–35 in *Toward a National Health Policy.* Friedman, K. and Rakoff, S., eds. Lexington, Mass.: D.C. Heath, 1977b.

Federal Register, Vol. 45, pp. 41794–41818, June 20, 1980.

Federal Register, Vol. 48, pp. 299–315, January 4, 1983.

Federal Register, Vol. 51, pp. 22010–22052, June 17, 1986.

Foster, J.T. States are Stiffening Licensure Standards. *Modern Hospital* 105:128–132, 1965.

Fry, H.G. *The Operation of State Hospital Planning and Licensing Programs.* American Hospital Association Monograph Series, No. 15. Chicago, Ill.: American Hospital Association, 1965.

GAO (General Accounting Office). *The Medicare Hospital Certification System Needs Reform.* HRD-79-37. Washington, D.C.: General Accounting Office, 1979.

Greenfield, S., Lewis, C.E., Kaplan, S.H., et al. Peer Review by Criteria Mapping: Criteria for Diabetes Mellitus: The Use of Decision-Making in Chart Audit. *Annals of Internal Medicine* 83:761–770, 1975.

Greenfield, S., Nadler, M.A., Morgan, M.T., et al. The Clinical Investigation and Management of Chest Pain in an Emergency Department: Quality Assessment by Criteria Mapping. *Medical Care* 15:898–905, 1977.

Greenfield, S., Cretin, S., Worthman, L.G., et al. Comparison of a Criteria Map to a Criteria List in Quality-of-Care Assessment for Patients With Chest Pain: The Relation of Each to Outcome. *Medical Care* 19:255–272, 1981.

HCFA Task Force (Health Care Financing Administration). HCFA Task Force Recommendations. Unpublished document in files of the Health Standards and Quality Bureau, Health Care Financing Administration, Baltimore, Md., 1982.

HCFA. Appendix A, Interpretive Guidelines—Hospitals. Pp. A1–A165 in *State Operations Manual: Provider Certification.* Transmittal No. 190. Health Care Financing Administration. Washington, D.C.: U.S. Department of Health and Human Services, 1986.

Health Insurance Benefits Advisory Council. *Report Covering the Period July 1, 1966—December 31, 1967.* Washington, D.C.: Social Security Administration, 1969.

Hess, A.E. Medicare: Its Meaning for Public Health. *American Journal of Public Health* 56:10–18, 1966.

IOM (Institute of Medicine). *Improving the Quality of Care in Nursing Homes.* Washington, D.C.: National Academy Press, 1986.

Jacobs, C.M., Christoffel, T.H., and Dixon, N. *Measuring the Quality of Patient Care: The Rationale for Outcome Audit.* Cambridge, Mass.: Ballinger, 1976.

JCAH (Joint Commission on Accreditation of Hospitals). *Standards for Hospital Accreditation.* Chicago, Ill.: Joint Commission on Accreditation of Hospitals, 1965.

JCAH. *1970 Accreditation Manual for Hospitals.* Chicago, Ill.: Joint Commission on Accreditation of Hospitals, 1971.

JCAH. *The PEP Primer: Performance Evaluation Procedure for Auditing and Improving Patient Care.* Chicago, Ill.: Joint Commission on Accreditation of Hospitals, 1975.

JCAH. Guidelines Set for AMH Revision. *JCAH Perspectives* 1(5):3, 1981.

JCAH. New QA Guidelines Set. *JCAH Perspectives* 2(5):1, 1982.

JCAH. New Quality and Appropriateness Standard Included in 1984 AMH. *JCAH Perspectives* 3(5):5–6, 1983.

JCAH. JCAH Board Approves New Medical Staff Standards. *JCAH Perspectives* 4(1):1,3–4, 1984a.

JCAH. Quality Assurance Standards Revised. *JCAH Perspectives* 4(1):3, 1984b.

JCAH. "Implementation Monitoring" for Designated Standards. *JCAH Perspectives* 5(1):3–4, 1985.

JCAH. Monitoring and Evaluation of the Quality and Appropriateness of Care: A Hospital Example. *Quality Review Bulletin* 12:326–330, 1986.

JCAH. *Hospital Accreditation Program Scoring Guidelines: Nursing Services, Infection Control, Special Care Units.* Chicago, Ill.: Joint Commission of Accreditation of Hospitals, 1987.

JCAHO (Joint Commission on Accreditation of Healthcare Organizations). Overview of the Joint Commission's "Agenda for Change." Mimeo. Chicago, Ill.: Joint Commission on Accreditation of Healthcare Organizations, 1987.

JCAHO. *An Introduction to the Joint Commission: Its Survey and Accreditation Processes, Standards, and Services.* Third edition. Chicago, Ill.: Joint Commission on Accreditation of Healthcare Organizations, 1988a.

JCAHO. Rules Change on Monitoring and Evaluation Contingencies. *Joint Commission Perspectives* 8:5–6, 1988b.

JCAHO. *Medical Staff Monitoring and Evaluation: Departmental Review.* Chicago, Ill.: Joint Commission on Accreditation of Healthcare Organizations, 1988c.

JCAHO. Proposed Clinical Indicators for Pilot Testing. Chicago, Ill.: Joint Commission on Accreditation of Healthcare Organizations, 1988d.

JCAHO. Field Review Evaluation Form: Proposed Principles of Organizational and Management Effectiveness. Chicago, Ill.: Joint Commission on Accreditation of Healthcare Organizations, 1988e.

JCAHO. Hospital Accreditation Program Surveyors, September 1988. Chicago, Ill.: Joint Commission on Accreditation of Healthcare Organizations, 1988f.

JCAHO. *1990 Accreditation Manual for Hospitals.* Chicago, Ill.: Joint Commission on Accreditation of Healthcare Organizations, 1989.

Jost, T.S. The Joint Commission on Accreditation of Hospitals: Private Regulation of Health Care and the Public Interest. *Boston College Law Review* 24:835–923, 1983.

Lohr, K.N. Outcome Measurement: Concepts and Questions. *Inquiry* 25:37–50, 1988.

Longo, D.R., Wilt, J.E., and Laubenthal, R.M. Hospital Compliance with Joint Commission Standards: Findings from 1984 Surveys. *Quality Review Bulletin* 12:388–394, 1986.

McNerney, W.J. *Hospital and Medical Economics*. Chicago, Ill.: American Hospital Association Hospital Research and Educational Trust, 1962.

Palmer, R.H. and Reilly, M.C. Individual and Institutional Variables Which May Serve as Indicators of Quality of Medical Care. *Medical Care* 17:693–717, 1979.

Phillips, D.F. and Kessler, M.S. Criticism of the Medicare Validation Survey. *Hospitals, Journal of the American Hospital Association* 49:61–62, 64, 66, 1975.

Roberts, J.S. and Walczak, R.M. Toward Effective Quality Assurance: The Evolution and Current Status of the JCAH QA Standard. *Quality Review Bulletin* 10:11–15, 1984.

Roberts, J.S., Coale, J.G., and Redman, R.R. A History of the Joint Commission on Accreditation of Hospitals. *Journal of the American Medical Association* 258:936–940, 1987.

Sanazaro, P.J. Quality Assessment and Quality Assurance in Medical Care. *Annual Review of Public Health 1980* 1:37–68, 1980.

Schroeder, S.A. Outcome Assessment 70 Years Later: Are We Ready? *New England Journal of Medicine* 316:160–162, 1987.

Silver, L.H. The Legal Accountability of Nonprofit Hospitals. Pp. 183–200 in *Regulating Health Facilities Construction*. Havighurst, C.C., ed. Washington, D.C.: American Enterprise Institute for Public Policy Research, 1974.

Somers, A.R. *Hospital Regulation: The Dilemma of Public Policy*. Princeton, N.J.: Industrial Relations Section, Princeton University, 1969.

Stephenson, G.W. College History: The College's Role in Hospital Standardization. *Bulletin of the American College of Surgeons* (February):17–29, 1981.

Taylor, K.O. and Donald, D.M. *A Comparative Study of Hospital Licensure Regulations*. Berkeley, Calif.: School of Public Health, University of California, 1957.

Vladeck, B.C. Quality Assurance Through External Controls. *Inquiry* 25:100–107, 1988.

Worthington, W. and Silver, L.H. Regulation of Quality Care in Hospitals: The Need For Change. *Law and Contemporary Problems* 35:305–333, 1970.

8

The Utilization and Quality Control Peer Review Organization Program

Kathleen N. Lohr and Allison J. Walker

INTRODUCTION[1]

In the early 1980s, the Utilization and Quality Control Peer Review Organization (PRO) program replaced the Professional Standards Review Organization (PSRO) program as the Medicare peer review effort. As with the PSROs, the purpose of the PROs is to ensure that services rendered through Medicare are necessary, appropriate, and of high quality. PRO activities extend well beyond those emphases into many aspects of the Medicare program, including implementation of the Medicare diagnosis-related groups (DRG) prospective payment system (PPS) for hospitals. PROs serve different purposes for different parties, not all of whom have the same interests or concerns. In the words of one interested observer, " . . . PROs are quickly becoming all things to all people . . . " (Webber, cited in OIG, 1988b). The program is important to the Office of Inspector General (OIG) in the Department of Health and Human Services (DHHS), the Executive Office of Management and Budget, the Medicare beneficiary community (and consumer groups more generally), and providers of many sorts (especially local practicing physicians).

This chapter describes the development of the PRO program up until the summer of 1989, with most emphasis being placed on the required activities that reflect the considerable expansion and complexity of responsibility and activity of the program. For more extended discussions of the early implementation of the PRO program, see Lohr (1985) or Dans et al. (1985). Volume I, Chapter 6 is excerpted extensively from this chapter, although the committee conclusions and recommendations in that chapter are not given here.

PRO LEGISLATION AND REGULATIONS

Legislation

The role of Congress in the development of the PRO program should not be underestimated. Several pieces of legislation successively broadened the mandate of the program, often beyond the capacity of the Health Care Financing Administration (HCFA) to implement them as expected; they also attempted to turn the program toward a greater emphasis on quality of care. The key act was the Tax Equity and Fiscal Responsibility Act (TEFRA) of 1982 (more specifically, the Peer Review Improvement Act, Title I, Subtitle C of TEFRA), which amended Part B of Title XI of the Social Security Act. Other important legislation included the Social Security Amendments of 1983; the Deficit Reduction Act of 1984 (DEFRA); the Consolidated Omnibus Budget Reconciliation Act (COBRA) of 1985; the Omnibus Budget Reconciliation Acts (OBRA) of 1986, 1987, and 1989; and the Medicare and Medicaid Patient Program Protection Act of 1987.

TEFRA (P.L. 97-248) established the PRO program. It changed the funding arrangement from a system of federal grants to a 2-year fixed-price competitive contract, and it extended eligibility for the PRO program to for-profit groups and to payer organizations such as insurers and fiscal intermediaries (FIs) if there is no other available entity. It also strengthened the PROs' ability to sanction providers, thus improving the potential effectiveness of the program. The original 195 PSRO areas were consolidated into 54 areas.

The Social Security Amendments of 1983 (P.L. 98-21) established Medicare's PPS scheme for hospital payment, which increased the number of required activities of the PROs as well as their visibility. The legislation required each PPS hospital to contract with a PRO as a condition of participation in the Medicare program. PROs were assigned many mandatory review tasks, mostly relating to monitoring the behavior of hospitals following PPS; the most obvious concern was increased unnecessary admissions. Required activities of PROs were aimed chiefly at the necessity and appropriateness of admissions and invasive procedures rather than inadequate or poor technical care.

As part of DEFRA (P.L. 98-369), PROs became the quality and utilization monitors for the new reimbursement system established by the Social Security Amendments of 1983. This act provided for the continued funding of PSROs from the Medicare Trust Fund until PRO contracts could be signed. It also extended the deadline for hospitals to sign a contract with a PRO.

COBRA 1985 (P.L. 99-272) and OBRA 1986 (P.L. 99-509) considerably expanded PRO responsibilities. COBRA mandated pre-admission and pre-procedure review of certain surgical procedures (based on studies of medical practice variations) and pre-procedure review of cases requiring surgical assistants at cataract surgery. It also gave PROs authority to deny Medicare payment to physicians and hospitals for substandard quality (which would come to be known as "quality denials"). This authority was expected to complement, not compete with, the PROs' ability to sanction providers in other ways. OBRA 1989 clarified the quality denial activity somewhat.

OBRA 1986 considerably extended PRO review responsibility beyond the inpatient setting to include review of the following: ambulatory services; services provided in hospital outpatient departments and ambulatory surgical centers (ASCs); care rendered in skilled nursing facilities (SNFs); care rendered by home health agencies (HHAs); inpatient and outpatient care from Medicare risk-contract health maintenance organizations (HMOs) and competitive medical plans (CMPs); and all written complaints from Medicare beneficiaries. These activities were to be phased in over several years.

OBRA 1987 (P.L. 100-203) extended contract cycles from 2 to 3 years and allowed a contract extension (up to 2 years) for existing contracts to achieve more efficient renewals. Accordingly, a contract renewal phase-in schedule (generally referred to as the third Scope of Work) was developed in which one-fourth of the PROs began the new contract cycle on October 1, 1988, and the remaining PROs on April 1, 1989. OBRA 1987 made numerous other changes in the PRO program, including a mandated minimum level of on-site review of rural hospital care and greater emphasis on education and other instructional activities for rural practitioners.

The Medicare and Medicaid Patient Program Protection Act of 1987 (P.L. 93-100) expanded both sanction and civil monetary penalty authorities for those programs. It also required the reporting of disciplinary actions made by state medical licensure boards to the Secretary of DHHS, with the latter being responsible for disseminating information on these actions to state boards and to other state and federal officials. It did not, however, mandate that PROs report their disciplinary actions to state boards.

Regulations

Apart from legislative acts, numerous regulations and other directives govern the administration and operation of PROs. The Administrative Procedure Act (APA) requires that regulations be promulgated through notice and comment rulemaking procedures. HCFA considers the APA procedures to apply to some but not all of its directives and publishes in the *Federal Register* those procedures for which it seeks public comment. As an alternative or adjunct to the rather cumbersome regulatory rulemaking mechanism, HCFA also relies extensively on PRO *Manual* transmittals, contracts and contract modifications (and their Scopes of Work), and other, less formal instructions.

Administration

HCFA's Health Standards and Quality Bureau (HSQB) administers the PRO program. HSQB functions are carried out in both the Central Office (CO) and in the 10 HCFA Regional Offices (ROs). CO staff establish policies for the program, perform a great deal of data analysis, negotiate PRO contracts (with help from RO staff), and set evaluation criteria. RO staff have appreciable involvement in PRO activities. They transmit program requirements to PROs, oversee implementation of those requirements, evaluate, and generally provide oversight and technical assistance. Some of HCFA's guidance for the PRO program is promulgated in this way; thus, inconsistencies among the ROs in interpreting HCFA policies and guidelines can pose a considerable problem for the program (OIG, 1989).

PRO ORGANIZATIONAL CHARACTERISTICS

In organizing the PRO program, one change from the earlier PSRO program was to consolidate the many PSRO regions into 54 PROs (all the states, the District of Columbia, Puerto Rico, the Virgin Islands, and a combined area of American Samoa, Guam, and the Commonwealth of the Marianas). In a legislative attempt to retain some semblance of "local peer review," Congress specified that, to qualify as a PRO, a statewide organization must either demonstrate sponsorship by being composed of at least 10 percent of the physicians practicing in the area (physician-sponsored organizations) or have at least one physician in every generally recognized specialty in the area available for PRO review (physician-access organizations). Third-party payers can obtain PRO contracts if no other eligible organization is available; at the time of this study only one such organization had a PRO contract.

A PRO may not be a health care facility or other entity subject to review. This avoids financial conflicts of interest with providers that may be the subject of review. The contractor must have at least one consumer representative on its governing board and must operate with objectivity and without apparent or real conflict of interest.

PRO CONTRACTS

Unlike their PSRO predecessors, PROs are financed by contracts, not grants. In principle, contracts make the program more manageable centrally and more consistent nationally, because the contracting agency can specify in great detail precisely what it expects its contractors to do and can then evaluate them on how well they meet those contract specifications. PROs carry out a very complex set of review and intervention tasks that are specified in minute detail in their HCFA contracts. The contracting procedure is based on a formal Request for Proposal (RFP), which includes a "scope of work" (SOW) that becomes part of the contract between the government and the PRO.

PROs began with 2-year contracts, and an effort was made to have all PROs start more or less at the same time. This proved very difficult to implement. (The first contracts became effective over a 5-month phase-in period from July to November 1984 that corresponded to the implementation of Medicare's PPS.) Therefore, OBRA 1987 extended contract periods to 3 years, to permit somewhat more stability in anticipated financing and planning. Timing of PRO contract periods is now staggered so that HCFA does not have to negotiate 54 contracts simultaneously.

Contracts can be renewed triennially or canceled and put up for competitive bidding if the existing PRO is judged not to qualify for a noncompetitive renewal. In some cases these contracts have been won by the original PRO because no competition emerged or because the bidding process galvanized the existing PRO into a credible renewal effort.

PRO contracts may be terminated by either the PRO or the secretary of DHHS. The secretary may terminate or choose not to renew a PRO contract when officials determine that the PRO has not met or is not meeting its obligations in a satisfactory manner. A complex set of procedures is specified by which termination or nonrenewal can be accomplished. The secretary's decisions in this regard are not subject to judicial review, and the secretary has the absolute right to terminate a contract (rightfully or wrongfully) without the possibility of the decision being overturned later in court.

In addition to contracts between the PRO and DHHS, PROs must maintain written agreements with hospitals and with FIs and carriers. In hospital agreements, PROs must include their review plans, criteria, and procedures (including frequency of reviews, documentation to be required of the hospital, and time and location of reviews). The review process must be consistent with the requirements placed on PROs in their own contracts with HCFA, and the PRO-hospital agreements must be coterminous with PRO-HCFA contracts. The agreements may be revised as needed to conform with changes in statutes, regulations, and HCFA policies and directives for the PRO program, meaning that changes to the PRO program can directly and materially affect the hospital industry.

PROs must also enter into agreements with the FIs serving providers in their areas. These agreements specify procedures to coordinate review activities of the respective organizations. PROs are responsible for establishing procedures to collect and process data in order to assure that they are complete, accurate, and promptly reported. FIs must provide internally consistent and prompt data each month so that PROs can conduct timely reviews, and they are responsible for both the internal consistency and promptness in delivery of the information that they are required to produce. PROs are not permitted to collect or have collected for them any information that duplicates information that FIs are responsible for, although the PROs can negotiate to purchase data not currently collected by FIs.

These relationships among PROs, hospitals, and FIs emphasize communication and data sharing. PROs must determine the accuracy of information that hospitals provide to their FIs, and PROs and FIs must establish a system of data sharing that permits PROs to inform FIs of data lacunae and inaccuracies and then obtain completed and corrected information. After completing their various reviews, PROs must also report to both hospitals and FIs any claims that require payment adjustments.

PRO SCOPES OF WORK

The SOW details the specific obligations of the PRO that will be incorporated into its contract. It defines the duties and functions of the Medicare review for a specific contract cycle. The first SOW was used during the first contract cycle (1984–1986); the second during the 1986-1988 contract cycle; and the third covers the present period. No new SOWs are contemplated. To reinforce the sense of stability and common expectations for the program, all future changes will be made through a contract modification process. All PROs will be expected to implement changes at the same time. If HCFA considers the contract modification to be significant, the agency will publish it in the *Federal Register* 30 days in advance of its intended start date. In the event that the contract modification requires more funding, PROs and HCFA will have to agree on the additional level of support before the PROs begin the work.

Although most PRO activities have remained fairly constant over the three SOWs, some tasks have changed dramatically. For example, the first SOW emphasized controlling inappropriate utilization, whereas the second and third SOWs direct more attention to assuring quality. The second and third SOWs remained fairly similar as a result of efforts to achieve consistency with minimum disruption to ongoing review activities; much of the second SOW remains in the third, but with variations in the size of samples.[2] All three SOWs are described in the following sections, but the third SOW is described in greater detail because it is the current guide for PRO work. Table 8.1 outlines the main activities of the third SOW, and Table 8.2 compares the three SOWs on certain key review and other requirements.

TABLE 8.1 Elements of Required Peer Review Organization (PRO) Activities for the Third Scope of Work

I. Prospective Payment System (PPS) Hospital Cases[a]
   A. Random (the 3-percent sample)
   B. Transfers
      1. PPS to PPS hospitals
      2. PPS to exempt psychiatric units
      3. PPS to exempt swing beds
   C. Readmissions in less than 31 days from discharge from a PPS hospital with review of intervening care
      1. PPS hospital readmission
         a. Identifying all readmissions
         b. Review a random 25-percent hospital-specific sample
      2. Intervening care
         a. Identify all cases in the 25-percent sample with care rendered by skilled nursing facilities, home health agencies, or hospital outpatient departments
         b. Review a 20-percent sample of each hospital's intervening care universe for quality of care (not medical necessity or overuse of services), with HCFA's generic quality screens
   D. Focused DRGs (100 percent review of DRGs 385–391, 472, 474, 475; 50 percent review of DRG 468; 25 percent review of DRG 462)[b]
   E. Day and cost outliers (25 percent random samples)
   F. Medicare code editor (12 principal diagnoses)[c]
   G. Hospital adjustments (any adjustments to higher weighted DRGs)
   H. Noncovered admissions (with covered level of care later in stay)
   I. FI and HCFA regional office referrals

II. Specialty Hospitals
   A. Exempt units of PPS hospitals
   B. Exempt hospitals

III. Ambulatory Surgery [Hospital Outpatient Areas and Ambulatory Surgical Centers (ASCs)]

IV. Intensified Review

V. Pre-admission and Pre-procedure reviews
   A. Ten procedures[d]
   B. Assistants at cataract surgery

VI. Review of Freestanding Cardiac Catheterization Facilities

VII. Objectives (e.g., based on Generic Quality Screens)

VIII. Development and Use of Explicit Written Criteria

TABLE 8.1 continues

TABLE 8.1 Continued

    IX. Reconsideration and Review of DRG Changes and Preparing Appeals Folders

    X. Data
- A. Reports submitted to HCFA on completed reviews
- B. Profiling
  1. Hospital statistics (by 14 variables)
  2. Physician statistics (by 4 variables)
  3. Other provider statistics (HHA, SNFs, ASCs)
  4. Internal quality control (monitoring of review decisions)

    XI. Beneficiary Communications
- A. *Important Message to Medicare Beneficiaries* (from hospitals)
- B. Hospital notices of noncoverage
- C. Community outreach
  1. Hotline
  2. Written inquiries responses
  3. Education programs, seminars, and workshops
  4. Informational materials
  5. Coordination with beneficiary groups

    XII. Responsiveness to Inquiries and Complaints

    XIII. Interaction with Physicians and Providers
- A. Peer review
- B. Opportunity for consultation
- C. Education
- D. Criteria development and dissemination
- E. Communications
- F. Confidentiality and disclosure guidelines
- G. External relationships with concerned organizations
- H. Management responsibilities

    XIV. Sanctions

    XV. Confidentiality and Disclosure of Information

    XVI. Fraud and Abuse Review (of Cases referred by OIG or HCFA)

    XVII. Anti-Dumping Review (of Cases referred by HCFA)

    XVIII. Private Review

    XIX. Civilian Health and Medical Programs of the Uniformed Services (CHAMPUS)

    XX. Other Requirements
- A. Cooperation with HCFA
- B. Cooperation with the SuperPRO
- C. Private review
- D. Internal quality control

[a]The required review activities include: generic quality screens, discharge review, admission review, invasive procedure review, DRG validation, coverage review, and waiver of liability.

[b]The DRG categories are as follows: 385, neonates, died or transferred; 386, extreme immaturity, neonates; 387, prematurity with major problems; 388, prematurity without major problems; 389, full-term neonate with major problems; 390, neonate with other significant problems; 391, normal newborn; 462, rehabilitation; 468, unrelated operating room procedures; 472, extensive burns; 474, tracheostomy; and 475, mechanical ventilation through endotracheal intubation.

[c]Diabetes mellitus, without mention of complication; noninsulin dependent and insulin dependent; obesity; impacted cerumen; benign hypertension; left bundle branch hemiblock; other bundle branch hemiblock; positive SRL/VRL HL3; elevated blood pressure reading without diagnosis of hypertension; other and unspecified complications of medical care, not elsewhere specified; and cardiac pacemaker (fitting and adjustment).

[d]Carotid endarterectomy and cataract procedures are required. Eight of the following 11 can also be selected: cholecystectomy, major joint replacement, coronary artery bypass graft, percutaneous transluminal coronary angioplasty, laminectomy, complex peripheral revascularization, hysterectomy, bunionectomy, inguinal hernia repair, prostatectomy, and pacemaker insertion.

SOURCE: Attachment 33, HCFA, 1988.

FIRST PRO SCOPE OF WORK (1984–1986 CONTRACT CYCLE)

The first PRO contracts emphasized the detection of inappropriate utilization and payments under the new Medicare hospital PPS after October 1983. Contract activities, which concentrated on inpatient hospital care, included reducing unnecessary admissions, ensuring that payment rates matched diagnostic and procedural information contained in the patient records, and reviewing patients who were transferred or readmitted to an acute care hospital within 7 days of discharge. In addition, HCFA negotiated five generic "quality objectives" for each PRO: (1) reduce unnecessary hospital readmissions resulting from substandard care provided during the prior admissions; (2) assure the provision of medical services which, when not performed, have significant potential for causing serious patient complications; (3) reduce the risk of mortality associated with selected procedures and/or conditions requiring hospitalization (initially denoted "reduce avoidable death"); (4) reduce unnecessary surgery or other invasive procedures; and (5) reduce avoidable postoperative or other complications.

Corrective actions for physicians or hospitals included education and consultation, intensified review, and denial of payment for inappropriate or unnecessary admissions or readmissions. During the first SOW, PROs were

TABLE 8.2 Comparison of the Three Scopes of Work (SOWs) with Respect to Selected Utilization and Quality Control Peer Review Organization (PRO) Activities (Ordered by Tasks Pertaining to the Third SOW)[a]

I.   Prospective Payment System Hospitals Cases

Random Samples
    First SOW: 5-percent admission sample. DRG sample ranging from 3 to 100 percent based on hospital discharge size
    Second SOW: 3-percent sample (includes 1- and 2-day stays)
    Third SOW: Same as second SOW
Transfers
    First SOW: From PPS to another hospital, exempt unit, or swing bed
    Second SOW: Same as first SOW, but lower level of review
    Third SOW: PPS to PPS, 50-percent sample; PPS to psychiatric, 10 percent; and PPS to swing bed, 25 percent
Readmissions
    First SOW: All related readmissions within 7 days of discharge
    Second SOW: All related readmissions within 15 days of discharge
    Third SOW: 25 percent of readmissions within 31 days of discharge
Intervening Care
    First SOW: Not in scope of work
    Second SOW: Not in scope of work
    Third SOW: 20 percent of all cases receiving home health agency, hospital outpatient, inpatient, or skilled nursing facility (SNF) care between sampled hospital admissions less than 31 days apart
Focused DRGs
    First SOW: Review of DRG numbers 462 and 468
    Second SOW: Review of DRG numbers 462, 468, and 088
    Third SOW: Review of DRG numbers 462, 468, 385–391, 472, and 474–475[b]
Day and Cost Outliers
    First SOW: Originally 100 percent; reduced to 50 percent during contract period
    Second SOW: 50 percent of day and cost outliers
    Third SOW: 25 percent of day and cost outliers
Medicare Code Editor
    First SOW: 100 percent of 9 diagnoses with code editor rejects
    Second SOW: Same as first SOW
    Third SOW: 100 percent of 12 diagnoses with code editor rejects[c]
Hospital Adjustments
    First SOW: 100 percent of all cases adjusted to a higher-weighted DRG
    Second SOW: Same as first SOW
    Third SOW: Same as second SOW
FI and HCFA Regional Office Referrals
    First SOW: 100 percent review of cases referred by FI or HCFA regional office for determination of medical necessity
    Second SOW: Same as first SOW
    Third SOW: Same as second SOW

II.   Specialty Hospital Review
      First SOW: Proposed by each PRO
      Second SOW: 15 percent of all discharges
      Third SOW: 15-percent random sample for PPS-exempt hospitals and units
III. Ambulatory Surgery
      First SOW: Not in scope of work
      Second SOW: Not in scope of work
      Third SOW: 5-percent random sample of all cases
IV.   Intensified Review
      First SOW: Trigger; 2.5 percent or 3 cases reviewed (whichever is greater).
      Review increased to 100 percent or subsets.
      Second SOW: Trigger; 5 percent or 6 cases reviewed (whichever is greater).
      Review increased to 100 percent or subsets (two consecutive quarters)
      Third SOW: Same as second SOW
V.   Preadmission Review
      First SOW: 5 procedures proposed by each PRO
      Second SOW: Pacemaker plus 4 procedures proposed by the PRO
      Third SOW: 100 percent of 10 procedures (cataract extraction, cartoid
      endarterectomy plus 8 of 11 others specified by HCFA)[d]
VI.   Assistants at Cataract Surgery
      First SOW: Not in scope of work
      Second SOW: 100 percent review of cases for medical necessity of assistant
      at surgery
      Third SOW: Same as second SOW
VII. Objectives
      First SOW: Three admission objectives and five quality objectives. All
      proposed and validated by the PRO. Very limited areas for focusing
      objectives
      Second SOW: Five objectives based on PRO data from first 90 days of
      generic quality screen review. HCFA-identified mortality rate outliers
      Third SOW: Objectives based on data from generic screens. May be
      statewide, or focused by physician, DRG, provider, etc.
XI.   Hospital Notices of Noncoverage
      First SOW: 100 percent where patient or physician disagrees; 100 percent
      where patient is liable; 10-percent random sample
      Second SOW: Same as first SOW
      Third SOW: 100 percent where patient or physician disagrees; 100 percent
      where patient is liable
      Community Outreach
      First SOW: Not in scope of work
      Second SOW: Each PRO to propose its own program
      Third SOW: Minimum requirements to be met

---

[a]Roman numerals refer to parts in Table 8.1.
[b]For definitions, see Table 8.1.
[c]For definitions, see Table 8.1.
[d]For listing, see Table 8.1.

SOURCE: Adapted from unpublished HCFA documents.

authorized to recommend sanction of providers or physicians to the OIG in one of two instances: (1) cases of a "substantial violation [of their Medicare obligations] in a substantial number of cases"[3] and (2) single cases of a "gross and flagrant" violation.[4] These categories of sanctionable problems continue to the present. The sanction process per se, however, has become more complex in response to legal and political challenges.

SECOND PRO SCOPE OF WORK (1986–1988 CONTRACT CYCLE)

During the 1986–1988 SOW, eight PROs reviewed two areas and one reviewed three. The following PROs conducted reviews in two states: West Virginia for Delaware; Maryland for the District of Columbia; Hawaii for Guam–American Samoa; Indiana for Kentucky; Rhode Island for Maine; Iowa for Nebraska; New Hampshire for Vermont; and Montana for Wyoming. The PRO for Washington State also reviewed Alaska and Idaho (OIG, 1988b).

New or Expanded Responsibilities

The second SOW emphasized quality review in addition to the detection of inappropriate utilization. This SOW lowered the level of review for hospitals with acceptable performance and increased it for hospitals with unacceptable performance. Contract goals were developed as guidelines for focusing quality review activities; these objectives were based on actual results of the first 90 days of review using generic ("occurrence") screens that were applied to a 3-percent random sample of medical records.

Other new areas of activity in the second SOW included the following: reporting the results of review of short hospital stays in the routine sample; review of related readmissions to the same hospital within 15 days (up from 7 days in the first SOW); retrospective review of all sampled cases to assess the appropriateness of the discharge; review of hospitals that were high-mortality rate outliers in the first release of HCFA mortality rate data; an emphasis on statistically identifiable adverse outcomes such as premature discharge and death; and development of a community outreach program.

Generic Quality Screens

Hospital generic quality screens were the most visible addition to the second SOW (see Table 8.3). Generic screens are widely used to detect what are regarded as the most common causes or manifestations of quality problems, and were adopted for use in the PRO program for all charts under review by the PRO for any reason. HCFA introduced them in the fall of 1986 without pilot-testing and issued interpretative guidelines in May of 1987. PROs were also permitted to develop their own screens to cover "adverse occurrences" that may reflect regional variations in practice patterns (and some PROs did), but locally devised screens could not change the intent of the federal screens.

Generic quality screens are applied by nurse reviewers. They can either determine that no screen has been failed (or that a screen has been failed but that no potential quality problem exists) or refer the case to a physician advisor for further evaluation. Initially, nurse reviewers had to refer all screen failures to physician advisors; this produced considerable numbers of false-positive cases and appreciable frustration and anger for reviewers and the medical community. HCFA later permitted PRO nurse reviewers to use their professional judgment in not forwarding some screen failures for physician review. Only the physician advisor can "confirm" a quality problem.

The six required generic quality screens for the second SOW are as follows (see Table 8.3 for details and subitems):

1. adequacy of discharge planning
2. medical stability of patient at discharge
3. unexpected deaths
4. nosocomial infections
5. unscheduled return to surgery
6. trauma suffered in hospital

THIRD PRO SCOPE OF WORK (1988–1990 CONTRACT CYCLE)

The third SOW incorporates provisions from COBRA, OBRA 1986, and OBRA 1987. Phase-in of the third SOW took place over several months; all PROs were expected to be on the third SOW as of April 1, 1989. In making the shift to 3-year contracts, HCFA put PROs into one of four categories. Two of those categories (28 states in all) were to be awarded full 3-year contracts; the remaining categories (26 states and territories) were to be awarded either 6- or 12-month extensions before negotiation of their 3-year contracts. As of summer 1989, however, four PRO contracts had not been awarded.

Table 8.1 outlines the major required activities for care rendered in the fee-for-service (FFS) system, and some are described in more detail below. The focus is on inpatient hospital review, but the activities do not differ appreciably for nonhospital practitioners or settings.

Required Review Activities for Hospital Inpatient Care

The required PRO review activities for all inpatient hospital cases reviewed are (1) generic quality screening, (2) discharge review, (3) admission review, (4) invasive procedure review, (5) DRG validation, (6) coverage

TABLE 8.3 Generic Quality Screens—Hospital Inpatient

1. Adequacy of Discharge Planning[a]

No documentation of discharge planning or appropriate followup care with consideration of physical, emotional and mental status needs at time of discharge.

2. Medical Stability of the Patient at Discharge

    a. Blood Pressure within 24 hours of discharge (systolic less than 85 or greater than 180; diastolic less than 50 or greater than 100)

    b. Temperature within 24 hours of discharge greater than 101 degrees Fahrenheit (38.3 Centigrade) oral, greater than 102 degrees Fahrenheit (38.9 Centigrade) rectal

    c. Pulse less than 50 (or 45 if the patient is on a beta blocker), or greater than 120 within 24 hours of discharge

    d. Abnormal diagnostic findings which are not addressed and resolved or where the record does not explain why they are not resolved

    e. Intravenous fluids or drugs after 12 midnight on day of discharge

    f. Purulent or bloody drainage of wound or open area within 24 hours prior to discharge

3. Deaths

    a. During or following any surgery performed during the current admission

    b. Following return to intensive care unit, coronary care or other special care unit within 24 hours of being transferred out

    c. Other unexpected death

4. Nosocomial Infection[a] (Hospital-acquired infection)

5. Unscheduled Return to Surgery

    Within same admission for same condition as previous surgery or to correct operative problem

6. Trauma Suffered in the Hospital

    a. Unplanned surgery which includes, but is not limited to, removal or repair of a normal organ or body part (i.e., surgery not addressed specifically in the operative consent)

    b. Fall[a]

    c. Serious complications of anesthesia

    d. Any transfusion error or serious transfusion reaction

    e. Hospital-acquired decubitus ulcer and/or deterioration of an existing decubitus[a]

f. Medication error or adverse drug reaction (1) with serious potential for harm or (2) resulting in measures to correct

g. Care or lack of care resulting in serious or potentially serious complications

"Optional Screen"

Medication or treatment changes (including discontinuation) within 24 hours of discharge without adequate observation

[a]Peer review organization (PRO) reviewer is to record the failure of the screen, but need not refer potential severity Level I quality problems to physician reviewer until a pattern emerges.

SOURCE: HCFA, 1988.

review, and (7) determination of the application of the waiver of liability provision. These are described in more detail below.

The cases selected for review through the 3-percent random sampling process plus cases under review for other reasons constitute almost 25 percent of all Medicare admissions. A cumulative data summary of PRO activity to the end of February 1989 gives the following national figures for combined retrospective review and pre-admission and prepayment review: of a universe of bills and cases numbering 26,747,451, a total of 6,407,967 were selected for review (24 percent); 6,993,179 were reviewed (26 percent).[5] The estimated number of reviews for the third SOW totals 10,541,730, including 7,600,006 hospital reviews, 877,739 HMO and CMP reviews, and 2,063,985 ambulatory surgery reviews (HCFA, 1989b); the estimates are reached partly by projecting expected Medicare admissions in the many different categories and applying the review sampling percentages to those projections.

Generic Screens

In addition to the six generic screens from the second SOW, PROs can use an optional screen for medication or treatment changes (including discontinuation) within 24 hours of discharge without adequate observation. The third SOW has also added an adequacy-of-care screen to the set of "trauma" screens to cover inappropriate or untimely assessment, intervention, or management resulting in serious or potentially serious complications. As before, these are applied to every case under PRO review for whatever reason. Figures 8.1a and 8.1b illustrate the full process.

With respect to generic screens, most of the major changes (from scope to scope) occur in the interpretive guidelines for the screens rather than in

FIGURE 8.1a Overview of the Quality Review Process for Inpatient Hospital, Home Health Agency, and Outpatient Surgery Generic Screens[a]

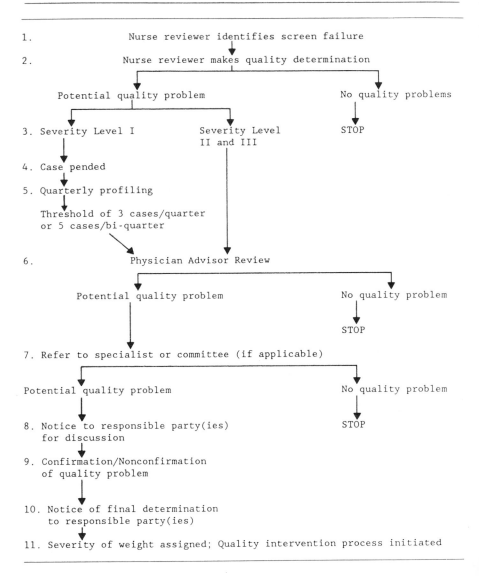

[a]Includes inpatient hospital screens 1, 4, 6b, and 6e and certain home health agency and outpatient surgery screens.

SOURCE: HCFA, 1989a.

FIGURE 8.1b Overview of the Quality Review Process for Other Generic Screens[a]

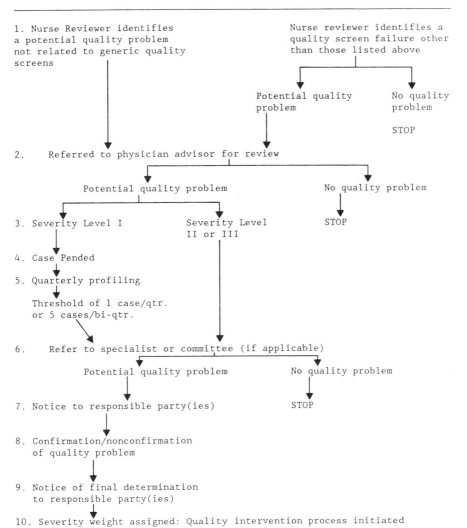

[a]Includes inpatient hospital, home health agency, and outpatient surgery generic screens not covered by the process in Figure 8.1a.

SOURCE: HCFA, 1989a.

the screens themselves.[6] Prompted by the finding that screens were not being uniformly applied across the country, starting in the fall of 1987 HCFA held a series of consensus-building meetings to discuss the use of inpatient hospital screens. The groups consisted of PRO medical staff, RO medical staff, and CO representatives. From this series of local meetings, two representatives from each meeting were asked to participate in a national task force. That group revised the screens, especially by adding clarifying guidelines, to bring more consistent definitions to the application of the screens. These refined screens were implemented in October 1988.

Other Required Review Activities

Discharge review identifies potential problems with premature discharge of two types: (1) the patient was not medically stable at discharge or (2) discharge was not consistent with the patient's continued need for acute inpatient care. This task relates in part to concerns about possible unintended consequences of DRG-based PPS.

Retrospective *admission review* identifies whether inpatient hospital care was medically necessary and appropriate; it involves reviewing reasons for admission against pre-established criteria devised or adopted by individual PROs and subjective physician review. Admission review in particular is a traditional utilization review effort that can be traced back to PSRO days and beyond. As a PRO requirement, it relates to concerns that PPS incentives would also induce hospitals to admit patients who were not sick enough to warrant hospitalization (i.e., for whom a full DRG payment would be made but who would require far less in hospital costs).

Invasive procedure review retrospectively examines the medical necessity of invasive procedures that affect the assignment of a case to one DRG rather than another (which means virtually all invasive procedures done in the hospital setting). The review is applied to cases already selected for review, not to additional cases. If the procedure is not medically necessary or is noncovered, and if the procedure was the sole reason for admission, then payments for the admission and the procedure are denied. If the procedure is not medically necessary and is noncovered, but other reasonable and necessary services were provided and the admission was medically necessary, then only the physician's payment for the procedure is denied and the DRG is changed.

Throughout the program, the purpose of *DRG validation* has been to assure that Medicare payments under PPS are correct, because it was immediately (and correctly) understood that DRG coding was susceptible to some manipulation and slow upward "creep" to higher-weighted DRGs over time (Simborg, 1981; GAO, 1988a; Hsia et al., 1988). A Registered Record Administrator or an Accredited Record Technician generally has the overall responsibility for the PRO's validation process. The result of DRG validation can be to leave the DRG unchanged or to upgrade or downgrade it, thereby affecting the hospital payment.

This activity also includes review to assure that the requirements for *physician attestation* are met. Physician attestation requires physicians to sign a statement certifying that their narrative descriptions of the principal and secondary diagnoses and the major procedures are accurate and complete to the best of their knowledge. Originally, physicians were expected to sign such a statement for every discharge, but it rapidly became clear that this was a considerable burden and an implicit indictment of physicians; the requirement is now that physicians sign a statement once a year and that hospitals keep that affirmation on file.

Coverage review determines whether items or services normally excluded from Medicare coverage are medically necessary. This review is performed only in instances when coverage can be extended for specific items and circumstances if certain medical conditions are met.

In PSRO days, hospitals and other providers were assumed to have a favorable *"waiver of liability"* status; waiver of liability meant that unless a hospital "knew or could reasonably have been expected to know" that the care it was providing was unnecessary, the costs of that care would still be reimbursed and the hospital was not financially liable. Only if the hospital's waiver was revoked or if the PSRO determined on a case-by-case basis that the provider could have been expected to know that the case was unnecessary would it become financially at risk for days of care or services provided to a beneficiary. Now, under the waiver of liability (also referred to as limitation of liability), the favorable presumptive status has been eliminated, and the PRO must determine whether the beneficiary or provider should be held liable for care not covered under Medicare because either the beneficiary or provider knew, or could reasonably have been expected to know, that such care was not covered.

Other Aspects of Hospital Inpatient Review

In addition to the above required review activities, several other hospital inpatient tasks are now either expanded or required. Each PRO will also be required to publish (at least annually) a report that describes their findings about care that was unnecessary, was inappropriate, was given in an inappropriate setting, or did not meet professionally accepted standards; this report is to be widely distributed to providers and practitioners whose services are subject to review.

Pre-admission and Pre-procedure Review

PROs are also required to review 10 procedures, generally on a pre-admission or pre-procedure basis, for necessity and for appropriateness of

setting (e.g., inpatient or ambulatory). They must review all proposed carotid endarterectomy and cataract procedures. In addition, they must either
pick an additional 8 procedures from a list of 11 supplied by HCFA or
document why a procedure not on the list should be subjected to 100 percent pre-admission review. The 11 conditions are cholecystectomy, major
joint replacement, coronary artery bypass graft, percutaneous transluminal
coronary angioplasty, laminectomy, complex peripheral revascularization,
hysterectomy, bunionectomy, inguinal hernia repair, prostatectomy, and
pacemaker insertion.

PROs establish their own prior-authorization criteria for this purpose,
sometimes in consultation with local or state physician specialty groups,
and some sharing of criteria does take place across PROs. Nevertheless,
PROs differ in the types of clinical factors or levels of patient functioning
that they require to be present (or absent) before they will approve the
procedure.[7]

Rural Providers

Rural providers have vigorously asserted that they are not reviewed by
"local peers" and that their style of practice and the constraints under which
they function are not well appreciated or taken into account. To respond to
these concerns and bring peer review more fully into areas that were rarely
visited, the third SOW mandates that at least 20 percent of all rural hospitals shall be reviewed on-site.

According to OBRA 1987, rural physicians (namely, those in counties of
70,000 or fewer residents or in officially designated rural health manpower
shortage areas) are also given special protection during the sanctioning
process. Except when the physician or provider is found to pose a "serious
risk" to Medicare enrollees, exclusions are to be put on hold until full
hearings before an Administrative Law Judge (ALJ) have been conducted.
Some effort is being mounted to extend these protections to all physicians
who live in counties of 140,000 or fewer residents, a move that would
effectively extend special appeal rights to about two-thirds of practicing
physicians (Vibbert, 1989d).

Nonhospital Review

Review of Skilled Nursing Facility and Home Health Agency Care:
Intervening Care

PROs have been directed to undertake review in several nonhospital settings. By and large, this review has not been very comprehensive. The
main effort to date has been in response to OBRA 1986 requirements for

PROs to assess the adequacy of post-acute care. PROs are expected to review a small sample of cases receiving "intervening care," mainly care delivered by home health agencies (HHAs) and skilled nursing facilities (SNFs) between two related hospital admissions up to 31 days apart. (Care rendered in hospital outpatient areas, or HOPAs, is also included.)

This effort had minimal pilot project pre-testing. Pilot studies in Massachusetts and Pennsylvania were conducted from mid-1987 and mid-1988, respectively. These efforts did not yield much in the way of quality deficiencies. By definition, this task does not cover the great bulk of post-acute care, because it focuses only on the interval between hospital admissions.

With respect to SNF review, little is being done in the PRO program, but some experience has been gained in this area. PSROs reviewed care provided in long-term-care facilities; at the peak, about 55 PSRO projects were under way in such facilities. A special effort assessed 10 PSRO demonstration projects in long-term-care review. The assessment included pre-admission, admission, and continued-stay review; quality assurance activities; Medical Care Evaluation studies (MCEs); and data systems development (Kane et al., 1979). The net conclusion of the evaluators was that the progress made by the 10 demonstrations justified optimism "that the PSRO has potential for affecting the appropriateness of utilization and the quality of nursing home care . . . [and that] it is imperative to preserve the incentive for PSROs to enter the long-term care review field" (Kane et al., 1979, p. vii).

Despite this injunction, PRO attention to this sector of the health care delivery system has been scant, in part because PROs (unlike PSROs) were mandated to review only Medicare (not Medicaid) services. PROs are allowed to contract with state Medicaid agencies to do Medicaid review, and as of mid-1989, 34 PROs had such contracts (H. Brook, personal communication, 1989). However, this does not represent a systematic federal effort by PROs to review the care of nursing home residents.

Review in Other Fee-for-Service Settings

Initiatives in the other settings, especially ambulatory physician office care, are getting under way mainly as pilot projects. Plans for these projects are described later.

Nonhospital Generic Screens

For the third SOW, generic quality screens have been developed to review care rendered in the following settings: (1) HHAs; (2) SNFs; (3) hospital outpatient departments (HOPDs); and (4) ambulatory surgery centers (ASCs) (see Table 8.4). Also under development are screens for reviewing

TABLE 8.4 Nonhospital Generic Screen Categories

Home Health Agencies

1. Adequacy of intake evaluation
2. Appropriate and timely interventions
3. Adequacy of restorative care (specialty therapies and nursing instructions)
4. Deaths within 48 hours of transfer to hospital
5. Possible indications of secondary infections
6. Issues related to patient care after the home health start of care
7. Documentation plan for appropriate follow-up care and discharge summary to physicians of record
8. Any other events or patterns of care resulting in adverse outcomes that should be evaluated

Skilled Nursing Facilities

1. Appropriateness of hospital discharge to SNF and appropriateness of admission to and continued stay in that SNF
2. Appropriate notification, response, and further evaluation within specified time frames (e.g., 4 hours to 24 hours) for a series of problems (e.g., medications, vital signs, fall, infection, hydration and nutrition, mobility, pressure sores, etc.)
3. Abnormal results of diagnostic services addressed, resolved, or explained
4. Assessment, plan of care, evaluation, and discharge plan for appropriate disciplines
5. Deaths following transfer to hospital
6. Any other events or patterns of care resulting in adverse outcomes that should be evaluated

Hospital Outpatient Departments

1. Intake assessment
2. Appropriate and timely interventions
3. Specialty therapies
4. Patient teaching
5. Death within 48 hours of admission to hospital
6. Issues related to provision of patient care
7. Documented plan for appropriate follow-up care or discharge
8. Any other events or patterns of care resulting in adverse outcomes that should be evaluated

Outpatient Surgery

1. Adequate pre-operative assessment
2. Appropriate and timely interventions during surgery for significant and sustained problems
3. Issues relating to post-operative care
4. Appropriate documented discharge plan with provision for follow-up care
5. Adequate patient education

SOURCE: Attachments, HCFA, 1988.

psychiatric care and rehabilitative services; the psychiatric screens were issued to all PROs in November 1989 and the rehabilitation screens are scheduled to be completed in fiscal year (FY) 1990.

The new screens are similar to inpatient generic screens, but they are supposed to be more relevant to the particular setting. For example, the SNF screens deal with polypharmacy (multiple medication) issues and the mental stability of the patient. Although the original set of generic screens was developed by the contractor for SuperPRO (SysteMetrics, Inc.) in conjunction with HCFA, providers were heavily involved in development of the new screens for use in nonhospital settings.

RESPONSES TO QUALITY OR UTILIZATION PROBLEMS: NOTIFICATIONS, CORRECTIVE ACTIONS, AND SANCTIONS

PROs can pursue several possible interventions when they have confirmed a quality or utilization problem. They can notify practitioners or providers of problems, put them on "intensified" review, require a wide variety of corrective actions, or institute sanction procedures. These responses to problems are described in connection with the quality intervention plan required by the third SOW, but they have been available since the start of the PRO program.

Quality Intervention Plan

The quality intervention plan (QIP) is "a prescribed blueprint which requires PROs to implement specific interventions in response to confirmed quality problems" (*Federal Register*, 1989, p. 1966). The QIP is new to the third SOW, was developed in an effort to achieve consistency among PROs, and is based on minimum requirements set by HCFA. It includes determination of the source of the problem; assignment of "severity levels" and weights to quality problems; establishment of a time frame for completion of the review process; profiling; and quality interventions that are related to severity levels.

Determination of the Source of the Problem

All initial case reviews are completed by a nurse reviewer. If a nurse reviewer identifies a potential quality problem, then a physician advisor reviews the case. The nurse reviewer can determine that a potential quality problem *does not* exist, but only a physician advisor can determine that a quality problem *does* exist. After the PRO decides a quality-of-care problem exists, it determines the source of the problem, such as an individual physician or hospital.[8] After an opportunity for discussion, the medical director or the quality assurance committee at the PRO assigns the severity level.

Assignment of Severity Levels and Weights

Severity levels are a way to categorize quality problems. They are assigned according to the nature of the problem and the potential for causing adverse patient outcomes. The relevant phrase, significant adverse effects, is defined as unnecessarily prolonged treatment, complication, readmission, or patient management that results in anatomical or physiological impairment, disability, or death. Weights (numerical points) assigned to severity levels indicate when PROs must take various corrective steps. The levels (with weights in parentheses) and definitions are as follows:

Severity Level I   (1): Medical mismanagement without the potential for significant adverse effects on the patient[9]

Severity Level II   (5): Medical mismanagement with the potential for significant adverse effects on the patient

Severity Level III   (25): Medical mismanagement with significant adverse effects on the patient

Time Frames for Quality Review

HCFA set a maximum time frame for quality review. If a potential Severity Level I problem exists, the case is held in a pending status until a pattern of problems emerges. For Severity Levels II and III, the maximum time frame for completion of the review is 135 days. To be timely, overall review must be completed within the specified periods.

Maximum time frames are as follows. For Severity Levels I to III, receipt of FI data tapes through the initial physician advisor-reviewer determination can take only 60 days. For Severity Levels II and III, there are three stages. Review by specialist or quality committee, if applicable, can take no more than 30 days. If the case has been determined to involve a potential quality problem, notification of the attending physician or provider (or both) and opportunity for discussion can take no more than another 30 days. Finally, confirmation or nonconfirmation of a quality problem and final notification to the attending physician or provider (or both) can take no more than 15 days. The sum (60 + 30 + 30 + 15) is 135 days.

Profiling

The purpose of profiling for the QIP is to identify areas for focused review or other corrective action. The PRO is required to produce a quarterly profile of every physician and provider for every case it reviews. It must also profile (1) potential quality problems with a Severity Level I, by the source of the problem (e.g., provider or physician), to determine whether the threshold levels of 1 case per quarter or 5 cases per 2 quarters (sometimes called a bi-quarter) are reached; (2) a weighted severity level score for confirmed quality problems, by the source of the problem (i.e., provider or physician); and (3) all confirmed quality problems, by source of the problem.

Quality Interventions

When a PRO identifies a quality problem resulting from case mismanagement, then the PRO develops a corrective action plan using a variety of interventions. The six types of interventions listed below must be included in its contract review plan, but the PRO may add more.

1. *Notification.* The notice of the final determination must include a description of the confirmed quality problem, what the appropriate action should have been, the severity level, and what interventions will be taken.

2. *Educational efforts.* These include telephone and/or in-person discussions with the responsible parties, suggested literature reading, continuing medical education (CME) courses, and self-education courses.

3. *Intensification* of review through 100 percent retrospective review of all cases or intensified review of a focused subsample.

4. *Other interventions* include concurrent or pre-discharge review; prior approval or pre-admission review; and referral to hospital committees (e.g., infection control, tissue, quality assurance committees).

5. *Coordination with licensing and accreditation bodies.* The PRO must disclose confidential information to state and federal licensing bodies upon request when such information is required by those entities to carry out their legal functions, and the PRO may do so even without a request (e.g., when a practitioner or provider has reached a weighted score of 25 points in 1 quarter).

6. *Sanction* plans (discussed below).

The PRO must use certain thresholds, called weighted triggers, to decide what intervention it should use. The threshold points are as follows:

1. Notification	1 per quarter or 5 per bi-quarter
2. Education	10
3. Intensification	15
4. Other interventions	20
5. Consideration of coordination with licensing bodies	25
6. Consideration of sanctions	25

When cases have multiple problems in more than one severity level, the PRO uses the highest severity level and weighted trigger. These scores are computed at least quarterly for each problem source (e.g., physician or hospital); they are simply sums of the total points of Severity Levels I, II, and III given earlier. For instance, three Level II problems would produce a total score of 15; three Level II plus six Level I problems would produce a total score of 21. The SOW allows the PRO some flexibility to take interventions before a trigger (e.g., a severity score of 25) is reached or to apply lower weighted interventions in special circumstances. For the last two interventions (coordination and sanctions), the PRO must consider but need not invoke them as long as it documents why it did not.

Sanctions and Other Interventions

The Secretary of DHHS, not the PROs, holds the authority to impose sanctions on Medicare providers, and the secretary has delegated that authority to the Office of Inspector General (OIG). The PROs' power lies in making sanction recommendations to the OIG. Figures 8.2a and 8.2b diagram this process.

PRO Responsibilities

The PRO recommends sanctions in either of two instances: (1) cases of "substantial violation" of a provider's Medicare obligations "in a substantial number of cases" and (2) a single case of a "gross and flagrant" violation. If a PRO recommends exclusion, and the OIG does not act on that recommendation within 120 days, the exclusion automatically goes into effect until a final determination is made.

No regulations define the criteria to be used by a PRO in determining whether a practitioner or provider has violated a Medicare obligation. The preamble to the PRO regulations states only that PROs must apply professionally developed standards of care, diagnosis, and treatment based on typical patterns of practice in their geographic areas (*Federal Register*, 1985). The PRO *Manual* also contains some material on the elements of a sanctionable offense.

For cases in which the PRO determines that the provider or physician has failed to comply substantially with a Medicare obligation in a substantial number of cases, it sends the practitioner or provider an initial sanction notice.[10] This notice gives the recipient 20 days to respond to the notification with additional information or to request a meeting with the PRO. If, after considering the additional information, the PRO confirms its original finding, it develops a corrective plan of action. If the practitioner or provider fails to comply with that plan, the PRO sends a second sanction notice. In such cases, the provider or practitioner has a second opportunity to submit additional information or discuss the problem with the PRO (within 30 days of the second notice).

If the concern is not resolved, the procedures at this point follow the pattern for gross and flagrant violations. Several specific procedures direct how the PRO should forward its recommendation to the OIG and how it should notify the individual or organization that is has done so, what the recommended sanction is, and how further information can be forwarded directly to the OIG (again within 30 days). The PRO must also give the practitioner or provider a copy of the material it used in reaching its decision. At this point, the responsible sanctioning party is the OIG, not the PRO.

OIG Responsibilities

The OIG must determine whether the PRO followed appropriate procedures, whether a violation occurred, whether the provider has "demonstrated an unwillingness or lack of ability substantially to comply with statutory obligations" (known as the "willing and able" provision), and ultimately whether it agrees with the PRO recommendation (OIG, 1988b). In these determinations, the OIG is expected to consider the type and severity of the offense, the previous sanction record, prior problems that Medicare may have had with the individual or institution, and the availability of alternative medical resources in the community. In response to the PRO recommendation, the OIG can sustain the finding, alter the recommendation, or reject it. (See OIG, 1988b for a more complete description of this process.)

If the OIG does not accept the PRO's recommendation, the sanctioning process stops. If the OIG does accept the PRO's recommendation, it must give notice that the sanction is to be imposed, effective 15 days after the notice is received by the practitioner or provider. The OIG notifies the public by placing a notice in a newspaper of general circulation in the individual's or institution's locality.[11] It also informs state Medicaid fraud control units and state licensing bodies, hospitals and other facilities where the practitioner has privileges, medical societies, carriers, FIs, and HMOs.

DHHS Responsibilities

The sanctioned provider or physician may appeal the OIG decision to an ALJ, who conducts a separate hearing starting essentially from scratch. The sanctioned individual or institution may call witnesses to testify under oath, cross-examine witnesses, submit documents and briefs, and present oral arguments. If practitioners or providers are not satisfied with the outcome of their hearing, they can request review by DHHS's Appeals Council

FIGURE 8.2a Overview of PRO/HHS Sanction Process for Substantial Violations[a]

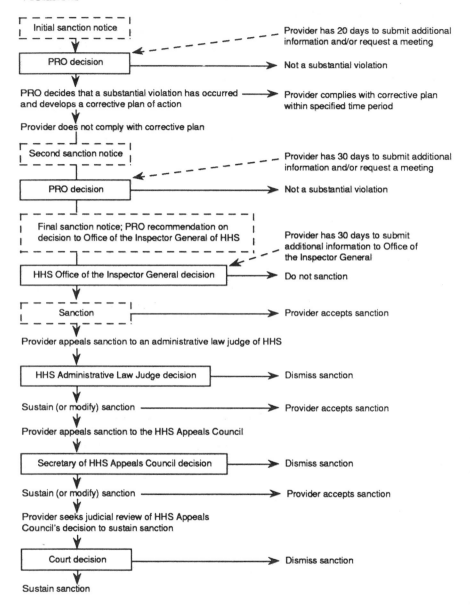

[a]A substantial violation is a pattern of care over a substantial number of cases that is inappropriate, unnecessary, does not meet recognized patterns of care, or is not supported by the documentation of care required by the PRO.

SOURCE: Adapted with permission from OTA, 1988.

FIGURE 8.2b Overview of PRO/HHS Sanction Process for Flagrant Violations[a]

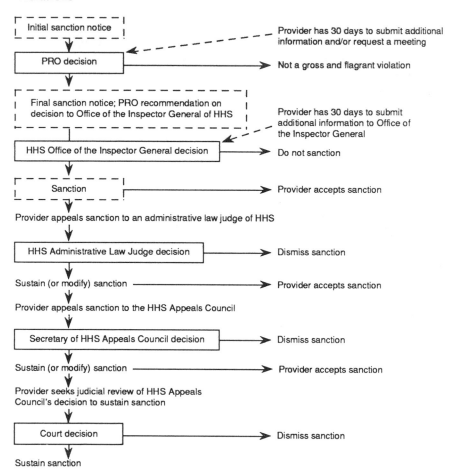

[a]A flagrant violation is a violation that has occurred in one or more instances and presents an imminent danger to the health, safety, or well-being of a Medicare beneficiary.

SOURCE: Adapted with permission from OTA, 1988.

and then still seek judicial review of the decision at the level of a federal district court.

If the OIG proceeds successfully through these steps, the Secretary of DHHS, through the OIG, can apply two kinds of formal sanctions: (1) exclusion from the Medicare program (which may be multi-year in duration); and (2) monetary sanctions (which at present cannot exceed the cost of the services that were rendered). Successfully sanctioned (i.e., excluded) hospitals and providers must petition to be reinstated in the Medicare program, and they can receive no payment for services rendered or items provided during the exclusion period.[12]

Historical Record of Interventions and Sanctions

The most frequent PRO intervention appears to be the formal letter of notification. By contrast, intensified review, formal education or similar programs, and sanction recommendations are used much less often, although during the second SOW more than 53 percent of hospitals were under intensified review for at least 1 quarter (HCFA, 1989c). PROs differ markedly in the rates at which they invoke various interventions. For instance, GAO (1988b) cites the following two ranges for letters of notification: 0 to 111 letters per 1,000 "new" physicians, and 0 to 396 letters per 1,000 "repeat" physicians.

PRO activity. Tables 8.5, a, b, and c, summarize intervention activity tabulated by HCFA for the second SOW, which is the most recent aggregate information. Of the more than 6.6 million completed reviews (mainly for the second SOW), PROs denied payment in over 4 percent of cases (including partial denials); the range across PROs was 1.2 to 25.5 percent. For about 33 percent of the denials the practitioner or provider requested a reconsideration (range, 0.6 to 69.6 percent). Of those reconsiderations, the denials were reversed in 44 percent of the cases (range, 15.1 percent to 100 percent); that is, the original decision was upheld 56 percent of the time.

Through early 1989, the PROs had identified more than 87,000 physicians with some level of quality problem (Table 8.5b). Over 81,400 of those problems had been resolved, presumably through the more than 70,000 quality interventions carried out (HCFA, 1989c).

HCFA data compiled from the start of the program through June 1989 shows that 43 PROs had sent a total of 1,065 first notices, the vast majority to physicians rather than hospitals (Table 8.5c). For physicians, more notices were for gross and flagrant violations than for substantial violations; the opposite was true for hospitals.

The PROs had also recommended a total of 119 sanctions to the OIG, the vast majority for gross and flagrant violations by physicians. Many of the

TABLE 8.5a Quality Intervention Activities of Peer Review Organizations (PROs) Through June 1989: Reconsiderations

Type of Action	Number	Percent of Completed Reviews	Percent of Denials	Percent of Reconsiderations Requested
Completed reviews	6,655,505			
Payment denials	278,294	4.2		
Reconsiderations requested	91,268	1.4	32.8	
Reconsiderations upheld	51,252	0.8	18.4	56.2

SOURCE: HCFA, 1989b.

TABLE 8.5b Quality Intervention Activities of PROs Through February 1989: Quality Interventions for Physicians

Category	Number of Cases	
	Newly Identified	Repeat cases
Physicians with quality problems	87,075	20,598
Physicians with quality problems resolved	81,440	19,888
Quality interventions taken	70,321	26,871

SOURCE: HCFA, 1989c.

TABLE 8.5c Quality Intervention Activities of PROs Through June 1989: Sanctions

Category of Activity	Number of	
	Physicians	Providers
First notices sent	907	158
Substantial violations	335	109
Gross and flagrant violations	572	49
Second notices sent[a]	68	17
Cases referred to the Office of Inspector General	109	10
Substantial violations	29	1
Gross and flagrant violations	80	9

[a]Second notices are sent only in cases of substantial violations.

SOURCE: HCFA, 1989b.

sanction cases date from earlier years of the program. The relatively lower numbers of sanction recommendations in more recent times has generated some debate and has been attributed to three factors: (1) revisions in procedures (prompted by the American Medical Association) that give practitioners the right to counsel during discussions with PROs of possible sanctions; (2) OIG directives that discouraged use of monetary fines as an alternative to exclusion; and (3) possibly the high reversal rate of the ALJs who had upheld only 8 of 18 sanctions on appeal during this period (McIlrath, 1989). In addition to these points, the growing confusion and tension caused by mixed signals from HCFA and the OIG concerning the relative emphasis to place on educational and disciplinary approaches to PRO implementation may have played a role in the sanction-recommendation picture.

OIG activity. From FY 1986 through FY 1988, the OIG reported it had received 197 referrals (150 gross and flagrant, 46 substantial, and 1 lack of documentation). Of these, 79 cases (40 percent) were rejected. Of the remainder, two cases were closed because the physician died, three physicians retired before exclusion, and three cases were pending. A total of 110 sanctions had been imposed (56 percent). Of the latter, 83 were exclusions (82 physicians; 1 facility) and 27 were monetary penalties (25 physicians; 2 facilities). In short, the OIG accepts about three in five sanction recommendations from PROs, a figure that has been fairly constant across the years. Of cases rejected, about two in five were because the case did not meet regulatory requirements, about two in five because the practitioner could show that he or she was willing and able to improve, and one in five because medical evidence was adequate. Of the sanctions imposed, the great majority were exclusions from the program.

Other PRO Required Activities

Beneficiary Relations

The PROs are required to act on behalf of Medicare beneficiaries in four ways not directly related to the technical quality of care rendered by providers or physicians. They must monitor hospital distribution of *An Important Message from Medicare* (concerning patients' rights to appeal denials of hospital care) and hospital notices of noncoverage, respond to beneficiary complaints, and carry on general community education and outreach.

Important Message to Medicare Beneficiaries. OBRA 1986 required all hospitals to provide Medicare patients (on or soon after admission) with a statement that explains (1) their rights to benefits, (2) their rights to appeal denials of benefits, and (3) the circumstances under which they will be liable for charges for those services (should a denial of benefits be upheld upon appeal). This two-page statement, *An Important Message from Medicare,* must conform to language specified in DHHS regulations except for minor changes in how receipt of the *Message* is acknowledged.

The PRO must monitor that all hospitals give beneficiaries the *Message.* Corrective action will be taken if the *Message* is not given to the beneficiary or his or her representative, if it is given to the beneficiary but not at or about the time of admission, or if its content is altered in any way. The SOW leaves the development of the monitoring plan for each hospital up to the PRO.

Hospital notices of noncoverage. A hospital can issue notices of noncoverage to Medicare beneficiaries when it determines that the patient's care is not (or will not be) covered because it is not medically necessary, is not delivered in the appropriate setting, or is custodial. These notices can be given before the patient is admitted or at any time during the hospital stay, according to a complex set of regulations. When hospitals issue such notices, beneficiaries are assumed to have knowledge that the services are not covered; they thus become liable for customary charges incurred after various periods of time have passed (e.g., at noon of the day following receipt of the notice of noncoverage). Similarly, providers who issue notices of noncoverage are assumed to know that the services furnished (or proposed) are not covered. In both these cases, issues relating to waiver (limitation) of liability come into play.

The hospital cannot issue these notices without the attending physician's concurrence. Either the attending physician or the patient, or both, may dispute the hospital's finding. The PRO must review cases in the following instances: (1) all hospital requests for PRO review when the attending physician does not agree that care is no longer required; (2) all cases where the patient disagrees with the notice issued by the hospital; (3) all cases where the patient is liable for charges for services furnished after notification; and (4) all cases where the hospital determined that the admission was noncovered.

When the attending physician disagrees with the hospital's desire to issue a notice of noncoverage and the hospital requests PRO review, the hospital must notify the beneficiary, in writing, that it has made that request. Before the PRO makes its review determination, it must make every effort to solicit the views of the patient, the physician, and the hospital. If the PRO concurs with the hospital, it issues a denial notice, which then becomes subject to reconsideration in accordance with the usual PRO reconsideration procedures.

Apart from responding to hospital or beneficiary requests for review of these notices, the main responsibilities of PROs in monitoring hospital notices of noncoverage are to track the content of the notice, the accuracy of the hospital's determination, and the conformance of the hospital to the specified process. The procedures, sample sizes, and other aspects of this monitoring are spelled out in the SOW.

Beneficiary complaints. All written complaints about the quality of care rendered by hospitals (inpatient or outpatient), SNFs, HHAs, ASCs, HMOs, and CMPs must be investigated by PROs. The focus is on care that does not meet professionally recognized standards. PROs do not review complaints involving underutilization, however, because that is the function of the FIs. Review of quality-related cases is to be based on medical record information, and procedures concerning disclosure of the review, the problem, and its disposition are specified in the SOW.

Community outreach. PROs must conduct programs to inform beneficiaries about Medicare PRO review and PPS; more specifically about the purpose of PROs and PPS, types of PRO review, and their right to appeal a PRO determination. PROs are also expected to devise ways to explain how they ensure the quality of care and respond to complaints from beneficiaries.

Each PRO must develop a detailed plan indicating how it will mount five community outreach activities. In addition, PROs are encouraged (not required) to use radio and television public service announcements. The minimum required areas of activity include the following:

1. Maintain a toll-free hotline to respond to beneficiary inquiries between 8:00 A.M. and 4:30 P.M. every working day.
2. Respond to written inquiries within 30 days of receipt. If this time frame cannot be met, an acknowledgement of receipt of the inquiry must be sent to the beneficiary within 10 days.
3. Conduct education programs, seminars, and workshops to inform beneficiaries about PRO review, PPS, and their appeal rights.
4. Develop and disseminate informational materials (e.g., brochures, slides, and tapes) that explain PRO review, PPS, hospital notices, and appeal procedures.
5. Coordinate with and involve concerned beneficiary and provider groups.

Provider Relations

The PRO program continues to stress peer review. In detailed specifications concerning what types of physicians shall review whom, the SOW appears to reflect HCFA's understanding of peer review.[13] It also calls for an "interaction plan" that will enhance the relationships between the PROs and providers, physicians, and other practitioners. That plan must give details concerning how physicians will be afforded opportunities to discuss problems or proposed denials and how the PRO will carry out educational efforts. The latter include informing physicians and other providers about PRO review, PPS, the rights of all parties under Medicare, and certain PRO confidentiality and disclosure guidelines.

The PRO is also required to publish and disseminate (at least annually) a report that describes what it has found about care that does meet Medicare obligations (i.e., necessary, appropriate, and of acceptable professional standards). This task mirrors the requirement that DHHS should submit to the Congress an annual report on the administration, impact, and cost of the program; such reports have not been published to date, however. In general, the outreach activities envisioned for providers are similar to those required for beneficiaries (seminars, informational material, etc.).

Data Acquisition, Sharing, and Reporting

PROs are required to exchange information with FIs and carriers, with other PROs, and with other public or private review organizations. (Sharing of information with FIs was briefly described in connection with PRO contracts and the conduct of review.) The rules governing acquisition, sharing, and disclosure are complex and open to some interpretation.

PRO access to information. HCFA regulations authorize PROs to have access to and obtain any records and information pertaining to health care services rendered to Medicare beneficiaries that are in the possession of any physician or provider in the PRO area. The PRO may require the practitioner or institution to provide copies of such information.

The preamble to the relevant regulations notes that quality problems that affect Medicare patients usually affect all patients, particularly in the context of acute care.[14] Often a quality problem may be adequately handled for Medicare patients only by addressing it for all patients. Thus, PROs may need to review both Medicare and non-Medicare patient records to resolve the problems for the former. The regulations thus provide that PROs may gain access to non-Medicare patient records if authorized by the physician or provider.

PROs are required to contact state medical licensing boards to establish mechanisms by which the state medical boards will send to the PRO the names of physicians against whom the board has taken disciplinary action. The PRO is then required to review all the cases of such practitioners (except for services provided in the physician's office) for the 3 months after notification by the board. Although this requirement has been in effect virtually since the start of the program, by the end of the second contract cycle fewer than half of the PROs had ever had any exchanges with their state boards, and fewer than one-quarter had more than two exchanges (GAO, 1988b).

The problems with information-sharing are bidirectional. Among the more common complaints that the Institute of Medicine (IOM) study committee heard during its site visits (from several different sources) was the lack of communication from the PROs about problem practitioners. The rules that govern information disclosure may play a part in this problem.

Disclosure of "confidential" information. Generally, information or records acquired by a PRO are confidential and not subject to disclosure. HCFA regulations distinguish between confidential[15] and nonconfidential information. They also limit the release of patient-identifying and physician-identifying information to that required for PRO review or for other statutorily required reasons. Disclosure of information that does not identify individuals is permitted.

PROs are required to disclose certain confidential information to appropriate agencies if the PRO believes that not to do so would pose a risk to public health. Confidential information must also be disclosed to federal and state fraud and abuse agencies and to state licensure or certification agencies upon those agencies' requests. Other disclosure of information with individual identifiers is allowed when such disclosure is required by judicial or administrative proceedings, when it is needed by the OIG and the General Accounting Office (GAO) in pursuance of their statutory responsibilities, or when it is necessary (because of a substantial risk to public health) to disclose the information to state or local public health agencies. Redisclosure by those agencies is permitted if information identifying patients and physicians is deleted. Persons who violate the disclosure provisions are subject to fines up to $1,000 or imprisonment for up to 6 months, or both, and must pay prosecution costs.

Among the more confusing aspects of data disclosure has been whether PROs may (or must) disclose to a hospital (or hospitals) the fact that they have confirmed a quality problem or are otherwise investigating or tracking the performance of a physician with privileges at the specific hospital (or at several hospitals). The early disclosure rules did not give unambiguous guidance on this point, and PROs apparently received guidance that varied among the HCFA ROs. Comments during study site visits also reflected complaints from hospitals that PROs never notified them of problem physicians.

In June 1989 (after study site visits were completed), HCFA clarified the rule, stating that information about a physician-specific quality concern, which can consist of as few as one confirmed quality problem, must be disclosed to the hospital if the hospital so requests and may be disclosed if the PRO so chooses even without a request (HCFA memorandum dated June 1, 1989). The PROs cannot, however, divulge to hospitals potential quality problems or the corrective actions being considered or taken. This clarification goes some way to meet the recommendations made in June 1989 by the Administrative Conference of the United States (ACUS, a federal advisory panel), namely that PROs should be required to send involved hospitals information about "confirmed violations of quality of care standards" by physicians and about the related corrective action plans (Vibbert, 1989c). It falls short by leaving the responsibility for requesting such information with hospitals (which can presumably register a blanket request with the PRO or otherwise develop cooperative relationships with the PRO so that the PRO will provide information even without a request) and by not including the corrective action information.

Finally, as noted above, PROs are expected to obtain information on disciplined physicians *from* various state authorities, but their responsibility to provide information on physicians who are involved in quality interventions (corrective action plans) or in sanction proceedings *to* such state agencies is not clear. Nor are PROs at present required to submit information about physician sanction recommendations to the National Practitioner Data Bank (which is being established through the Health Care Quality Improvement Act of 1986). Thus, another set of reforms suggested by ACUS specifies that sanction recommendations be forwarded to state medical boards and licensing authorities and possibly to the data bank as well (Vibbert, 1989c).

Disclosure of aggregate data. PROs must provide to agencies responsible for health planning certain summary utilization and demographic statistics. They may not include anything to identify patients or physicians. Various regulations provide for disclosure of nonconfidential aggregate statistical information, including PRO interpretations and generalizations about the quality of care. They specifically mandate PRO disclosure, upon demand, of information on quality and the appropriateness of health care services in individual hospitals. PROs may release information on average length of stay, death rates for individual departments and illnesses, the number and type of surgical procedures performed, and the number of patients in each category who required readmission.

Disclosure of hospital-specific information. Information that identifies hospitals is not considered confidential, and disclosure of information that identifies particular institutions is permitted. Provider institutions may disclose information about themselves as long as identifiers of patients and physicians are excluded.

To protect the rights and interests of hospitals, regulations require a PRO to notify a hospital when it intends to disclose information about that institution (other than routine reports sent to HCFA or FIs, information to or from PRO subcontractors, or information to or from the hospital itself). The PRO must notify the institution at least 30 days before release, supply the institution with a copy of the information to be released, and give the institution an opportunity to submit comments. If the disclosure concerns an investigation of fraud or abuse and the information relates to a potentially prosecutable offense, the PRO need not notify the institution before releasing the information. Investigative agencies other than the OIG or GAO must stipulate in writing to the PRO that the information they are requesting does relate to possible criminal prosecution.

Freedom of Information Act. PROs are granted by statute a flat exemption from requirements of the Freedom of Information Act (FOIA) and are not subject to FOIA disclosure requirements, but the situation is complex. As implied earlier, PROs must disclose all information to DHHS that the department requests. Because all agencies of the federal government are covered by the FOIA disclosure provisions, seemingly the information submitted by PROs *to* DHHS would be subject to disclosure under FOIA. However, the preamble to the relevant regulations notes that the information routinely provided to DHHS does not identify individual patients or practitioners, and DHHS regulations protect individual privacy. Also, the regulations provide that some information must be disclosed only on-site at the PRO. Furthermore, FOIA protects personal privacy by providing that information contained in personnel and medical files, the disclosure of which would constitute a clearly unwarranted invasion of personal privacy, is exempt from FOIA. In short, the protections favor nondisclosure of PRO information.

COSTS

The annual PRO program budgets have risen in absolute terms in the latter half of the 1980s, although in earlier years they did not keep pace with those of the PSRO program. According to HCFA, the PRO program is currently budgeted (excluding internal expenditures of HCFA) at approximately $300 million a year, up from $157 million a year for the first round of PRO contracts (FY 1984–1986) and $217 million a year for the second round of PRO contracts (FY 1986–1988).

In FY 1987, Part A Medicare benefits amounted to $50.8 billion and Part B outlays to $30.8 billion (for a total of $81.6 billion) (Committee on Ways and Means, 1989). For FY 1987 PRO outlays, the Congressional Research Service (CRS) gives $187.5 million for all PRO activities; GAO cites $155 million for inpatient review (GAO, 1988a). The first figure amounts to about 0.2 percent of all outlays, and the second approximates 0.3 percent of Part A expenditures.

For FY 1989, Parts A and B expenditures are estimated at about $98.5 billion[16]; the PRO budget was put at $300 million, about 0.3 percent of outlays. An estimate for FY 1990 puts expenditures at better than $112 billion and the PRO budget presumably remains at $300 million; equivalent estimates for FY 1991 are approximately $130 billion and $330 million, respectively (H. Brook, personal communication, 1989). Again, the PRO budgets amount to about 0.3 percent of Medicare outlays.

These appear to be large numbers for the PROs, and in some sense they are. It is instructive, however, to place them in the context of the expenditures on services, the quality of which the PROs are expected to ensure. Total Medicare expenditures are, of course, an imperfect denominator for gauging the adequacy of the Medicare quality assurance investment, but the ratio of PSRO and PRO dollars to total expenditures over time does indicate whether that investment is rising, falling, or remaining constant in the face of changing demands on the peer review program. As a proportion of Medicare expenditures, these figures are lower for the PRO program than for the PSRO program, although the emphasis has shifted over the years a little more toward quality assurance and away from utilization and cost control. Still, even if the $11 million intended for pilot projects were added to the estimates given above for the PRO program, its expenditures would not exceed those of the PSRO program as a percentage of expected Medicare outlays.

Given the expanded responsibilities of the PROs compared with the PSROs, the markedly changing environment of health care for the elderly, and the greater perception of threats to high-quality care in the future, some view this level of funding as parsimonious. Furthermore, even if the $300 million per year were adequate for all the varied activities presently required of PROs, the need for future congressional or executive branch assignments to be adequately budgeted should be clear.

Because PRO budgets are tightly tied to the number of expected reviews, which is driven by the numbers of Medicare enrollees in a given state, individual budgets for PROs range very widely. For instance, of the PROs awarded full 3-year contracts for the third SOW, the California PRO was awarded nearly $82,838,000, the largest award in the country and a record for the PRO program (Vibbert, 1989a); the PRO for Wyoming was awarded $1,210,000. Of PROs awarded extensions of existing contracts for 6 or 12 months, the largest award was to Texas (just over $16.1 million) and the smallest award was to American Samoa and Guam ($24,120) (unpublished HCFA data, April 11, 1989).

PRO budgets are based on negotiated costs for "simple," "complex," and

ambulatory reviews; for fixed administrative costs and some start-up costs
(largely accounting system updates); for photocopy and postage pass-through
costs; and for costs of Civilian Health and Medicare Programs of the Uni-
formed Services (CHAMPUS) review, for those PROs doing such review.
Costs per review average $17.03 for simple review (range, roughly $13 to
$32), $33.29 for complex review (range, nearly $27 to over $48), and $9.16
for ambulatory review (range, $4 to almost $15).

QUALITY REVIEW IN MEDICARE RISK-CONTRACT PLANS[17]

As of April 1989, 1 million Medicare beneficiaries were enrolled in 133
"risk contracts" held by HMOs and CMPs. That enrollment figure accounts
for about 3 percent of the Medicare population (O'Kane, 1989). The Medicare program has been experimenting for a decade with the concept of
enrolling Medicare beneficiaries into HMOs. In 1981, prepaid health plans
delivered care, on a cost-reimbursement basis, to nearly 600,000 beneficiaries. The Social Security Amendments of 1982 sought, through Section
1876, to expand participation of HMOs through risk-contracting. Also in
1982, TEFRA established the strategy of paying HMOs 95 percent of the
average adjusted per capita cost (AAPCC) of the Medicare program, but
implementation was delayed until 1985 until a means for computing the
AAPCC had been devised. By 1989, it seemed clear that the risk-contract
program had not been successful for many HMOs, owing to the extent of
financial losses (except in areas where the AAPCC is extremely high),
possible adverse selection because of the generosity of some benefit packages, and high use of Medicare beneficiaries who had previously been un-
derusing services because of financial reasons. Some HMOs withdrew from
the program; others stopped marketing to the Medicare population.

The history of quality review for the care rendered to such beneficiaries
by HMOs and CMPs is both complex and historic. It is historic chiefly
because it ushered in (1) ambulatory care review (i.e., review of care provided in private physicians' offices), (2) an attempt to review "episodes" of
care, and (3) an effort to design a way to reduce required review for providers having an adequate quality assurance plan of their own. Because of the
importance of these developments, the history and provisions of the HMO-
CMP portion of the PRO program are described in some detail.

History

Section 1876 of the Social Security Amendments of 1982 was the first
attempt to entice prepaid group practices into risk-contracting with Medicare, but the initial design of the program, particularly its payment provisions, was not attractive to the HMO community. To overcome these

drawbacks, TEFRA amended Section 1876 to create a new payment strategy based on the AAPCC. Implementation was considerably delayed while methods for computing the AAPCC were worked out. TEFRA did not specifically mandate PRO (or indeed any) review of quality of care per se, although it did call for monitoring the quality assurance *programs* of risk-contract HMOs and CMPs. (PROs were not required to review or monitor plans with cost-based contracts.)

During this time HCFA was attempting to design a strategy for reviewing capitated systems. The agency's "white paper" focused on the financial incentives of capitation (underuse, untimely care, and inappropriate settings), inpatient and outpatient care, consumer access, and medical review. The final TEFRA regulations, which became effective February 1985, included provisions requiring risk-contract HMOs and CMPs to comply with requirements for PRO review.

In short, before COBRA, no specific legislative requirements existed for the review of services provided to Medicare beneficiaries enrolled in risk-contract HMOs and CMPs, but review was nonetheless contemplated by HCFA. The HMO industry resisted the TEFRA provisions, arguing that review was unnecessary because all plans were required to have an internal quality assurance program in order to qualify for a risk contract. Additionally, the industry argued that if quality review was to be external, then using existing PROs would be inappropriate because they are staffed primarily by fee-for-service (FFS) physicians (i.e., not by "peers").

Nevertheless, given the regulations promulgated after TEFRA, some common understanding needed to be reached. HCFA thus convened a meeting that led to the designation of a PRO-HMO Ad hoc Committee that would draft an industry proposal for HMO review by PROs.[18] It was envisioned that this collaborative effort would guide the design of HMO-CMP review for Medicare.

The industry proposal had the following main elements. First, a new national quality review organization (similar to the existing National Committee for Quality Assurance [NCQA], an HMO industry body) would be established. It would have the following functions: (1) establish screening criteria for the quality review process; (2) establish qualifications of physician reviewers; (3) define review, analysis, and reporting activities for each PRO's (to be established) HMO committee; (4) train HMO and CMP physician reviewers; and (5) render technical advice to PROs and to HMOs and CMPs on proper interpretation and application of review criteria. Further, each PRO would create a committee of HMO and CMP physicians. This committee would be responsible for quality review and would (1) perform reviews, (2) analyze data to identify areas of concern, (3) validate areas of concern through chart review, and (4) recommend corrective actions.

The PRO-HMO Ad Hoc Committee's proposed scope of PRO review

was quite broad. It included (1) examination of the validity and effectiveness of internal quality assurance programs at HMOs and CMPs (using NCQA standards); (2) monitoring plans, with review based on screening criteria developed by the national committee and focused review of potential problems; (3) medical record review of areas of concern; and (4) recommendations for corrective action to be made to the HMO and CMP. Both institutional and ambulatory settings would be covered. The committee proposed to develop an approach to ambulatory review based on 15 "sentinel conditions" as screens for possible inadequate ambulatory care.[19]

In the midst of this activity, the executive Office of Management and Budget (OMB) overruled HMO review, citing the lack of legislative authority. In the aftermath, the work of the PRO-HMO Ad Hoc Committee was effectively lost.

Because of continuing concern for underutilization in risk-contract programs, OBRA 1986 solved the legislative-authority problem by mandating review of care rendered in HMOs and CMPs effective for services provided after January 1, 1987. "Comparable review"[20] was to focus on quality, especially appropriate treatment and setting, access and timeliness of services, and the potential for underutilization of services. The review process was heavily oriented toward medical record review and required a considerable volume of review. The basic approach was modified, at the instigation of the executive OMB, to permit a level of reduced review (which came to be known as "limited review") for those HMOs and CMPs that requested such status and could demonstrate they had properly functioning internal quality assurance programs.

Rather than use existing models developed by NCQA, the Joint Commission on Accreditation of Healthcare Organizations (the Joint Commission), and similar groups, HCFA defined de novo a set of "areas of focus" by which HMO and CMP internal programs would be evaluated. Characteristics of concern to HCFA were whether the plan (1) reviews individual cases of patient care, (2) reviews all settings, (3) includes physician review of medical records, and (4) uses reasonable sampling methods to select cases for review; whether the plan has been operating long enough for it to be able to demonstrate actual performance; and whether physicians make final decisions on quality issues. The industry widely regarded these concerns as rather old-fashioned and lacking in an understanding of what HMO and CMP quality assurance plans actually do.

One other factor complicated the implementation of this review. OBRA 1986 allowed review of HMO and CMP services by entities other than PROs in the area as a means of stimulating competition among review organizations. These other entities are referred to as Quality Review Organizations (QROs). QRO contracts were limited to no more than half the states, covering half the Medicare population. In March 1987, a Request for Proposals was issued for QRO review of HMO and CMP services in 25 states.[21] Quality Quest (a subsidiary of InterStudy, located in Minneapolis, Minnesota) was awarded the review contracts for the states of Illinois, Kansas, and Missouri; California Medical Review was awarded the review for Arizona and Hawaii.[22] All remaining HMO and CMP reviews is done by PROs in the state itself.[23] Hereafter, PRO is understood to include the QRO.

Three Types of HMO and CMP Review

HMO and CMP review[24] has three levels of review: limited, basic, and intensified (outlined in Table 8.6). Basic review is the core approach to HMO review. Limited review is intended to reduce the volume of active

TABLE 8.6 Summary of Activities for Health Maintenance Organization (HMO) and Competitive Medical Plan (CMP) Review, by Requirements for Limited, Basic, and Intensified Review

Type of Review	Sample Size for Review		
	Limited	Basic	Intensified
Thirteen sentinel conditions[a]	50% - RS[b] (of only 4 conditions)	50% - RS	100%
Hospital admissions	3% - RS	3% - RS	6% - RS
Transfers[c]	100%	100%	100%
Readmissions within less than 31 days	25% - RS	50% - RS	100%
Nontrauma deaths in all care settings	5% - RS	10% - RS	100%

[a]These conditions, which are defined by ICD-9-CM codes, include: diabetic complications (ketoacidosis, hyperosmolar coma, other coma, and hypoglycemic coma); acute appendicitis with generalized peritonitis or peritoneal abscess; hypertensive problems (several categories, including occlusion and stenosis of precerebral arteries and transient cerebral ischemia); gastrointestinal catastrophes (acute, chronic, or unspecified gastric ulcer with hemorrhage without obstruction; chronic duodenal ulcer with hemorrhage without obstruction; unspecified intestinal obstruction); gangrene of the extremity; operations for breast malignancy (including certain biopsies and unilateral radical mastectomy); malignant neoplasm of the genitourinary organ; adverse drug reactions (several categories, mainly poisoning by specific pharmacologic agents); other cellulitis and abscess; malignant neoplasm of colon; hypokalemia; septicemia; and pulmonary embolus.

[b]RS is random sample.

[c]Transfer category eliminated August 1989.

SOURCE: HCFA, 1988.

PRO review for the plan, mainly by requiring smaller sample sizes than are prescribed for basic review. Intensive review has the same general meaning as in FFS settings (i.e., it is invoked when a threshold for a quality problem is reached), and sample sizes are larger than for the other two levels of review (usually in 100 percent of relevant cases). The three levels are not a true continuum, however, because for plans on limited review, quality problems that reach specified thresholds trigger intensified, not basic review.

Limited Review

Limited review is available only to those HMOs and CMPs that request it and pass an assessment of their internal quality assurance program to determine that it has the capacity to identify and correct quality problems. It has two main components.

First, if the PRO judges the risk-contract plan's quality assurance program adequate according to the "areas of focus" mentioned above, then it reviews a subsample of cases already reviewed by the plan to validate the plan's judgments. This is done when the plan is first assessed, and quarterly thereafter. The purpose is to monitor the plan's internal program, not to provide a generalized statement about the quality of care provided.

One of four "outcomes" for the subsample review effort is possible:

1. According to the PRO, care was deficient (in quality, appropriateness, or access) and the plan had not made this determination.
2. Care was deficient and the plan had already so determined. If a pattern is identified, the PRO would then monitor the plan's corrective action activities.
3. Care was not deficient and the plan had so decided.
4. Care was not deficient and the plan had previously found that it was.

If a pattern of problems (relating to Outcomes 1 and 4 above) becomes apparent, the PRO then monitors the plan's corrective actions and may assign the HMO to intensified review.

Second, medical record review is required in four main areas[25]: (1) a 50-percent random sample of four conditions selected from among 13 specified "sentinel" conditions,[26] (2) a 3-percent random sample of inpatient admissions, (3) a 5-percent random sample of nontraumatic deaths in all health care settings, and (4) a 25-percent random sample of readmissions within 31 days. For the 13 sentinel conditions, both pre- and post-hospitalization ambulatory care is reviewed through the use of criteria developed by HCFA and the PRO. A fifth area is focused review of ambulatory care, for which PROs were given 6 months to develop a methodology. In addition, beneficiary complaints are also reviewed, and PROs must perform community outreach activities for risk-contract enrollees similar to those for FFS beneficiaries.

For plans on limited review, the total number of cases selected for the random validation subsample plus the total number selected for the remaining reasons for review cannot exceed the number that would have been reviewed under the basic plan.

Basic Review

Plans not opting for, or not eligible for, limited review are placed on basic review. It includes the same five areas covered by the second component of limited review but uses larger samples, and it requires the beneficiary complaints and outreach activities. *Not* included in basic review is the first component of limited review; that is, the extra quarterly review of charts.

Intensified Review

If a plan comes under intensified review, the sample of cases reviewed is again larger: 6 percent of all admissions, 100 percent of all cases among any of the 13 conditions, 100 percent of nontrauma deaths, and 100 percent of all readmissions. Plans on limited review move to intensified review in one of two instances: (1) if 5 percent or 6 cases selected for the subsample validation review in a quarter have Outcome 1 (in which the PRO found a problem but the plan did not); and (2) if 5 percent or 6 cases of all other cases reviewed have problems related to standards of quality, appropriateness of care, or access. Basic plans are put under intensified review only in the second instance. Intensified review continues for 6 months before the plan's status is reviewed.

The Review Process

By and large, the process for reviewing care rendered to Medicare beneficiaries in risk-contract HMOs and CMPs is similar to the process for reviewing care in traditional FFS settings (e.g., use of generic screens, assignment of severity levels, physician or plan notification, and the like). That process has already been described.

The main difference is that HMO-CMP review has attempted to implement episode-of-care review based on two types of cases, simple and complex. A "simple case" is one in which services being reviewed were provided in only one setting and during only one admission (if inpatient)—for instance, those in the 3-percent inpatient sample. A "complex case" is one in which services being reviewed were provided in more than one setting or involve more than one hospital stay; for example, cases selected under the 13 sentinel conditions would normally be classified as complex. For complex cases, PROs are expected to review the care rendered in all relevant settings (ambulatory, hospital, and post-acute).

Arguably the most significant step is the requirement for ambulatory review, which leaves to each PRO the responsibility of developing a focused review methodology and establishing clinical screening criteria to be used in reviewing the 13 sentinel conditions. Because the HMO industry, the PRO community, and HCFA believed that the possibility of dozens of different approaches to ambulatory review was not an attractive proposition, these groups agreed that an industry-PRO task force would develop model methods to offer the PRO community. Because of the lack of uniform data among PROs, the task force recommended a random sample of HMO Medicare enrollees for this "focused ambulatory review" activity. As of mid-1989, experience with focused ambulatory review was limited, but the process of collaboratively developing acceptable tools for such an effort was considered valuable (O'Kane, 1989).

CURRENT AND FUTURE INITIATIVES OF THE PRO PROGRAM

Uniform Clinical Data Set

HCFA began in 1987 a complex project to develop a data set and accompanying decision rules for use by PROs and the wider research community that would contain far more detailed clinical data than was heretofore available in the HCFA data files. Known as the Uniform Clinical Data Set (UCDS), this project is one of a number of steps intended to expand and improve the ability of the agency to assure the quality of care delivered to Medicare beneficiaries, using the PROs as the principal mechanism.

The genesis of the UCDS was in the recognition that the way PROs make judgments about the necessity, appropriateness, and timeliness of care varies and is too subjective. One objective of the UCDS, therefore, was to put in place a mechanism to make PRO review more systematic. The basic principle is to screen cases by applying a uniform set of computerized decision rules that are based on more complete clinical data. Such a common set of guidelines would also permit a more effective assessment of the work and performance of PROs.

The second purpose of the UCDS is to permit the development of more and better information about the practice of medicine, so that PROs, among others, will be able to base decisions about quality, appropriateness, and medical necessity of care on systematically and objectively evaluated collective data rather than on individual experience. The availability of the extensive clinical information collected in the UCDS formats would support more thorough and detailed analysis of patterns of interventions and outcomes than is possible simply with billing data. Thus, for patients with particular medical problems, a large body of information about alternative interventions could be made available to PROs and the medical community. The agency plans to make the UCDS data available for intramural and extramural analysis.

The basic operating premise of the UCDS is that relevant clinical data will be abstracted from medical records of all inpatient admissions reviewed by the PROs for whatever reason. (This amounts to about 20 to 25 percent of all Medicare admissions in a year, or approximately 2.0 to 2.5 million admissions; of these, about 3 percent are a truly random sample of admissions, and the remainder are cases mandated for review for specific reasons, largely related to the probability of problems related to PPS fiscal incentives or to quality of care.) Quality-of-care algorithms have been developed to screen cases for potential quality problems automatically. Nurse reviewers who flag instances of potential quality deficiencies for more in-depth review will have more organized, objective, clinical information before them, and physician reviewers likewise will have better organized information on which to base their decisions. More broadly, HCFA hopes to be able to set national and individual PRO goals for improving quality of care and to measure the success of PROs in reaching those goals (Morford, 1989a, 1989b).

The total number of data elements available on the UCDS is about 1,600, although not every data element is needed or relevant for every case. The contents of the UCDS fall into 10 major categories (for details, see Table 8.7):

    I. Patient Identifying Information
   II. Patient History and Physical Examination and History and Physical Exam Findings
  III. Laboratory Findings
  IV. Imaging Findings and Other Diagnostic Test Findings
   V. Endoscopic Procedures
  VI. Operative Episodes
 VII. Treatment Interventions
VIII. Medication Therapy in Hospital
  IX. Recovery Phase
   X. Patient Discharge Status and Discharge Planning

Medical records will be abstracted by PRO abstractors either on-site or at a central office; data will be entered via desktop or laptop computers. At present, data abstraction requires about 1 hour per case, but that time requirement is expected to decline as software is improved and experience is

TABLE 8.7 Elements of the Uniform Clinical Data Set

I. Patient Identifying Information

Patient's Medical Record Number
Health Insurance Claim Number
Provider Number
Physician Number
Date of Admission
Date of Discharge
Patient's Date of Birth
Patient's Sex
Source of Admission (location of patient just before admission to inpatient bed)
Readmission Code
Ambulatory Care
Care-giver on Admission
Patient's Race
Patient's Occupational Status
Patient's Insurance Coverage

II. Patient History and Physical Exam

Part 1. (Source of data: physician and nursing notes)

    Activities of Daily Living Prior to Admission (continence; mobility)
    Patient Weight
    Patient Height
    Vital Signs (temperature, pulse, respiratory rate, blood pressure)
    Current Medications
    History of Drug Reaction
    History of Drug and Substance Use
    Medications Administered in Emergency Department
    History of Total or Partial Excision of Major Organ
    History of Amputation of Major Limb
    History of Replaced Body Structure (e.g., cardiac valve; hip)
    History of Organ Transplant
    History of Congenital Absence of Organs

Part 2. (Source of data: all available information concerning findings documented within the first 24 to 48 hours following admission or up to 6 weeks before admission, with emphasis on whether the patient is "under current management or monitoring")

    History of chronic neurological disease(s)
    History of neurological surgery
    Current neurological examination findings (e.g., Glasgow Coma Score; cerebrovascular accident; speech deficit; syncope)
    History of chronic cardiac disease(s) (e.g., chronic hypotension)
    History of chronic vascular disease
    History of cardiovascular surgery (coronary artery surgery or bypass graft; angioplasty; intracardiac surgery; vascular surgery; peripheral vascular surgery)

Current cardiovascular exam findings (22 findings such as shock, pulmonary edema, peripheral edema, arrythmia, stasis ulcers, or steady chest pain)

History of chronic pulmonary disease(s)

History of pulmonary surgery

Current pulmonary findings (e.g., tachypnea; cyanosis, cough, stridor)

History of chronic immunological disease (e.g., HIV positive; other autoimmune disease; systemic infection)

History of endocrine disease(s) (e.g., diabetes mellitus; hyperthyroidism)[a]

History of endocrine system surgery (e.g., thyroidectomy)

History of cancer[a]

History of chronic gastrointestinal disease (upper GI disease, lower GI disease, hepatobiliary disease, pancreatic disease, GI bleeding, colicky pain, weight loss)[a]

History of gastrointestinal surgery

Current gastrointestinal findings (e.g., ascites; GI bleeding; abdominal distension, rigidity; rectal blood, mass; recent persistent nausea, vomiting, etc.)

Current cutaneous findings (e.g., skin ulcer; burn, cellulitis)

History of musculoskeletal surgery (spine, hips/knees, and long bone fracture considered separately)

Current musculoskeletal findings (e.g., congenital deformity; fracture; soft tissue trauma)

History of chronic urologic conditions[a]

History of urologic surgery (prostate, bladder, ureter, kidney)

Current urologic exam findings (e.g., enlarged prostate; flank or genitalia tenderness)

History of chronic psychiatric disorders

Current psychiatric exam findings (e.g., suicidal; major affective disorder; dementia or mental retardation)

History of chronic ob/gyn disorders

History of gynecologic surgery (in relation to pregnancy and to other gynecologic conditions)

Current ob/gyn findings (pregnant; not pregnant)

Current neonatal exam findings (e.g., gestational age; Apgar)

III. Laboratory Findings

(Listed laboratory values at three points in time: first (or worst) within 24 hours of admission (or pre-admission up to six weeks before admission), worst interim value, and last test)

Chemistry/hematology (26 tests such as alkaline phosphatase, bilirubin, creatinine, glucose, hematocrit, platelets, potassium, and white blood cell count; plus 7 additional tests within 48 hours, including CPK, SGOT, and thyroid tests)

Urinalysis: microbiology (e.g., protein, red cells, bacteria)

Microbiology - cultures (e.g., blood, cervix, cerebrospinal fluid, sputum, stool, urine)

Cytology/histology (e.g., bronchial wash, aspirates; joint fluid)

TABLE 8.7 continues

TABLE 8.7 Continued

IV. Imaging and Other Diagnostic Test Findings

(Dates of examination and specific findings are recorded; pre-admission tests up to six weeks before admission are acceptable.)

Chest x-ray (with or without contrast)
Upper GI, barium enema/swallow, gallbladder
KUB/abdominal x-ray
IVP/urogram
Ultrasound
Extremity/skeletal/spinal x-ray or myelogram
CT scan (head and neck; spine; chest; body)
Magnetic Resonance Imaging (head and neck; spine; chest; body)
Nuclear medicine/isotope studies (thyroid, lung, bone, hepatobiliary, cardiac)
Electrocardiogram
Cardiac catheterization, ventriculogram
Echocardiogram
Arteriogram, angiogram
Electroencephalogram
Pulmonary function test
Gastrointestinal motility (manometric)

V. Endoscopic Procedures

(Dates of examination and specific findings are recorded; pre-admission tests up to six weeks before admission are acceptable.)

Procedures: arthroscopy, cystoscopy/cystogram; upper GI endoscopy, lower GI endoscopy, endoscopic retrograde cholangiopancreatography (ERCP), laparoscopy, hysteroscopy, bronchoscopy and laryngoscopy.

Also recorded: anesthesia type; anesthesia risk grade; and unexpected intra-endoscopic events (e.g., apnea, hemorrhage, cardiac arrest, perforation)

VI. Operative Episodes

All procedures recorded (using ICD-9-CM codes)
Also recorded:
anesthetic type
anesthesia risk (American Society of Anesthesiologists classification system)
vascular access line surgical wound classification (clean, clean-contaminated, contaminated, dirty)
tissue findings
occurrence of unexpected intra-operative events (e.g., respiratory arrest, acute myocardial infarction, blood loss, stroke)
return to operating room

VII. Treatment Interventions

(This section covers various data items relating to noninvasive procedures.)

Blood products

Inhalation therapy

Professional services (e.g., physiotherapy, respiratory therapy, social work, psychiatric counseling, pastoral care)

VIII. Medication Therapy in Hospital

Current medication at admission (See Section II, Part 1)

Medications administered in the hospital (this section covers name of medication, route of administration, and dates medication was initiated, stopped, or route changed; dosage is not recorded.)

Medication at discharge (name)

Adverse reactions to medications during hospital stay (e.g., abnormal drug reaction; expected toxic side effect)

Delivery systems for medications (i.e., other than oral)

IX. Recovery Phase

Special care unit days (e.g., coronary care, general intensive care, neurosurgical)

Do not resuscitate order (date)

Unexpected inpatient events (a lengthy list of major or catastrophic complications with possible outcome of death or chronic disability, such as myocardial infarction, pulmonary embolism, acute bowel obstuction, septicemic shock, respiratory failure, wound infection, urinary retention, pneumonia)

Trauma suffered in hospital (e.g., fall or accidental injury with significant untoward effect; decubitus ulcer, attempted suicide)

Nosocomial infections

Prolonged stay (e.g., awaiting placement into chronic care facility; inability or refusal of family to care for patient)

X. Patient Discharge Status

Discharge vital signs

Discharge physical exam findings (cardiovascular, neurological, pulmonary, gastrointestinal, cutaneous, urologic, last chest x-ray, last abdominal x-ray)

Last EKG

Discharge Activities of Daily Living (urinary incontinence; walking; alimentation, elimination)

Other discharge therapies (medications, IV therapy other than alimentation, oxygenation, monitoring, mechanical implants, dialysis)

Discharge plan (care-giver; follow-up)

Discharge disposition (e.g., home, transfer, home health service, died)

Full and final listing of diagnosis (first 15 final diagnoses in ICD-9-CM codes)

---

[a]Resource manual refers abstractors to separate lists that are embedded in the software and called up on the computer screen for reference.

SOURCE: "Resource Manual for Uniform Clinical Data Set (U.C.D.S.)," prepared by Case Mix Research, Queen's University, Department of Community Health and Epidemiology, Kingston, Ontario, Canada, in association with the Wisconsin Peer Review Organization (WIPRO), Madison, Wisconsin, 1988.

gained with this approach. The detailed guidelines that describe precisely the data to be acquired (for an example, see Table 8.8) have been developed by Case Mix Research, Queen's University, Ontario, Canada, in association with the Wisconsin Peer Review Organization, Madison, Wisconsin.

The computer algorithms fall into several categories (for details, see Table 8.9): surgery (12 specific procedures), specific diseases (12 conditions), organ systems (10 systems), generic quality screens (6 classes of problems), and discharge screens. They have been developed with the help of a task force of clinicians; initial programming was done in part through KePRO, the Pennsylvania PRO.

As of April 1989, the UCDS project was in a small pilot-test phase. Field testing of the whole approach, including use of algorithms to assist in the selection of cases for physician review, is expected to begin during the winter of 1989–1990. An assessment and recommendation about whether to go forward with this approach as an integral part of the PRO quality review task is expected late in 1990.

Pilot Projects for PROs

Apart from the UCDS activity, HCFA and the PRO community are embarking on a series of pilot projects designed to begin the implementation of several new review activities required by legislation (e.g., OBRA 1987). These are all projects that should form a bridge to a more comprehensive quality assurance program in the future. These efforts fall into two categories: (1) reduced hospital review (sometimes referred to as alternative hospital review) and (2) noninstitutional setting review, specifically outpatient (physician office-based) review and post-acute (HHA and SNF) review.

Approximately $9 to 11 million in Medicare Trust Fund monies will be set aside over 3 years to pilot new review methods. Only PROs will be eligible for funding through contract modifications, although they can and will subcontract with each other and with outside research and academic groups for needed technical assistance. Two formal requests for contract modification proposals (for noninstitutional and alternative hospital review methods) were released in May and July 1989.

Noninstitutional Review

A pilot project on noninstitutional review began on December 1, 1989, in response to the request issued in mid-May 1989. The emphasis is on ambulatory (office-based) care. The Wisconsin PRO serves as the lead PRO; six other PROs are included in the effort. The project will evaluate approaches to monitoring and assessing care in the office setting, taking four factors into account: (1) severity of illness, sequence and patterns of care, variety

TABLE 8.8 Example Of Data Element Recorded for Uniform Clinical Data Set: Cardiac Catheterization and Ventriculogram

---

Formal report of the first cardiac catheterization and/or ventriculogram performed during the admission or up to 6 weeks before admission; if more than one test, use the one closest to admission. Catheterization takes precedence over ventriculogram. Any procedure done in an operating room, minor treatment room, at the bedside, or in the radiology suite can be included. All approriate categories of specified findings are checked.

The general rules for recoding information for the UCDS are to change default values on the computer screen ("F") to "T." The specific findings to be recorded for catheterization or ventriculogram are the following. The reviewer changes F to T unless a percentage is called for, in which case the worst percentage is recorded, or other information is specified.

Normal
AV shunt
Ventricular/atrial septal defect

Valvular defects:
    Aortic stenosis (<1 sq cm)
    Aortic regurgitation (moderate or severe)
    Mitral stenosis (<1 sq cm)
Stenosis: left main (%)
Stenosis: left anterior descending (%)
Stenosis: circumflex (%)
Stenosis: right (%)
Cardiac output (liters/minute) (%)
LV ejection fraction (%)
Abnormal chamber size/wall motion
Ventricular aneurysm
Congenital anomalies (patent ductus, ventricular septal defect)
Aortic aneurysm
Dissecting aortic aneurysm
Other abnormal findings

Coronary artery grafts—number
Number with >70% stenosis

Pressures
    Left ventricular—systolic; diastolic
    Aortic—systolic; diastolic; mean
    Pulmonary artery (including Swan-Ganz)—systolic; diastolic

SOURCE: "Resource Manual for Uniform Clinical Data Set (U.C.D.S.)," prepared by Case Mix Research, Queen's University, Department of Community Health and Epidemiology, Kingston, Ontario, Canada, in association with the Wisconsin Peer Review Organization (WIPRO), Madison, Wisconsin, 1988.

TABLE 8.9 Selected Categories of Quality-of-Care Algorithms for the Uniform Clinical Data Set

I. Surgery Algorithms

Prostatectomy
Major joint replacement
Gastrointestinal surgery
Cardiac revascularization
Cholecystectomy
Hernia repair
Vascular bypass and endarterectomy
Hysterectomy
Mastectomy
Cataract surgery
Laminectomy
Thoracotomy

II. Disease-Specific Algorithms

Ischemic myocardial disease and chest pain
Cardiac pump failure
Acute lower respiratory infection
Ischemic cerebrovascular disease
Obstructive airway disease and respiratory failure
Cardiac dysrhythmia
Diabetes mellitus
Urinary tract infection
Malignant pulmonary neoplasm
Septicemia
Thrombophlebitis and pulmonary embolism
Malignant neoplasm of female breast

III. Organ System Algorithms

Cardiac system
Vascular system
Pulmonary system
Gastrointestinal system
Genitourinary system
Bone, joint, and muscular system
Neurological system
Infectious diseases
Endocrine system

IV. Generic Quality Screen Algorithms

Adequacy of discharge planning
Medical stability of patient at discharge
Deaths
Nosocomial infection
Unscheduled return to surgery
Trauma suffered in hospital

V. Discharge Screens

Discharge status/disposition

of treatments associated with various medical specialties, and the continuum of care (rather than specific encounters); (2) methods for retrieving appropriate details from office medical records; (3) methods for organizing and integrating such information with other data (e.g., the Medicare claims files); and (4) the impact of care on the patient's condition over time. The aim is to be able to evaluate the effectiveness of the care and to test the practicality and usefulness of the techniques available for making that evaluation. HCFA had called for two general approaches. The first is a statistical assessment of the "impact of the physician's services on the condition of his overall patient population"; the second is an evaluation of cases with unexpectedly adverse risk-adjusted outcomes.

Reduced Hospital Review

The first pilot projects in this category were intended to develop alternative mechanisms by which hospitals can be put on "reduced review"; that is, be "focused out" of the level of review they presently experience. This effort reflected two factors: (1) the wide recognition that the volume of hospital review, especially for hospitals with good performance records, is too burdensome; and (2) the judgment that the old PSRO approach of "delegating" review to hospitals was not entirely successful and would probably not be practical in today's more data-intensive review world.

The main purpose of this set of projects was to test alternative review methods for hospitals that are based on outcomes. Hospitals would provide information on their patients that would let HCFA track risk-adjusted outcomes. The hospitals would provide information to the PROs; with outside expert assistance in epidemiology and statistics, the PROs were then supposed to assess hospital performance on the basis of risk-adjusted outcomes. Although an RFP was published in July 1989, no contract modifications were made.

This proposed activity was questioned because it appeared to call for "delegated review" similar to that of the PSRO program (which presently is forbidden by HCFA regulations). Although hospitals can be expected to be responsive—if they believe it will help reduce the review burden for hospitals with low rates of payment denials or quality problems—opposition from Congress, presumably owing to disappointment about PSRO performance in this arena, was expected (Vibbert, 1989e).

Appropriateness Guidelines

One of the more dramatic developments in the health sector in the late 1980s has been the acceptance of, and indeed the call for, national practice guidelines, appropriateness indicators, and similar utilization management instruments (PPRC, 1988, 1989; IOM, 1989). These tools serve various purposes, such as providing guidance for decisions about pre-procedure and pre-admission review and for understanding whether large variations in population-based rates of use of services reflect large variations in appropriateness or quality of care.[27]

HCFA will consider pilot projects designed to develop appropriateness indicators and practice guidelines through the PROs. Such projects could update existing procedure-specific guidelines or indicators (such as those developed in the mid-1980s by The RAND Corporation) or develop and test similar tools for other procedures and services. As with the other projects, one PRO will be the lead PRO, will negotiate a contract modification, and will subcontract with other PROs or academic and research institutions as necessary.

Other Activities

Small Area Variations. Perhaps the most ambitious PRO project currently under way is a small area analysis of variation in utilization and outcomes of hospital care being conducted by the American Medical Review Research Center (AMRRC). The project began in October 1987 and is expected to continue until June 1990. It will compare rates of use of hospital services in 1984–1986 in approximately 4,800 hospital market areas. Using these data, project investigators will (1) develop and disseminate information on use and outcomes of hospital care; (2) engage 12 PROs in a complex pilot education program to review, interpret, and feed back information to physicians on identified practice patterns; (3) improve the use of small area analysis methods as an operational tool for PROs; and (4) examine various intervention strategies to determine how they might best be applied in both the public and the private sectors.

The 12 PROs involved in the educational component of the project, known as Medical Assessment Program (MAP) pilots, are located in the following states: Arizona, Arkansas, Colorado, Connecticut, Illinois, North Carolina, Ohio, Pennsylvania, Texas, Utah, Virginia, and Washington. The physician study group phase will include five surgical conditions (coronary artery bypass graft, cardiac catheterization, carotid endarterectomy, male reproductive organ operations, and small and large bowel operations) and five medical diagnoses (chronic obstructive pulmonary disease, pneumonia, bronchitis and asthma, acute myocardial infarction, and diabetes). All PROs are to receive data, technical training in small area analysis methods, and necessary computer software.

Uniform needs assessment. OBRA 1986 mandated the development of a "uniform needs assessment instrument" to be used to evaluate the needs of patients for post-acute care such as home health services or other health-related long-term-care services. This instrument is to be used by discharge planners, hospitals, nursing facilities, HHAs, and other providers, as well as by FIs—to make decisions about postdischarge needs and payment for services provided to Medicare beneficiaries.

The instrument was to be developed in consultation with an advisory panel. The panel was chartered in May 1987 and its members appointed in March 1988. It met several times to review preliminary drafts of the instrument and consider recommendations for its use. An extensive effort was made to solicit review and comment on the final draft before formal publication, which was expected in July 1989. (Table 8.10 indicates the major dimensions of the draft instrument.) HCFA plans to develop a users' manual and a standard training process and to field test the instrument for reliability, validity, and administrative feasibility.

EVALUATING PRO ACTIVITIES

HCFA has three mechanisms to monitor and validate PRO medical review activities: (1) the PRO Monitoring and Protocol Tracking System (PROMPTS-2); (2) the SuperPRO; and (3) the monthly and quarterly data

TABLE 8.10 Content of the Uniform Needs Assessment Instrument

---

  I. Sociodemographics

 II. Health Status
     Physical Health
     Mental Health

III. Functional Status
     Activities of Daily Living (ADL)
     Instrumental Activities of Daily Living (IADL)
     Medical restrictions on ADLs or IADLs

 IV. Environmental Barriers to Post-discharge Care

  V. Nursing and Other Care Requirements
     Skilled observation
     Monitoring/supervision/evaluation
     Therapeutic needs
     Educational needs
     Therapy/service needs
     Durable medical equipment needs

 VI. Family and Community Support

VII. Patient/Family Goals and Preferences

VIII. Summary of Assessment of Needs for Continuing Care

---

reports that PROs must submit. Some observers also attempt to draw conclusions about PROs' effectiveness from their record of bringing successful sanction recommendations (which are discussed elsewhere). Sanctions data, however, ignore the far greater number of corrective action plans required by PROs for less serious problems; thus, counting sanctions is a very limited way to evaluate PRO activities. In an effort to provide additional and more rounded information about the PRO experience, the American Medical Peer Review Association (AMPRA, the national PRO association) mounted a survey of its membership in mid–1989.

PROMPTS, SuperPRO, and AMPRA activities are described in some detail below; data reporting is discussed in the next section. These approaches are oriented more toward evaluation of the performance of individual PROs than of evaluation of the impact of the PRO program. No overall evaluation has been undertaken to determine what effect the program itself has had on maintaining or improving the quality of care for Medicare beneficiaries.

PROMPTS-2

The PROMPTS-2 system, developed under the second SOW, provides information about how well PROs have fulfilled their contractual obligations. HCFA uses such information to determine each PRO's status at the time of contract renewal (for a description and evaluation, see OIG, 1989). Specific attention is given to timeliness and accuracy of medical review, responsiveness to beneficiary and provider inquiries, personnel requirements, report generation, and cost-effectiveness through a series of yes/no questions and some rereview of cases. Thus, the focus is more on "process" aspects of performance than on "outcomes," and more on contract deliverables and cost-containment efforts than on quality of care. The 400 points to be assigned to four categories of PRO activity (utilization review, quality review, data, and management) are allocated evenly (100 each) across the categories.

PROMPTS-2 review is required twice during a contract cycle and is completed by RO staff. Staff select a random sample of cases from various review categories (i.e., readmissions, transfers, outliers, etc.) and determine whether the PRO is correctly applying generic screens and other review procedures. The minimum number of cases to be rereviewed is generally 25 per review category unless the PRO performs a larger volume of reviews, in which case larger rereview samples will be chosen. The RO staff record the results of the rereview, indicating the number of cases for which they disagree with the initial PRO determination.

PROMPTS-2 does not generate information on the types of quality problems the PROs detect (or fail to detect). It does alert HCFA to possible problems with PRO performance of medical review activities and contract compliance. The process largely duplicates the SuperPRO effort, although on a considerably smaller scale. Questions have also been raised about inconsistency across ROs, the expertise of their medical reviewers, and the validity of their decisions, as well as about the ability of data so generated to discriminate adequately among PROs (OIG, 1989). A new PROMPTS is being developed to ensure consistency among regions (H. Brook, personal communication, 1989).

SuperPRO

The SuperPRO (SysteMetrics, Inc.) reviews records previously examined by each PRO to make independent judgments about necessity, appropriateness, and quality of care. HCFA then compares SuperPRO findings with results of the PROs to determine whether either the PRO program or individual PRO performance need improvement or modification. More specifically, the basic objectives of SuperPRO are as follows:

1. To validate the determination made by the PROs, specifically on admission review, discharge review, and DRG validation;
2. To validate the medical review criteria being used by nonphysician reviewers for admission review;
3. To verify that nonphysicians are properly applying the PRO's criteria for referring cases to physicians for review;
4. To identify quality issues that should have been addressed by the PRO.

Original Procedures

During the first few years of SuperPRO, the process was essentially the following. For each review cycle (13 in a year), SuperPRO received 400 hospital medical records randomly selected by each PRO from among the cases it reviewed during that cycle. SuperPRO used the same generic screens initially applied by the PRO to judge each case. SuperPRO nurse reviewers first reviewed the case and referred those not passing the screens on to SuperPRO physician advisors; no information was sought directly from the providers whose care may have been in question. Unlike the PRO nurse reviewers, SuperPRO nurses had more leeway in referring cases for physician review. Cases identified by SuperPRO as having quality problems were reported to the PRO, which could further review the cases, appeal the judgment of SuperPRO, and provide additional information in its rebuttal. Approximately 25 percent of PRO appeals led to reversals of decisions in favor of the PRO (data provided by HCFA reviewer of this chapter; see also GAO, 1988a).

SuperPRO reports were, until mid-1989, considered advisory and did not affect payment of claims for Medicare services. For PRO evaluation, HCFA reviewed SuperPRO findings and took necessary action to follow up identified problems.

Early Results

HCFA believes that SysteMetrics would have identified more quality problems than the PROs did, had it (rather than the PROs) been conducting all the review nationally (Morford, 1989a). SuperPRO data indicate that approximately 10 to 15 percent of hospital admissions were unnecessary; that is, the services could have been performed in alternative settings. For instance, for Cycle 6 of SuperPRO review (dated mid-December 1988), PROs collectively had a denial rate (based on lack of medical necessity) of 2.7 percent. Depending on what cases were included or excluded in the calculations, SuperPRO had denial rates of 6.5 percent, 10.1 percent, and 13.9 percent.

SuperPRO contends that approximately 5 percent of the cases it rereviews have quality problems. Of this 5 percent, approximately 3.5 percent represent potential harm to patients; 1 percent represent minor, reversible harm, and 0.5 percent represent irreversible or life-threatening harm.[28] Cycle 6 data showed that the PROs had a rate of quality problems of 1.3 percent as contrasted with the SuperPRO rate of 4.8 percent (or about 3.8 times the average PRO rate). The discrepancies for individual PROs were considerable, however. The SuperPRO problem rate was 44 times higher than that for one PRO but only 1.4 times higher than the rate for another PRO.

Nevertheless, these rates of problem detection (or the prevalence of quality problems they might imply) cannot be compared directly with each other because the review methodologies and data (particularly the level of information from the attending physicians or hospitals) are not the same for PROs and SuperPRO. Moreover, SuperPRO reviews do not provide information about the incidence of quality problems in the Medicare population (because it only rereviews cases already reviewed by the PRO), nor do these reviews make determinations about how cases are selected by the PRO or whether cases not reviewed by the PRO should have been.

The OIG notes that "it is impossible to assess a particular PRO's performance based on SuperPRO data" (OIG, 1989, p. 12), citing two reasons. First, no criteria have been established for assessing the seriousness of discrepancies between PRO and SuperPRO findings. Second, no national analyses of the variations in quality problems have been undertaken. The OIG thus calls for an evaluation of the appropriateness of SuperPRO reviewers and criteria, an examination of how SuperPRO activities complement or duplicate the PROMPTS-2 process, and an assessment of how several SuperPRO procedures might be improved (OIG, 1989).

Future Plans

HCFA issued a new competitive contract for SuperPRO in mid-1989 and awarded a 42-month contract for more than $5.6 million to SysteMetrics, beginning October 1, 1989. The contract calls for approximately 60,000 rereviews of PRO cases (Vibbert, 1989f). It also makes several changes to the current SuperPRO efforts (information provided at HCFA Data Conference, June 14, 1989), although it is not clear these address the issues raised by the OIG. First, HCFA (rather than the PROs) will select the random sample of cases, now to number 600 per 6-month cycle (217 inpatient admissions, 195 HMO cases, and 188 ambulatory surgery cases). Second, if the PRO disagrees with the SuperPRO decision and sends a rebuttal, SuperPRO will do a rereview that may include "local" criteria. HCFA intends that the PROs and SuperPRO should be on a "level playing field" and that SuperPRO should use the same information that the PRO originally had in making quality judgments—that is, the material reviewed by SuperPRO in making its decision is the information the PRO obtained from the hospital or physician in reaching its final decision. Nevertheless, SuperPRO will still not seek additional input from the hospital or physician whose care is under question. (This can be the point at which PRO and SuperPRO procedures differ most, if the additional information used by the PRO physician reviewer in deciding that the quality of care was acceptable is not fully documented or available to the SuperPRO, perhaps because it was gained through face-to-face discussion with the physician in question. This divergence can produce a systematic bias against PROs, insofar as the PRO may determine on the basis of that information that the quality of care was in fact acceptable, whereas the SuperPRO will decide that the quality of care was not acceptable.) Third, and most important from HCFA's point of view, the agency will now use SuperPRO results as a formal rather than advisory part of its evaluation of PROs (Vibbert, 1989c)—hence the strengthening of the rebuttal process.

Because HCFA expects PRO–SuperPRO disputes to arise, the agency will establish a referee in the form of a nationwide "Physician Consultant" contract. PROs will be able to appeal to this entity when they and the SuperPRO disagree about at least three cases with a common clinical cause. Appealable disagreements can include issues of necessity of admission and levels of quality-of-care citations but not DRG validation (Vibbert 1989c). Another option for adjudicating PRO–SuperPRO disputes is to ask the HCFA ROs to resolve such differences (OIG, 1989), although variable RO performance for PROMPTS-2 may call this option into question. The physician consultant contract may be a way to provide the necessary physician backup to the ROs if they are used when third opinions are needed in PRO–SuperPRO disputes.

AMPRA 1989 Impact Survey

Neither PROMPTS-2 nor the SuperPRO evaluation provides any concrete assessment of how well PROs are doing in improving the quality of care rendered under Medicare, and no formal evaluation similar to HCFA's intensive 1979 evaluation of the PSRO program has been undertaken. To provide some information about impacts on quality and what PROs are doing to accomplish them, in mid-1989 AMPRA began the first of several contemplated surveys on the impact of PROs. Results were expected by late 1989.

The first survey was intended to document PRO experience in the acute care setting for the first two contract cycles (i.e., roughly through 1988). Data were sought for five major dimensions of PRO review: (1) the effect of Medicare's PPS on quality of care and the kinds of problems PROs found during hospital review; (2) rates of hospital use for certain procedures and medical conditions; (3) PRO quality objectives; (4) DRG validation; and (5) educational activities and successful quality interventions. A sixth part of the survey focused on desirable improvements to the PRO review program.

DATA COLLECTION, MANAGEMENT, AND REPORTING REQUIREMENTS

HCFA collects an enormous amount of data through the PRO program. The SOW requires specific areas of review responsibilities, and the data compiled or reported by the PROs reflect these responsibilities. This section briefly outlines three types of data generated by the PROs on a periodic basis: profiles, PRO files (or PROFs), and management information reports. At fixed intervals (either monthly or quarterly), PROs electronically submit information to HCFA on each completed review, including the review determination. Owing to the large amount of data required, the PRO does not have to generate hard copies of all reports. Although the interval and method for submission vary depending on the number and type of cases reviewed by the PRO, the record format is standard and has been defined by HCFA. The data elements in the record constitute a minimum data set that must be collected for each review.

Profiles

PROs develop numerous provider- and practitioner-specific profiles for several purposes: to identify areas for focused review or objectives, to monitor PRO performance, to assess internal staff, and to identify aberrations in utilization or quality of care for further study. Those outlined in Table 8.11 are required as a minimum and must be produced quarterly. Under the first and second SOWs, the PRO was required to develop a profile of each provider, and for the immediate past 2-year period, to include variables that can be computed using PRO or HCFA data. The aim is to identify aberrant providers and physicians so that the PRO can focus its activities where it expects potential problems. Profiling includes averaging hospitals and physicians so that those falling two standard deviations from (above or below) the norm (for length of stay, death rates, readmission rates, and transfer rates) can be identified. In addition to the provider profiles, the PRO is to use its own experience in review and data analysis to design and produce profiles that will assist in the review process.

PROFs

A new system of reporting has been developed using the following seven PRO files, or "PROFs." PROFs 1 to 4 are produced monthly, the remainder quarterly.

PROF 1, Pre-admission and Pre-discharge Review Record, collects all pre-admission review cases in which a final decision has been made; it includes all PRO interventions subsequent to notifying the provider or practitioner that a confirmed problem exists. This record also captures cases where review is performed before discharge. *PROF 2*, Universe Data Record, collects data on the universe of cases from which the random samples are drawn. *PROF 3*, Completed Review Record, collects the completed results of all cases reviewed either prepayment or retrospectively. *PROF 4*, Ambulatory Surgery Record, reports data on ambulatory surgery performed in HOPDs and ASCs, and it will reflect review of the required 5-percent random sample. *PROF 5*, Quality Interventions Record, collects data on the number and sources of problems (e.g., physician, provider, other) where the quality intervention is education, intensification of review, other interventions, coordination with licensing and accrediting bodies, or sanction. (Notification of a quality problem does not require generation of a record to HCFA.) *PROF 6*, Cost Report Data, summarizes each PRO's accrued costs during a contract cycle, divided into costs related to review and costs not related to review. Costs for reviewing each type of case are also included in the report. *PROF 7*, Dynamic Objectives, summarizes new objectives

TABLE 8.11 Profiles that Peer Review Organizations (PROs) Must Perform

---

A. Profiles of hospital statistics by:

Average length of stay per diagnosis-related group (DRG) per quarter
Average number of discharges per DRG per quarter
Frequency of procedures identified for quality objectives
Frequency of specific diagnoses identified for quality objectives
Noncompliance with PRO review procedures
Cases that fail admission and quality objectives
Cases that fail generic screens, by screen and physician
Mortality rates
Day and cost outlier rates
Transfer rates to other acute care facilities and exempt units
Pre-admission denials
Readmission rates
Admission denial rates

B. Profiles of physician statistics by:

Denial rates
Admissions
Readmissions
Mortality rates
Length of stay for premature discharge

C. Profiles of other provider statistics, for example:

Home health agencies, skilled nursing facilities, ambulatory surgical centers

D. Profiles for internal quality control:

Review determination denials, DRG validation findings, and audit
Review decisions by:
    Physician reviewers
    Review coordinators

SOURCE: HCFA, 1988.

that are proposed during the PRO contract and approved by the HCFA RO for resolution of utilization and quality problems.

Management Information Reports

Management information reports have two purposes. The first is to help the PRO achieve efficient and effective operations, and PRO staff are to use the reports for decision making and monitoring contract compliance. Specific reports are supposed to be developed throughout the life of the contract in order to meet the changing needs of the particular organization. They are not regularly submitted to HCFA.

The second purpose is to monitor review selection requirements. For example, the PRO is required to review a 3-percent random sample of all cases. To determine whether selection requirements have been met, the PRO needs to know the total number of and the percentage of cases selected each month. Management reports thus are supposed to reflect the same time periods as the related PROF report; for example, PROF 1 should be consistent with the PRO management report on pre-admission activities.

PRO/FI Data Exchange Reports

Data exchange reports are produced monthly and monitor the frequency, volume, and effectiveness of the tape submission process from FIs. Information in these reports includes whether the tapes are processed within the 15-day requirement; whether the correct number of cases has been selected; error rates; types of errors; and whether all hospitals are reporting, and if not, why not. An *adjustment report* is also produced monthly to monitor the number of adjustments in data generated, forwarded, pending, and returned to the FI.

Medical Review Activities

Medical review activities generate four types of management information reports, which are produced on a monthly basis. *Timing of review reports* are used to monitor the adherence of the review process to required time frames. The number, type, location, and age (length of time in the pending category) of all pending cases by review category are included in the report. *Review results reports* monitor the nature and results of review determinations. Data on who is making the determinations, final determinations, and reconsiderations are included. *Pre-admission review reports* assist the PRO in monitoring the operation of the pre-admission review process through the identification of the number of phone calls expected and received, and the decision made by the type of procedure. Finally, *sampling reports* are initially generated on a monthly basis, but then only as needed once the sampling process has been determined to be adequate. The report includes the number of cases received for each review category, the number of cases selected, and the percentage selected.

Quality Control

The final category of required PRO management information reports includes three types of reports. Monthly *correspondence control reports* monitor the number and type of beneficiary complaints and inquiries to determine if a pattern is developing in a particular facility or with a particular physician. *Quality intervention reports* monitor the various stages of quality interventions. These reports include the numbers of physicians or providers for which some intervention has been set in motion, the numbers of notifications, and the numbers of cases under formal education, intensified review, and sanction, as well as the numbers that have been sent to the OIG. Finally, *internal quality control* reports, produced quarterly, concern information about the accuracy of decisions made by nurse reviewers and physician advisors that would enable PROs to identify problems in management.

CONTROVERSIAL OR PROBLEMATIC ASPECTS OF PRO QUALITY-RELATED ACTIVITIES

Issues Relating to PRO Activities in All Systems or Settings

Generic Screens

The initial experience with inpatient generic screens has come under considerable scrutiny and criticism. Recall that the screens are: (1) adequacy of discharge planning; (2) medical stability of the patient at discharge; (3) deaths; (4) nosocomial infections; (5) unscheduled return to surgery; and (6) trauma suffered in the hospital.

Issues include extreme variation across PROs in rates of screen failures and confirmed quality problems, the low yield of confirmed quality problems among cases reviewed, and the value of generic screening for cases that are already under review for other quality-related reasons. Several groups have compiled data on generic screening, including the OIG, GAO, the Prospective Payment Assessment Commission (ProPAC), and HCFA.

For instance, the OIG calculated that the rate of screen failures ranged from 0.1 percent (for screens 1, 3, and 5) to 43 percent (for screen 2) and that the rate of confirmed quality problems ranged from 0 percent (screens 1 and 5) to 99 percent (screen 4) (OIG, 1988a). GAO calculations indicated that in the first 6 to 9 months of use ". . . in several PROs, less than 5 percent of cases failed any screen, while in others, more than 40 percent failed. The percent of confirmed quality problems found in cases with screen failures ranged from less than 5 to over 70 percent; about half of the PROs fell in the 20 to 50 percent confirmed failure confirmation range" (GAO, 1988a, p. 47). HCFA itself noted that, after a year of experience, it had become apparent that the screens were not being uniformly applied. They found, for instance, that in some PRO areas the percentage of screen failures to confirmed problems was close to 100 percent for certain screens (e.g., the discharge planning screen) whereas in other PRO areas it was considerably lower. They concluded that the differences between PROs were too disparate to be attributable to differences in medical practice (H. Brook, personal communication, 1989).

In a separate report, GAO also noted that the PROs themselves rate generic screens behind nurse judgments and profiling and tied with intensified review in terms of their effectiveness in identifying cases with possible quality-of-care problems (GAO, 1988b). In this same report, GAO repeated its conclusion that the PROs vary considerably in the rates at which review coordinators fail cases and especially in the rates at which physician advisors confirm the quality problems.[29]

These aspects of generic screens were evidently still an issue through the period of this study. Calculations based on data compiled by HCFA through June 1989 reflect the wide variation across PROs in the incidence of screen failures and confirmed quality problems; depending on the specific screen, screen failures among cases reviewed ranged from 0.2 percent to 38.6 percent, and confirmed problems from 0 percent to 100 percent (Table 8.12).

One drawback of these rate calculations is that the percentages of confirmed problems are based on a denominator of referred screen failures, not on the universe of cases reviewed. PROs that look quite different on the two measures may actually be detecting fairly similar rates of problems.

What fraction of all charts reviewed actually reflects a true quality problem? Table 8.13 gives the average rates of screen failures and confirmed problems among screen failures through June 1989. The upper panel is based on more than 6.3 million cases reviewed. The first two columns clearly reflect the highly dissimilar rates of screen failures and confirmed problems as a percentage of screen failures. The third column, which gives the percentage of confirmed problems among all cases reviewed, shows the very low overall yield of the screens. The most productive screens relate to adequacy of discharge planning and nosocomial infections.

Another question sometimes raised about generic screens is related to the fact that they are applied to cases targeted for review for many reasons. A purer test of their usefulness might be to examine their yield in just the 3-percent sample, which can be said to represent the universe of Medicare admissions. The lower panel of Table 8.13 reports on data for just the 3-percent random sample of all Medicare admissions. The yield for just that sample is roughly the same as that from all sources of reviewed cases. ProPAC (1989, Table 1.20) had earlier reported percentages of confirmed failures for the 3-percent sample that were lower than those among failures for all cases. The latter includes, of course, the randomly selected cases, cases selected for expected quality problems, and other cases picked for review that do not relate, presumptively, to quality problems (e.g., those required for review by virtue of being 1 of 12 Medicare Code Editor princi-

TABLE 8.12 Range of Generic Screen Failures and Confirmed Problems (in Percentages), by Type of Screen

Generic Screen	Range of	
	Screen Failures	Confirmed Problems
Adequacy of discharge planning	0.2–19.1	2.1–100.0[a]
Medical stability of patient at discharge	1.4–38.6	0.1–68.5
Deaths	0.4–5.8	0.0–37.1
Nosocomial infections	1.1–20.4	0.4–95.7[b]
Unscheduled return to surgery	0.2–2.6	0.0–66.7
Trauma suffered in hospital	1.0–24.1	2.2–65.8

[a]Four Peer Review Organizations (PROs) reported numbers that yielded a figure above 100%, the highest one equalling 109.1%.

[b]One PRO reported numbers that yielded a figure of 106.8%.

SOURCE: HCFA, 1989b.

pal diagnoses). The data suggest, however, that even if the smaller numbers in the random sample are taken into account, using generic screens on just that sample will not produce quality problems with any greater regularity than screening all cases reviewed.

Another, and perhaps more pressing, issue is why PROs differ so dramatically in the rate of referrals and confirmed problems. The process is supposed to be quite standardized (witness the evolution of interpretative guidelines described earlier). Nonetheless, the data strongly suggest that process does vary from PRO to PRO and from HCFA region to region. Believing that vagaries of smaller PROs might account for some of these differences, we analyzed data through June 1989 for just the eight largest PROs (tables available on request). Calculations were done as before for screen failures as a percentage of total cases reviewed, confirmed problems as a percentage of screen failures, and confirmed problems as a percentage of total cases reviewed.

Several issues emerge from an examination of these numbers. The first issue is low yield. For instance, for the eight largest PROs, screen 1 failures as a percentage of total cases reviewed ranged from less than 1 percent to less than 8 percent (national average, 3.05 percent); for screen 2, the range was from about 3 to 29 percent (national average, 12.47 percent). Further, confirmed problems as a percentage of screen failures was as low as 2 percent in several of the eight PROs (against a national average of 28.54 percent).

The relatively low yields of screen failures and confirmed problems (although comforting in terms of the implications about quality of care that might be drawn) combine to produce very small yields of quality problems among all cases reviewed. For these eight PROs, screen failures and confirmed problems ranged from a low of 0.01 percent (for several screens) to a high of about 8.3 percent (for nosocomial infections in one PRO). In short, differences across all PROs do not seem to be a product of peculiarities of only the very small ones.

A second issue is that of variability across screens. The figures for screen failures and confirmed problems by screen for the largest eight PROs show that the percentage of failures for individual screens range from less than 1 percent to more than 100 percent, again demonstrating the variability across PROs and across screens.

Another facet of the differences across all PROs is that of quality problems never detected (and hence never addressed) in any formal way. ProPAC

TABLE 8.13 Percentages of Cases Failing Generic Screens and with Confirmed Problems, by Generic Screen and Universe of Cases

Generic Screen and Universe of Cases	Percent Failing Screen Review	Percent Confirmed Problems Among Failures	Percent Confirmed Problems Among Reviewed Cases
All cases[a]			
Adequacy of discharge planning	3.05	71.27	2.18
Medical stability of patient at discharge	12.47	10.60	1.32
Deaths	1.49	7.50	0.11
Nosocomial infections	7.84	35.67	2.80
Unscheduled return to surgery	0.99	7.56	0.08
Trauma suffered in hospital	4.92	20.82	1.03
Cases in the 3-percent sample[b]			
Adequacy of discharge planning	2.93	79.52	2.33
Medical stability of patient at discharge	12.87	10.76	1.39
Deaths	1.24	8.45	0.11
Nosocomial infections	6.53	31.84	2.08
Unscheduled return to surgery	0.62	7.07	0.04
Trauma suffered in hospital	4.05	21.46	0.87

[a]Number of all cases reviewed: 6,309,839.
[b]Number of cases reviewed in 3-percent sample: 705,983.

SOURCE: HCFA, 1989b.

(1989), for instance, cited one study in which researchers estimated that as many problems were present among cases not flagged by screens (e.g., in about 5 percent of the cases reviewed) as were identified by the screens. The problems allegedly related more to insufficient attention or response to medical problems than to poor care actually provided.

Several factors may account for these differences. For instance, nurse reviewers may differ in how narrowly or expansively they interpret the screens regardless of interpretative guidelines. What may be a failure for some may not be for others; nurse reviewers within PROs, and even individual nurse reviewers from day to day, may differ on what they see or do not see in a given medical chart. Moreover, because of the required case selection specified in their contracts' SOWs and the close relationship of the budgets to those required types of review, PROs may not select "extra" providers, physicians, or problems for review that they suspect may be delivering substandard care. (This may have been more true in the first and second SOWs than the third, because as of now HCFA will pay for reviews conducted for these reasons.)

Furthermore, PROs will differ in the collection of cases to which they apply generic screens because they will have hospitals and physicians on 100-percent intensified review for different reasons and problems and because they will have different mixes of hospital transfers to other types of units.[30] Finally, some cases are targeted for review precisely because a quality problem is considered more likely (e.g., day or cost outliers; the first of a pair of admissions within 31 days; and most cases on intensified review). The question thus becomes the *marginal* productivity of the screens given that there is already reason to believe a quality problem might be present.

The PRO community initially argued for this type of review tool to be used nationally (Lohr, 1985), and a majority of PRO officials and HCFA staff believe that screens have been at least moderately effective (GAO, 1988b; OIG, 1988a). Nevertheless, they have not proven to be entirely successful in efficiently identifying quality problems, and criticisms can be raised in three areas: their value overall; their productivity for detecting problems in a random set of admissions, which appears to be lower (or at least no better) than for a pool of cases where quality problems are already suspected; and their incremental utility in those latter, "suspicious" cases.

Other difficulties remain. Their application is highly labor-intensive. Apparently they still result in considerable false-positives, regardless of the relaxation of the requirement that nurse reviewers must refer failures for physician review, and they have a nontrivial false-negative rate as well. Revisions to the generic screens that are incorporated into the third SOW are essentially untried as of this date. Furthermore, some PROs have found that their own additional screens do as good a job or better than the HCFA screens.[31] Finally, there are numerous reasons why PROs can legitimately differ in the rate of cases detected by the screens, making conclusions about the uniformity of this tool difficult to draw.

Thus, standard, well-known generic quality screens might permit HCFA and the public to track quality problems nationally (depending on how much one can assume about the reliability and validity of these, or any, generic screens). Less certain is whether they can or should be used to compare the performance of PROs. If the quality assurance process were expected to become more alike across the review entities (e.g., more national and more centrally directed), then the factors discussed above would have to be addressed. If, however, the quality assurance program were to remain more responsive to "local" needs and circumstances, then flexibility and local autonomy about these elements of the review process are both more important and more acceptable. Whether generic screens are a strong and reliable tool on which to base a considerable part of the Medicare quality assurance effort seems problematic, and a rigorous evaluation of their utility and productivity is probably warranted.

This experience with inpatient generic screens underscores the need for rigorous pilot-testing of similar instruments designed for nonhospital settings, where there is much less experience with them. Perhaps more importantly, this experience argues for considerable testing and review of the computerized screening algorithms now being developed in the UCDS, in part because they are very different from what the PROs have used so far and in part because of the likely cost of implementing such an extensive data collection effort.

Pre-procedure Review

Whether PROs should be doing pre-procedure authorizations is part of a complicated issue concerning what entities should be doing physician review. It has generated considerable debate for the Physician Payment Review Commission (PPRC, 1989). The debate reflects confusion in at least two areas. First is which entities (carriers, FIs, and/or PROs) have the most experience in prior authorization of procedures and are in the best position to carry it out on a wide scale. Carriers and FIs have a history of prepayment review of physician services more extensive than that of PROs.

The second is whether this is first and foremost an exercise in utilization and cost control or in quality assurance. It may never be possible to draw a firm distinction between prior authorization activities (prospective utilization management as contrasted with retrospective utilization review) that serve a quality assurance function and those that control use of services. To the extent that the latter purpose is the preeminent one, however, the question can be raised whether it detracts from the purported greater emphasis on quality intended for the PROs.

Reviewing Physician Office-Based Care

According to PPRC (1989), the following entities carry out the following tasks. *Carriers* process claims, conduct utilization review, and initiate sanctions for substandard or abusive practices (for inpatient physician visits and procedures, ambulatory physician visits and procedures, durable medical equipment, and diagnostic testing). Carrier reviews of submitted claims involve both prepayment and postpayment review, and medical reviews are done with close consultation of their own medical staffs. *FIs* do the same set of tasks, as well as limited quality review, for inpatient hospital care, outpatient hospital care, SNF and HHA care, hospice care, outpatient rehabilitation facility care, and Part B outpatient physician therapy. *PROs,* of course, do utilization review, quality review, verify bill and DRG data, and initiate sanctions for substandard care for inpatient hospital care, TEFRA HMOs and CMPs, ASCs, and "intervening" HHA and SNF care, with their role regarding physicians' services in office settings to be determined (PPRC, 1989, p. 239).

In short, the three groups have overlapping, or possibly conflicting, responsibilities. They operate in different ways, with different data bases and different rules, such as when (before or after hearings) they can deny payment and what information about review criteria and screen thresholds must be made public. They also collectively leave a big gap. According to PPRC (1989), none of these entities has specific responsibility for reviewing most Part B services for *quality of care,* although carriers have authority to deny payment and initiate sanctions for substandard, unnecessary, or inappropriate care. PROs, however, are charged with reviewing office-based (ambulatory) care, which they do not yet do (although the pilot project on office-based care has begun). In short, the picture of which agencies have what authority to review outpatient care for quality of care and to take action in the face of instances of poor care remains clouded.

PPRC (1989) made four recommendations concerning Part B carrier and PRO utilization and quality review. First, HCFA should establish procedures to encourage input from carriers and PROs in designing utilization and quality criteria, in developing physician profiling methods, and in investigating physicians suspected of providing inappropriate or substandard care or of billing inappropriately. Second, HCFA, carriers, and PROs should work together to delineate future roles of PROs in ambulatory care review. Third, PROs and carriers should consult with appropriate medical organizations when developing review criteria (over and above what they are required to do now). Fourth, HCFA should designate a single entity to support research, demonstrations, evaluations, and technical assistance for all three entities doing utilization and quality review.

Peer Review

In spite of the historical emphasis on peer review in federal programs and in the PRO SOW, physicians and hospitals heard from during this study widely contend that PRO reviewers are not "peers." The points in contention concern rural practitioners and providers, physicians fully in private practice reviewed by physicians only partly still in practice (e.g., because they are semiretired), specialists not being reviewed by members of their own specialty, and physicians for whom the relatively low reimbursements for PRO review are an important portion of their income. Physicians in prepaid group practice settings reviewed by those in FFS settings are discussed later. HCFA does require PRO physician reviewers to be in active practice and have admitting privileges in one or more hospitals in the PRO area.

PROs we visited acknowledged the problems concerning rural areas and specialists but generally defended their record of using peers. They cited budget constraints as playing a large role in these problems: among these were not being able to maintain regional offices in rural areas and not being able to reimburse reviewers at competitive levels. The emerging debate about "quality denial letters" discussed elsewhere in this chapter is expected to add to the problems of recruiting specialists and, especially, subspecialists.

Sanctions

Retention of PRO sanction authority. The role of PROs in the sanctioning process, and the role of sanctions in the quality assurance efforts of PROs, have both been misunderstood over the course of the program. With regard to the former, several points need to be emphasized. First, PROs can only recommend sanctions to the OIG, not invoke or enforce them. Second, in principle (although perhaps not in practice), practitioners and providers have a considerable number of due process steps open to them before a sanction is actually imposed. Consequently, PROs have little influence over the outcomes of a full sanction process, even when they have provided full documentation of their reasons for recommending a sanction.

Nevertheless, PROs are virtually uniform in their view that having the sanction-recommendation capability is an indispensable tool in their dealings with providers and practitioners whose performance is unacceptable (OIG, 1988a). For instance, GAO reported that almost 70 percent of PROs rated sanctions as very or extremely effective for correcting quality problems; the next most useful intervention was counseling, with about 45 percent of PROs rating this as very or extremely effective; about 30 percent of PROs gave those ratings to formal education and to communication with quality assurance committees and with hospitals (GAO, 1988b).

In short, PROs would not be willing to relinquish the sanctioning authority they now have in favor of simply greater educational or persuasive interventions. William Moncrief, M.D., representing AMPRA at a hearing before the Committee on Governmental Operations in April 1989, testified that the "PRO sanction activity is important to the effectiveness of the program," describing it as "a careful and extensive" process involving "extended consultation and due process procedures." This was also the view of those PRO officials who provided information to this study through the public hearings and site visits, although some cited the costs (in terms of financial and human resources) as a significant barrier to their effective pursuit of all but the most egregious cases.

Elimination of PRO sanction authority. The most radical suggestion about the PRO authority to recommend sanctions is to eliminate it. Several arguments have been advanced for this view (Jost, 1989). Critics believe that the educational and enforcement dimensions of the program are not compatible and that PROs have overemphasized one function or the other. Others argue that PROs lack legal expertise, which has led to inadequate protection for the due process rights of sanction targets.

Thus, one proposal is to turn the sanction function over entirely to the OIG.[32] PROs would continue their quality assurance functions by monitoring medical records, investigating complaints, and requiring corrective action where quality problems were identified; they could put into effect other interventions that they currently use, such as limiting practice, mandatory consultation, preceptorships, attendance in residency programs, obtaining board certification, and requiring oversight in surgery (Jost, 1989). When, however, they discover problems on which formerly they would have taken sanction actions, now they would refer the matter without recommendation to the OIG for investigation and possible action.

The OIG, either with its own medical resources (which it would have to develop) or with experts borrowed from the PRO (or perhaps elsewhere, such as HCFA ROs or the FIs), would build its case, decide on an appropriate penalty, and present the case to a specially trained ALJ. The ALJ would decide whether to impose a sanction and the nature and extent of the penalty (Jost, 1989). The OIG would, however, be given summary suspension power where the situation indicated that, because the practitioner poses an immediate risk to beneficiaries, immediate action is warranted (Jost, 1989).

This revised system allegedly has several advantages. It would allow the PRO to concentrate solely on its primary function, peer review. It would simplify the currently complicated procedures and remove PROs from the disputes about due process (Jost, 1989). It would also be preferable from the perspective of practitioners who may be subject to investigation and sanction, because they would receive a hearing before an impartial ALJ before any sanction could be imposed (Jost, 1989); this improvement, however, could be made without changing the PROs' sanction authority. In short, it is claimed that the revised system would permit the PROs to carry out their most important function—promoting quality of care for Medicare beneficiaries—by threatened action (i.e., referral to the OIG) against offending practitioners and providers while avoiding much of the hostility and mistrust that the provider community currently feels toward them.

This proposal has met significant opposition. The PROs fear the loss of some of their enforcement powers. The administrative conference (ACUS) has rejected it (Jost, 1989). In view of the difficulties of the PSRO program—which did not have the same sanctioning (or related regulatory) powers that the PRO program has—weakening these powers for the PRO program does not seem to be an attractive option. Correcting some of the other problems of the entire sanctioning process, however, does appear to offer ways to strengthen the government's ability to protect the quality of care delivered to Medicare beneficiaries.

Monetary penalties. PROs strongly advocate that a broader, or more finely tuned, set of sanction recommendations be open to them, viewing the choice of exclusion of the provider or a nearly meaningless monetary penalty as essentially no choice at all. That is, no viable sanction measure short of exclusion has really been available to them.[33] (In the visits to PROs as part of this study, this issue tended to be seen as part of a larger need to strengthen all the intervention options open to PROs, not just the sanction capabilities.)

In its 1988 review, the OIG recommended that the monetary penalty option be strengthened by allowing PROs to propose a fine of up to $10,000 per violation of Medicare obligations (i.e., the provision of substandard, unnecessary, or uneconomical care). GAO seconded this stand by recommending that the relevant congressional committees enact legislation setting a fixed upper limit to monetary policies in place of the present cost-based limit. HCFA agreed to assist the OIG in drafting such legislation. The ACUS also recommended that DHHS be permitted to assess "a substantial" fine against providers and practitioners (Vibbert, 1989c). Countering these proposals were recommendations from the House Commerce Committee to cap the monetary fines at just $2,500 (Vibbert, 1989d), a step that would effectively nullify the effort to shore up the monetary penalty option of sanctions. Exactly how this issue would be resolved was uncertain at the time this report was completed.

The "unwilling and unable" provisions. The requirement that a provider or practitioner be found "unable or unwilling" to meet their Medicare obligations (in addition to finding that they have not in fact complied with those obligations) has caused unending confusion and frustration with the sanction process. Among other things, it effectively required that PROs demonstrate that a doctor or institution was unable to conform to a corrective action plan, because the physician or institution can claim that it was both able and willing to meet the specified obligations or corrective action. Thus, although the "unable and unwilling" provision can be seen as a desirable aspect of due process for physicians or institutions, it is a nearly impossible task and one that can take a very long period of time (during which the practitioner or provider could continue to provide services).

Providers, for their part, have complained that PROs do not explain the basis for the "unwilling or unable" finding and do not give physicians a chance to respond to such determinations before the PROs impose sanctions. In one case (*Lavapies v. Bowen*), the federal district court held that the matter of the practitioner's alleged unwillingness or inability to comply was a serious question and that she had been denied an opportunity to present her side of the case under existing procedures; on that basis, the court issued a preliminary injunction against the OIG's sanction.

The problems were sufficiently apparent and persuasive toward the end of 1988 that the OIG recommended that DHHS submit a legislative proposal to the effect that failure to comply with patient care obligations was sufficient basis for sanctioning (OIG, 1988b). The ACUS has endorsed a recommendation that would remove this requirement to prove that a physician or institution is "unwilling and unable" to meet Medicare obligations before sanctioning. Because this seemingly constricts due process, the ACUS has also suggested that all physicians now be afforded the opportunity to seek pre-exclusion stays (not just physicians in rural areas, as is the case in mid-1989). Such stays mean that sanctioned providers can have exclusions lifted pending the outcome of a full evidentiary hearing. The ACUS would, however, require that the burden of proof in such hearings be shifted from the government (to prove that the sanction should be upheld) to the sanctioned physician (to prove that it should not).

Such stays may not be regarded as sufficient protection for sanctioned practitioners, however, and the American Medical Association is expected to push for the retention of the "unwilling and unable" provisions (Vibbert, 1989c). Moreover, the House Commerce Committee has recommended that the time during which a physician can claim to be willing and able be expanded (Vibbert 1989d). Hence, as with monetary penalties, the question of whether PRO sanction capabilities will be strengthened or weakened remains open.

Timing of sanctions before hearings. Practitioners and providers sanctioned by the OIG are excluded from the Medicare program before they can obtain an ALJ hearing. They have argued that the procedures to safeguard their rights are inadequate to protect their constitutional rights under the Due Process clause of the Fifth Amendment. Although many courts have agreed that either a constitutionally recognized property interest or liberty interest is implicated in this exclusionary process, they have uniformly held that the government's interest in expediting procedures to protect Medicare patients outweighs the physician's or the institution's interest in increased procedural protection. The multiple levels of case review before the OIG imposes sanctions are seen as affording substantial protection already.

Adequacy of notice of grounds for sanction. The concept of not meeting "professionally recognized standards of care" has evidently been confusing to some parties (from PROs to ALJs). Despite specific requirements in the regulations that the practitioner or provider be informed of the nature of the violation, the basis for the PRO determination, and the procedure rights due, PROs have in some cases issued vague charges and in other instances raised new issues at sanction meetings that were not reflected in the original notice (Jost, 1989). One possible result has been a high rate of reversals of OIG sanction actions by ALJs (10 of 18 cases by one recent count) (Vibbert, 1989b). In addition, in an effort to correct this problem, HCFA has issued model notice letters for PROs to use (Jost, 1989), but because of their legalistic and punitive tone, these are not universally liked in the PRO community.[34]

Denials for Substandard Quality of Care

COBRA and OBRA 1987 allow PROs to deny Medicare payment for substandard quality of care, although the provisions of the legislation were not implemented awaiting final regulations; a draft proposed rule to effect these requirements was published in January 1989 (*Federal Register*, 1989). It required payment to be denied when substandard care resulted in actual, significant adverse effects on the beneficiary or placed the beneficiary in imminent danger of health, safety, or well-being (i.e., places the beneficiary in a situation that constitutes a "gross and flagrant violation"). The former condition (actual . . . effects) was defined quite broadly, as including unnecessarily prolonged treatment, medical complications, readmission, physiological or anatomical impairment, disability, or death.

To protect the concept of peer review, the proposed rule specified that physician advisors engaged in initial denial determinations of substandard quality be specialists in the same field as the attending or consulting physician whose care is under question. The requirement could be met by having the initial determination made by a physician reviewer who is actually in the same specialty, by having a second level review by such a specialist when the original determination was made by a physician in a different specialty, or by having a committee of specialists, at least one of whom is in the same field. This requirement could be relaxed, however, when meeting it would compromise the effectiveness or efficiency of PRO activities.

The proposed rule further provided that hospitals would be held financially liable even if they did not contribute directly to the substandard care rendered by the physician. Thus, any denial of physician payment on these grounds would also result in a denial of reimbursement to the hospital. Furthermore, physicians may not charge patients for the care denied for these reasons and, if they have done so, must refund those payments to the beneficiary.

The proposal then specified that the PRO shall notify the patient when such payment has been denied on the basis of substandard care. The key section was to read: "Our determination [concerning denial of Medicare payment of a hospital admission or physician services provided in connection with that admission] is based on a review of your medical records, which indicates that the quality of services you received does not meet professionally recognized standards of health care. Denial decisions are made by the PRO physician. Your attending physician and hospital were given an opportunity to discuss your case with the PRO before the denial decision was made . . . " (*Federal Register*, 1989, p. 1966).

In the initial proposal, this letter would have been sent *before* providers were able to exercise their rights to appeal (i.e., to have the case reconsidered), rather than after a final determination had been made. The notion that the initial denial determination would (supposedly) have been made by a physician in the same specialty as the physician whose care was being denied and the fact that there was a 30-day opportunity to discuss it was evidently considered sufficient protection for that practitioner whose patient would receive such a letter.

The entire quality denial process prompted much debate, especially during the time this study was being conducted. Among the concerns was the lack of protection for physicians if they could not invoke their full due process rights to reconsideration before their patients are notified of such denials, especially because of the high proportion (more than 45 percent) of denial decisions that are now overturned by the PROs after reconsideration (Vibbert, 1989b). The "same-specialty" requirement does not, in many observers' minds, adequately mitigate this problem.[35] Most professional and consumer interest groups thus support early opportunities for appeal. The ACUS has recommended that DHHS proceed expeditiously to implement PRO quality denial authority, but with appeals *before* patient notification (Vibbert 1989c).

Another criticism centered on the impetus such letters might provide for increased malpractice suits filed by beneficiaries and the impact of higher litigation on PRO activities. There are also concerns about the expected increased difficulties in recruiting the specialists that will be needed to participate in these reviews and decisions. A fourth concern focused on how much specific information the PRO should have to put in the letter to the beneficiary. Some wanted to keep the letters general but specify that care was substandard, others wanted more specificity about what was discovered that led to that decision, and yet others wanted the letters to say only that care did not meet Medicare payment guidelines (and not refer to the denial as a quality denial) (Vibbert, 1989b).

OBRA 1989, passed in late November 1989 (after the main part of this study had been completed), addressed some of these issues (Congressional Record, House, November 21, 1989). First, it protected the physician or institutional provider from unwarranted notices to patients. Specifically, it provided that the PRO should not notify beneficiaries until after the PRO had notified practitioners or providers of its determination about the quality problem and their right to a reconsideration; if the practitioner or provider requests such a reconsideration, then one would be conducted before any notices to beneficiaries. Second, it softened the wording of the beneficiary notice, by saying that the letter need only state: "In the judgment of the peer review organization, the medical care received was not acceptable under the Medicare program. The reasons for the denial have been discussed with your physician and hospital" (p. 9380).

Administrative Procedures and Public Oversight

As noted at the outset of this chapter, the authority for PRO activities resides in several legislative acts; in a broad array of regulations, guidelines, and directives; and in various documents such as the PRO *Manual,* the contract SOWs, and periodic instructions. The practice of relying on *Manual* transmittals, contracts, and other less formal instructions, instead of promulgating regulations through "public notice and comment" rulemaking as required by the APA, has raised serious questions. This is not unique to the PRO program, however, as DHHS has frequently sought to carry out its regulation of the Medicare and Medicaid programs by means less formal than this relatively burdensome rulemaking method.

The APA requires that the public be given an opportunity to comment on proposed rules, that the comments be considered by the agency, and that the final rules be published at least 30 days before their effective date. Section 603 of the APA requires regulatory flexibility analyses, and executive orders require that the OMB review some rules. All these make notice and comment rulemaking under the APA time-consuming and burdensome, and it is not unusual for the promulgation of a rule to take a year (Jost, 1989).

Experts argue, however, that sound policy reasons support using the more cumbersome rulemaking process (Jost, 1989). It promotes public participation and fairness to parties who will be affected by the rules; it also forces the agencies to consider their proposals with greater care and to express them clearly. In foregoing the rulemaking process, HCFA has opened the door to accusations that it is attempting to govern the PRO program through "a continual and confusing stream of instructions [that has] severely hampered their ability to carry out their mandate" (Jost, 1989) and earned the hostility of those governed by the program.

Legal suits[36] and legislation in the last few years have clarified the situation somewhat. OBRA 1987 calls for substantive changes in PRO contract provisions to be published in the *Federal Register,* although not necessarily according to APA procedures. Section 4035(a) specifically provides that "no rule, requirement, or other statement of policy (other than a national coverage determination) that establishes or changes a substantive legal standard governing the scope of benefits, the payment for services, or the eligibility of individuals, entities or organizations to furnish or receive services or benefits under this title shall take effect unless it is promulgated by the Secretary by regulation . . . ."

Nevertheless, the question of public access to, understanding of, and ability to comment on the myriad rules governing the PRO program remains important. One commentator suggests that in view of congressional deadlines, DHHS should whenever possible publish PRO SOWs and any changes or modifications made during the contract cycle for an abbreviated period for comments and should publish final provisions at least 30 days before their effective date (Jost, 1989). Others have urged DHHS to make PRO contracts, interpretive rules, statements of policy, and guidelines of general applicability available in places of easy public access and to publish updated lists of these materials every three months (Jost, 1989). The ACUS contends that DHHS should use formal rulemaking procedures "when seeking PRO program changes except when the agency has 'good cause' to believe the process is 'impracticable, unnecessary, or contrary to the public interest'" (Vibbert, 1989c, p. 6), should publish SOW rules in the *Federal Register* with 30 to 45 days for public comment, and should publish PRO contracts, *Manual* instructions, and other guidelines quarterly in the *Federal Register* (Vibbert, 1989c).

Although steps such as these might be seen as markedly constraining the ability of HCFA to administer the PRO program, the gains in terms of useful and timely reaction *beforehand* to proposed changes and modifications to the program might be substantial. It might facilitate decision making as to when new program initiatives (e.g., new review or data collection instruments or methods) should be extensively pilot- and field-tested and when such rigorous examination can be foregone. Moreover, the increased sense that program administration is open to public scrutiny might be a considerable benefit to a program that is often poorly understood by beneficiaries and health care providers alike.

Evaluation

Considerable criticism can be leveled at how the PRO program itself is evaluated, especially in terms of its impact on the *quality* of care. Virtually no reliable or comprehensive examination of PRO program impact has been done within DHHS. The several careful external investigations by the OIG and GAO have tended to focus on specific operational aspects (e.g., usefulness of generic screens; structural aspects of PROs). How HCFA evaluates individual PRO performance can also be criticized. Existing tools such as PROMPTS-2, although in transition to improved efficiency, have not been especially successful at providing a coordinated approach to evaluation (although PROMPTS-2 evidently is more productive that the SuperPRO effort). The OIG in particular has criticized HCFA's ability to assess PRO performance (OIG, 1989). When combined with the lack of public oversight and accountability noted above, these problems appear to have high priority for attention and correction.

Collectively, these efforts underscore the need for considerably more innovative and comprehensive review of the impact of the PRO program on quality of care (as contrasted with narrow evaluations of how well individual PROs appear to be applying review methods or complying with contract specifications). The requirement in the third SOW for PROs to publish an "annual report" may prove to be a useful step in that direction. The changes in PROMPTS-2 and perhaps the SuperPRO effort may also prove useful over the longer run.

Another step that some have recommended is to appoint a "national council" of outside experts that could oversee the operations of the PRO program and report periodically (e.g., annually) to the Secretary of DHHS or to the Congress, or both, on the progress, successes, and problems of the program. Such a council might also be very useful in solving some of the public oversight and administration issues noted above. Precedent for such a step might be found either in the former PSRO National Council or in the appointment of the advisory commissions established since the advent of PPS, namely ProPAC and PPRC.

Congress established ProPAC in 1983 in response to concern about the need to monitor and update the PPS system. The 17 members of ProPAC are appointed by the director of OTA for a 3-year term. The commission has two major responsibilities; first, it recommends annual changes in the hospital payment rates to the Secretary of DHHS and, second, it recommends changes in the DRG classifications. It has discharged these responsibilities through regular commission meetings, which are generally open to the public, and detailed annual reports and technical documents. The statute limits the number of staff to 26, and the annual budget for the ProPAC activities approaches $4 million.

Physician payment under Medicare has come under close scrutiny in the last several years, and Congress established PPRC in 1986 to advise on reforms to the physician payment system under the Medicare program (PPRC, 1988, 1989). PPRC is modeled on ProPAC (e.g., members appointed by the director of OTA for a 3-year term, and a staff limited to 26 persons). This commission plays four major roles (PPRC, 1988). First, it provides advice to the Secretary of DHHS. Second, it seeks the views of physicians, beneficiaries, and others concerning its recommendations. The conduct of analyses to form the basis for policy decisions is the third role of the commission. Finally, it undertakes the work necessary to implement the recommended policy changes.

PPRC has initiated several research projects to develop a Medicare fee schedule for physician payment based on the relative value of resources used by the physicians to produce the services rendered to the patient (see Hsiao et al., 1988). The implementation of such a system, however, will not take place for several years. PPRC has also taken the lead in calling attention to the need for "practice guidelines" to help physicians understand better when services, especially procedures, are appropriate and when they are not.

Issues Relating to HHA Review

PROs that had begun HHA review during the site visits for this study noted two significant problems. First, selecting an appropriate sample for this task requires that hospitals bill for the two admissions in a reasonably timely way. At least one PRO noted, however, that some hospitals bill for two admissions more than 31 days apart (which would not constitute a reviewable readmission); only much later would the hospital bill for the admission that occurred within 31 days of the first admission (which would be a reviewable readmission). This practice severely complicates the identification of 31-day readmissions and hence of cases that would constitute the potential pool of HHA care. A related sampling problem is simply that the pool of HHA cases for readmissions only is itself small, and whether it is representative of all HHA care is unknown.

Second, at least one PRO noted that the HHA sector is undergoing great growth and change, which includes the emergence and disappearance of "fly-by-night" agencies. An agency might be out of business by the time the PRO knew what cases of HHA intervening care had fallen into its sample. Review in that case probably would be impossible and certainly would be moot. Other technical problems involving data and records have also been noted (Vibbert, 1989d).

Issues Relating to HMO-CMP Review

Peer Review

Physicians in prepaid group plans have always argued that physicians in FFS practice are not well placed (and historically not well disposed) to judge the care from HMOs and similar plans on a "peer basis"; the premises underlying prepaid practice and the resulting styles of practice are simply too different. This perception reflects the historic concern of the HMO community that their care will be unfairly and improperly judged by the standards of the larger and more powerful FFS community. These concerns are heightened by the reliance to date on implicit physician review of cases referred to them through the nurse-reviewer screening process rather than on more explicit quality-of-care criteria developed with some appreciation of the different practice styles of the prepaid setting. Thus, there is some concern that using "local standards of care" may perpetuate existing practice patterns and vitiate the potential of prepaid systems for innovation and improved service to the Medicare population.

To meet this objection from the HMO industry, the HMO-CMP SOW requires the PRO to use HMO-CMP physicians to perform reviews whenever possible. In addition, conflicts of interest can arise in several instances: when only FFS physicians review HMO-CMP care, when HMO-CMP physicians review care rendered by a plan from which they may receive financial benefit, and when HMO-CMP physicians review care from a competing plan. Thus, PROs are required to develop a means of addressing these possible situations. In addition, PROs are expected to develop a quality control mechanism that will protect the integrity of the review process as it is applied to HMOs and CMPs (e.g., by creating a committee whose membership includes one representative from each plan under review in the state).

Records and Case Selection

Cases for inpatient review are to be selected on the basis of claims (the UB-82 Medicare hospital bill) submitted to FIs that are aggregated into a file (the "UNIBILL" file) forwarded to the PROs; the PROs in turn select their samples from this file. For the FFS system, this procedure works well; because payment is tied to the submission of a bill, this record of hospital admissions can be assumed to be quite complete.

For the HMO and CMP system, this process does not work well at all and results in a very inadequate "universe" of inpatient claims for several reasons. HMOs and CMPs (and the hospitals with which they have various payment arrangements when they do not own their own) have no particular incentive to file such claims because payment is not related to them. Moreover, in many cases FIs were not processing UB-82s submitted by risk-contractors or their affiliated hospitals or were not forwarding the UNIBILL file on to the PROs. Although efforts were made to force hospitals to prepare and submit these bills to the FIs, HCFA estimated that still only about half are being submitted (O'Kane, 1989).

To overcome this still inadequate pool of cases from which to select samples of cases for review, HCFA now requires HMOs to keep a separate record of all admissions; those not reflected in UNIBILL data will be subjected to their own random sampling procedure so that the required level of review will be reached. Because HMOs and CMPs will differ in the proportion of their total hospitalizations subject to this form of random sampling, an additional source of variability has been added to review in the risk-contracting segment of the Medicare program.[37]

Apart from the problem of identifying which cases to review is the considerable set of obstacles that exist to acquiring the charts. Obtaining hospital charts is not appreciably more difficult for the HMO and CMP sector than for the FFS sector, and both systems contend that low reimbursement of copying costs (just over $0.049 per page) and lack of reimbursement for administrative costs are problems.[38] For outpatient records, however, the problems can be extreme, when records for one plan must be retrieved from numerous health centers. Although the problem is manageable for most group- and staff-model HMOs and even for group network models, it presents independent practice associations (IPA-model HMOs) with extraordinarily complex logistics, because large plans of this sort may have hundreds of physicians practicing in individual offices. HCFA has indicated it would support legislation to allow HMOs to be reimbursed for administrative costs of retrieving such records, which should alleviate the problem to some degree.

Limited Review

One of the more contentious issues in HMO-CMP review has been the limited success of so-called limited review (only 11 of 133 risk contractors are currently on limited review), and several factors seem to be at work. First, the notion of reviewing an HMO's own quality assurance plan was unfamiliar to PROs, and HMOs may thus have been reluctant to put themselves in the position of having their internal programs subjected to an unpredictable and uneven evaluation process. Second, PROs are expected to review all care rendered in a case that falls into the limited review sample, even if, in the HMO's own program, only selected parts of that care were subject to review (e.g., as part of a focused audit study of some particular problem that the HMO was evaluating in depth). The HMO thus becomes liable for a failure ("Outcome No. 1," a quality problem found by the PRO but not by the HMO) relating to care it had never reviewed as part of a quality assurance plan that the PRO had found acceptable.

Third, the main argument for limited review was that it reduced the number of cases subject to review; in practice, however, HMOs subject to limited review can end up having as many cases reviewed (but no more than) as HMOs on basic review. Finally, because of the second factor (the scope of PRO review versus that of HMO review under its own quality assurance program), the HMO under limited review in theory can run more of a risk than the HMO under basic review of being subjected to intensified review on the basis of PRO findings on the "validation subsample" (i.e., cases having been reviewed by the HMO pursuant to its own quality assurance plan).

Ambulatory Care Review

With respect to ambulatory review, the interesting question is how physicians will respond to review of the care they provide in their own offices. In the HMO environment, physician resistance might add to the incentive for plans to withdraw from the risk-contract program, especially if the requirement for office-based review in the FFS setting is not fully implemented for some years. As noted earlier, FFS office-based review is expected to be started as a pilot project. Given the lack of experience and proven tools for ambulatory review, this is arguably a good strategy for the PRO program. It does, however, place the HMO community in a position that they can understandably regard as unfair.

Accountability

Who is responsible for quality problems is a question that arises in any health care delivery system, but it is especially salient in the complex world of prepaid group practice arrangements. For instance, for HMOs that do not own their own hospitals, that contract for certain types of care (e.g., subspecialty care), or that cover their members on a FFS or contractual basis for out-of-plan (e.g., out-of-region) care, the issue of whether they are accountable for care well beyond their ability to oversee or control becomes very complicated. In situations when an HMO's patients are not concentrated in only a few hospitals or are otherwise widely dispersed across practitioners, the HMO can find itself held responsible by the PRO program for quality problems but without any authority or ability to monitor or control the performance of those providers, except over the very long run when a sufficient number of patients have had experience with those providers.

The question of accountability may be more complicated by legal precedent and rulings concerning whether entities that employ physicians and other professionals are held to different standards than those that only contract with physicians (essentially the distinction between group and staff models on the one hand and IPA-type models on the other). Some IPA physicians hold that they should not be subject to review until such time as all physicians who contract with Medicare (presumably meaning all FFS physicians) are reviewed. This may be especially salient in the light of a case (*Harrell v. Total Health Care, Inc.*)[39] in which the court held that an HMO as a corporate entity could be liable for the negligence of contracting referral physicians.

Other Issues Relating to HMO-CMP Review

PROs differ dramatically in the proportions of quality problems they find in HMOs; one accounting showed a range of 1.8 percent in one state to upwards of 30 percent in three states (HCFA data cited by O'Kane, 1989). Although it may be the case that HMO quality differs as much as 15-fold across the states, variations of that magnitude call into question more than the true quality of the care being rendered, most especially the validity of inferences drawn about comparisons of HMOs with each other and with the FFS system. It also raises the issue of whether HMOs operating in several or many states are subjected to the "same" review, because the PRO in each state is responsible for the state-specific portion of the HMO risk-contract care.

In the site visits for this study, multistate HMOs had different views on this issue. At least one felt very strongly that it wished to deal with only a single PRO because it was experiencing considerable, unexplainable variation in review from the different PROs in the different states in which it operated. By contrast, at least one other plan found PRO review sufficiently nontroublesome that differences across PROs were either not noticeable or not a problem.

The question of valid comparisons is especially problematic for those states with only a single risk contractor, because information about numbers of cases reviewed and numbers and percentages of quality problems cannot be protected from public disclosure. For an HMO with an "unblemished" record, this obviously poses no problems, but for an HMO with a "poor" record the risk to its competitive position (vis-à-vis other HMOs in the state) could be considerable.

CONCLUDING REMARKS

This chapter has presented information on the current Medicare PRO program. It is intended mainly as a reference document for Volume I, Chapter 6, of the IOM study committee's report. The history of the program for review of care rendered in both FFS and prepaid group practice settings is recounted with emphasis on the most recent (third) SOW. Some problems related uniquely to HMO and CMP review are described, in addition to current special projects and other activities of the PROs (or HSQB and HCFA).

Among the issues discussed are the following: the usefulness of hospital generic screens, the practical question of ensuring review by peers, the limitations of the current sanctioning process and denials for substandard care, the adequacy of public oversight and administrative procedures for the program, and the lack of any systematic program evaluation to date. In formulating its mission of a model quality assurance program, the IOM study committee took many of these issues under advisement, intending that its proposed program overcome some of the more troublesome drawbacks (e.g., the adversarial "regulatory" aspects of the program and the lack of public accountability) while building on the considerable expertise, skills, and experience of the PRO community.

NOTES

1. The authors wish to acknowledge the perceptive and timely assistance of Alan Kaplan, a Washington, D.C. attorney and consultant, at various stages of the preparation of this overview of the PRO program. Harvey Brook and John Spiegel of the Health Standards and Quality Bureau were always responsive to questions and requests for data, and we thank them and their staff for a detailed and helpful review of this chapter. We also thank Andrew Smith and Maxwell Mehlman, authors of a related background paper for this study, for important legal and regulatory information on which this chapter in part relies. Finally, the commissioned paper on the history of and current issues relating to PRO review of risk-contract prepaid group practices, by Margaret O'Kane, was a valuable background document.

2. The OIG (1989) notes that HCFA appears not to have formally published the rationales for the sampling methods imposed on PROs. They also contend that HCFA apparently sets most of the specific requirements for review internally, usually without pilot-testing.

3. A "substantial violation in a substantial number of cases" is a pattern of care that is inappropriate, unnecessary, does not meet recognized professional standards of care, or is not supported by documentation required by the PRO.

4. "Gross and flagrant violation" means a violation of an obligation (in one or more cases) that represents an imminent danger to a Medicare beneficiary's health, safety, or well-being, or that places a beneficiary at an unnecessarily high risk.

5. More cases are shown as reviewed than as selected for review. This may be an artifact of counting practices. For instance, transfer and readmission categories in the reviewed classification actually involve two or more cases, and Medicare code editor cases are reported under both pre-admission–prepayment and retrospective review (HCFA, 1989b).

6. Interpretative guidelines for generic screens include two features, exclusions and explanatory notes. For example, exclusions for adequacy of discharge planning include death, transfer to an acute short-term general hospital or swing bed status, or patient left against medical advice. Explanatory notes for nosocomial infection are another example. They state: "A screen failure is not necessarily a confirmed problem. A screen failure occurs when more than one indicator of an infection is identified more than 72 hours after admission. Indicators [are]: temperature elevation of 101 degrees Fahrenheit or greater (oral) (38.9 Centigrade); elevated white blood cell and/or left shift; isolation of organism from body fluids or specimens; appropriate radiographic imaging abnormalities; purulent draining; heat, redness, focal tenderness and/or pain; pyuria, dysuria; and productive cough. When the case has two or more indications of a nosocomial infection (i.e., a screen failure), you are encouraged to refer to the CDC's [Centers for Disease Control] guidelines to determine whether there was a nosocomial infection. The presence of a nosocomial infection is always a confirmed quality problem. Treatment of the nosocomial infection does not negate the confirmed quality problem."

7. Prior-authorization criteria vary by PROs. For cataracts, for instance, the Delmarva PRO indications for the procedure require visual acuity of 20/50 or worse in the affected eye for distance, or visual acuity of 20/40 or worse in the affected eye for near vision. Three other criteria are also (ambiguously) stated: visual acuity is interfering with the patient's lifestyle; cataracts are causing another ocular disease; and cataracts are preventing treatment for another disease. (Another set of specifications serve as indications for admission for the procedure.) The New York PRO indications for the procedure require the patient to meet one specific criterion (cataract removal will improve the patient's visual performance for daily activities, employment, and/or recreation) and one of a number of others, including vision in the operative eye less than 20/60, or the nonoperative eye is phakic and visual acuity is less than 20/40.

8. This chapter refers in various places to practitioners and providers; the distinction is a term of art for the PRO program in that practitioners would be used to refer to physicians or other individual clinical caregivers, and providers to facilities and institutions such as hospitals, SNFs, HHAs, as well as HMOs and CMPs.

9. Comments to study site visitors from PRO officials indicated that many Severity Level I cases ultimately turn out not to be quality problems as defined, because they are related to poor documentation. The "quality problem" is not confirmed when the target physician or provider provides satisfactory additional information.

10. HCFA prescribes the format and wording of these initial sanction notices (apart from the specifics of the case at hand). Presumably for legal reasons, they are very formal in tone and must contain the following information: (1) the obligations involved; (2) description of the activity resulting in the violation; (3) the authority and responsibility of the PRO to report violations of obligations; (4) a suggested

method and time period for correcting the problem (at the discretion of the PRO); (5) an invitation to submit additional information or discuss the problem with the PRO within 20 days of the notice; and (6) a summary of the information used by the PRO in reaching a determination.

11. As part of a case (*American Medical Association v. Bowen*) settled 3 years ago, the OIG committed itself to seek a regulatory alternative to the practice of newspaper notices. It was intended to permit sanctioned physicians to inform their Medicare patients personally that Medicare would no longer pay for the physicians' services (e.g., by mailing notices to individual patients).

12. Payment cannot be made to another party where services or items have been ordered by an entity excluded by sanction when that order was necessary as a precondition of payment. Payment may be made for services provided up to 30 days after the effective date of the exclusion (1) when the recipient of the services or items is an inpatient in a hospital or SNF and was admitted before the effective date or (2) when home health care services are delivered under a plan established before the exclusion.

13. The relevant passages defining peer review include: ". . . whenever possible, the contractor [i.e., the PRO] [shall] use physician reviewers who practice in a setting similar to that in which the physician whose services are under review practices. In . . . initial review of psychiatric and physical rehabilitation services, the contractor must arrange for review (to the extent possible) by a physician who is trained in the appropriate discipline. . . . In addition, the contractor would be required to use board certified or board eligible physicians or dentists, in the appropriate specialty, to make reconsideration determinations, wherever practicable. . . . The contractor would consult with other health care practitioners (e.g., podiatrists) when appropriate (e.g., when reviewing services rendered by that type of practitioner)" (HCFA, 1988). The qualifiers ("whenever possible," "to the extent possible," "wherever practicable") appear to give the opportunity to dilute the emphasis on peer review, although HCFA argues that the term "whenever possible" is used for cases where it is not administratively feasible for the PRO to use a specialist. Examples of such situations include (1) when the specialist is located on the other side of the state or (2) when the specialty is so unique that it is not possible to locate a specialist reviewer in the field.

14. Consistently throughout this study, respondents at site visits confirmed the observation that quality problems tend to affect all patients, not just the elderly. Especially in hospitals and prepaid systems, it was noted that most quality problems tended to be with "systems" that cut across units and patient age groups. Moreover, facilities and groups with well-established internal quality assurance systems deliberately did not single out "the elderly" or "Medicare patients" for specific quality assurance attention (except insofar as they needed to meet PRO demands for records and similar requirements), believing that a more efficient and ultimately more successful approach to quality improvement would involve the entire institution, its entire staff, and its entire patient census.

15. Regulations define "confidential information" as information that explicitly or implicitly identifies an individual patient, practitioner, or reviewer; sanction reports and recommendations; quality review studies that identify patients, practitioners, or institutions; and/or PRO deliberations. "Implicitly identifies" means data

sufficiently unique or numbers so small that identification of an individual patient, practitioner, or reviewer would be obvious.

16. Estimates for Medicare outlays are from the Committee on Ways and Means (1989, Table 15, p. 152), where slightly different figures are given depending upon whether the estimates are from the Congressional Budget Office (CBO) or from HCFA (CBO estimates tend to be higher). The figures cited here are roughly midway between the CBO and HCFA numbers. Estimates for PRO budgets are from HCFA staff (H. Brook, personal communication, 1989).

17. Material for the Medicare risk-contract section is based in part on a paper prepared for this study, "PRO Review of Medicare Health Maintenance Organizations and Competitive Medical Plans," by Margaret E. O'Kane, Director of Quality Assurance, Group Health Association, Washington, D.C., May 1989.

18. The PRO-HMO Task Force had three representatives each from three organizations, the Group Health Association of America, the American Medical Care Review Association, and the American Medical Peer Review Association; the first two are prepaid group practice trade organizations, and the latter is the PRO national association.

19. The 15 sentinel conditions for ambulatory care review were diabetic coma or acidosis, ruptured appendix, stroke with hypertension, bleeding or perforated ulcer, gangrene, breast cancer, cancer of cervix, drug overdose/toxicities, mal-union of fracture of hip, cellulitis, bowel obstruction, bleeding secondary to anticoagulation, hypokalemia, septicemia, and pulmonary emboli.

20. The "comparable review" language for risk contracts was interpreted to mean that the number of cases reviewed must be at the same level as was occurring under PPS in the FFS system; this in turn implied a substantial level of record review. The legislation did not provide for pilot projects or staged implementation.

21. The 25 states for QRO review of HMO and CMP services were Alabama, Arizona, California, Georgia, Hawaii, Illinois, Indiana, Iowa, Kansas, Kentucky, Maryland, Massachusetts, Missouri, New Jersey, New Mexico, North Carolina, Pennsylvania, South Carolina, South Dakota, Tennessee, Texas, Virginia, Washington, West Virginia, and Wisconsin.

22. As of December 1989, Quality Quest is the QRO only for Missouri. The Illinois PRO (Crescent Counties Medical Foundation) is the QRO for Illinois. The QRO contract for Kansas had not yet been awarded.

23. Each month, the PRO (or the QRO) receives a copy of the "Monthly Report of Medicare HMO/CMP Contracts and Applications." This list is reconciled against a list of established risk-based HMOs and CMPs to identify new plans in the area. For each new plan that requests "limited review," the PRO (QRO) performs an initial analysis to determine whether this level is appropriate. Absent such a request, the plan is automatically placed on basic review.

24. The SOW for QRO review is sufficiently similar to that for PROs that it is not described more fully here.

25. An additional requirement for HMO and CMP review, 100 percent of hospital transfers, was eliminated in July 1989.

26. The 13 "sentinel" conditions for HMO and CMP review include: diabetic complications (ketoacidosis, hyperosmolar coma, other coma, and hypoglycemic coma); acute appendicitis with generalized peritonitis or peritoneal abscess; hy-

pertensive problems (several categories, including occlusion and stenosis of precerebral arteries and transient cerebral ischemia); gastrointestinal (GI) catastrophes (acute, chronic, or unspecified gastric ulcer with hemorrhage without obstruction; chronic duodenal ulcer with hemorrhage without obstruction; unspecified intestinal obstruction); gangrene of the extremity; operations for breast malignancy (from other biopsy through unilateral radical mastectomy); malignant neoplasm of the genitourinary organ; adverse drug reactions (several categories, mainly poisoning by specific pharmacologic agents); other cellulitis and abscess; malignant neoplasm of colon; hypokalemia; septicemia; and pulmonary embolus. These are very similar to the 15 conditions proposed by the PRO-HMO Ad Hoc Committee; mal-union of fracture of hip is missing and bowel obstruction was evidently subsumed under GI catastrophes. For limited review, one of the four conditions reviewed must be the hypertensive problems. In addition, two of the four must be selected from among the following conditions: diabetic complications, gangrene, adverse drug reactions, other cellulitis and abscess, hypokalemia, septicemia, or pulmonary embolus.

27. In 1988, HCFA proposed an Effectiveness Initiative intended to bring the resources of Medicare to bear on the question of what works in the practice of medicine (Roper et al., 1988; IOM, 1989). Information generated from that initiative was expected to provide an expanded basis of knowledge for the development of practice guidelines and similar work, even if HCFA was not directly involved in that development. The UCDS was seen as an integral part of the initiative. At HCFA's request, the IOM convened one workshop of clinicians to advise on appropriate clinical conditions most appropriate for priority attention in such research; that study recommended five conditions: stable and unstable angina, acute myocardial infarction (AMI), breast cancer, congestive heart failure, and hip fracture. HCFA then asked the IOM to convene three "research strategies" workshops on breast cancer, AMI, and hip fracture to advise on key patient management issues that should be addressed first; these workshops were conducted between February and July 1989 (IOM, 1990a–d).

Because of greatly heightened interest in effectiveness and outcomes research on the part of Congress and DHHS, considerable attention was placed in mid-1989 on exactly where in the department resources for this work should be placed. OBRA 1989 (P.L. 101-239) created the Agency for Health Care Policy and Research in the Public Health Service to conduct such work, and relatively little would be done in HCFA. Consequently, the fate of the Effectiveness Initiative as envisioned by HCFA was unclear as of this writing, although it was expected that the PRO pilot projects relating to practice guidelines could proceed independently and that the UCDS might be a source of clinical data.

28. Figures cited in the text concerning the rates of quality problems found by the SuperPRO are from the oral testimony of Christy Moynihan, Ph.D., of SysteMetrics, Inc., at the October 21, 1988, public hearing of the IOM Study to Design a Strategy for Quality Review and Assurance in the Medicare Program.

29. PROs sometimes negotiate review objectives with HCFA on the basis of their experience with generic screens, with the idea of specifying a target problem reduction level. Discharge planning is the most popular screen on which such objectives are based, and it plus hospital-based trauma are areas in which PROs are most successful in reaching or exceeding their targets (GAO, 1988b). Discharge

planning and falls (as part of hospital-based trauma) are the two screens for which nurse reviewers need not refer cases to physician advisors.

30. In its cumulative data summary, HCFA (1989b) notes that "totals for all reviews for the generic quality screen data should not be used to project national rates of occurrence" of the various problems identified through the screens. The reason is that national totals include problems detected through focused review, which (if it is being conducted as intended) should detect more than the usual number of quality problems. Hence, the total rates of occurrence, if projected to all discharges without accounting for the higher rates among focused review, might yield rates higher than are actually the case.

31. With respect to additional screens developed by the PROs, the Peer Review Organization of Washington (PRO/W) reported that some of its specially developed screens identify more failures and/or confirmed problems than do the HCFA screens.

32. An ancillary proposal is that the OIG be given the authority of a "national medical board" to protect beneficiaries. States have not been very effective in exerting discipline over the medical profession, and some suggest that such a national system would permit uniformity and greater protection for Medicare beneficiaries (Jost, 1989).

33. The OIG had advised PROs in July 1987 not to recommend fines unless they could demonstrate that they would be cost-effective. Apart from perhaps contradicting legal requirements that PROs bring sanction recommendations against all providers that have violated their Medicare obligations, this advisory discouraged PROs from recommending monetary penalties and decreased the number of sanction filings. This situation was to have been remedied by Spring of 1989 by a change in policy from the OIG to the PROs (McIlrath, 1989; Vibbert, 1989a).

34. Smith and Mehlman (1989) provided the basis for much of the discussion in this entire section.

35. The site visits for this study took place during the time that the proposed rule was published for public comment, and thus PROs were just beginning to analyze how it would affect their local operations. A major problem mentioned to the site visitors was that implementation of quality denials as planned, particularly the allegedly harsh language required for the letters to beneficiaries, would seriously erode the ability of PROs to attract the necessary specialist physician advisors who would be expected to make the initial denial decisions. Moreover, PROs believe that the relatively low rates they can pay physician advisors, often only between $55 and $65 an hour, already markedly hampers their recruitment efforts, especially of certain kinds of specialists and subspecialists; implementation of the quality denials, with the heavy reliance on specialists as described, was expected to exacerbate the problem.

36. Early in the PRO program the American Hospital Association (AHA) charged that HCFA's administrative practices violated the APA and requested that DHHS promulgate comprehensive PRO regulations (i.e., in accordance with APA requirements). This request was not met, and the AHA filed a lawsuit (*American Hospital Association v. Bowen*) claiming that DHHS had failed to meet its statutory duties under the APA. The district court for the District of Columbia agreed with AHA. DHHS appealed the decision, and the court of appeals reversed the district court ruling. The majority opinion held that the contracting process, the issuance of the

SOWs, and *Manual* transmittals were all covered by exceptions to the APA (Smith and Mehlman, 1989).

37. Vibbert (1989c) reported that some legislative language may require that DHHS make HMOs, not hospitals, responsible for assuring that PROs obtain the inpatient discharge abstract information needed to draw the relevant review samples. The rationale was that the current random analysis approach is ineffective and intrusive (a point with which HMOs might well agree); nevertheless, this option would not appear, from the point of view of the HMO industry, to overcome that particular problem.

38. The issue of reimbursing hospitals for costs incurred in photocopying medical records has been especially contentious since 1985. A court order in mid-1989 required that HCFA reimburse hospitals retroactively for costs incurred in photocopying; the American Hospital Association argues in favor of a $0.12 per page reimbursement level. Recently hospitals gained class action status in a federal suit involving photocopying costs (Vibbert, 1989g).

39. No. WD39809 (Mo. Ct. App. 1989). The Missouri Court of Appeals found that the doctrine of "corporate negligence" is not limited to treatment settings because it is based on common law principles of negligence. Moreover, it determined that the defendant (the HMO) had a duty of care to protect members from unreasonable risk of harm by exposing them to unqualified or incompetent physicians (and the HMO had not done so because it had failed to make any investigation of the background of the physician in question).

REFERENCES

AHA v. Bowen, 640 F. Supp. 453 (D.D.C. 1986).

AMA v. Bowen, Civil Action No. 87-995 (D.D.C. 1987).

Committee on Ways and Means. *Background Material on Programs Within the Jurisdiction of the Committee on Ways and Means. 1989 edition.* Committee Print WMCP 101-4, March 15, 1989. Washington, D.C.: Government Printing Office, 1989.

Dans, P.E., Weiner, J.P., and Otter, S.E. Peer Review Organizations: Promises and Pitfalls. *New England Journal of Medicine* 313:1131–1137, 1985.

Federal Register, Vol. 50, pp. 15364–15389, April 17, 1985.

Federal Register, Vol. 54, pp. 1956–1967, January 18, 1989.

GAO (General Accounting Office). *Medicare Improving Quality of Care Assessment and Assurance.* PEMD-88-10. Washington, D.C.: General Accounting Office, May 1988a.

GAO. *Medicare PROs Extreme Variation in Organizational Structure and Activities.* PEMD-89-7FS. Washington, D.C.: General Accounting Office, November 1988b.

HCFA (Health Care Financing Administration). 1988–1990 PRO Scope of Work. Baltimore, Md.: Health Care Financing Administration, Department of Health and Human Services, 1988.

HCFA. Request for Proposal for the SuperPRO Contract, Attachment II. Baltimore, Md.: Health Care Financing Administration, Department of Health and Human Services, 1989a.

HCFA. Peer Review Organization Data Summaries dated February, May, and August 1989, and Technical Notes to the Data Summaries. Baltimore, Md.: Office of Peer Review, Health Standards and Quality Bureau, Health Care Financing Administration, 1989b.

HCFA. Utilization and Quality Control Peer Review Organizations Second Scope of Work. Executive Data Summary. Report through March 1989. Report dated July 5, 1989. Baltimore, Md.: Health Care Financing Administration, 1989c.

Hsia, D.C., Krushat, W.M., Fagan, A.B., et al. Accuracy of Diagnostic Coding for Medicare Patients Under the Prospective-Payment System. *New England Journal of Medicine* 318:352–355, 1988.

Hsiao, W.C., Braun, P., Yntema, D., et al. Estimating Physicians' Work for a Resource-Based Relative Value Scale. *New England Journal of Medicine* 319:835–841, 1988.

IOM (Institute of Medicine). *Effectiveness Initiative: Setting Priorities for Clinical Conditions.* Washington, D.C.: National Academy Press, 1989.

IOM. *Effectiveness Initiative: Setting Priorities for Research in Breast Cancer.* Washington, D.C.: National Academy Press, 1990a.

IOM. *Effectiveness Initiative: Setting Priorities for Research in Acute Myocardial Infarction.* Washington, D.C.: National Academy Press, 1990b, forthcoming.

IOM. *Effectiveness Initiative: Setting Priorities for Research in Hip Fracture.* Washington, D.C.: National Academy Press, 1990c, forthcoming.

IOM. *Effectiveness and Outcome Research: Proceedings of a Conference.* Washington, D.C.: National Academy Press, 1990d, forthcoming.

Jost, T. *Administrative Law Issues Involving the Medicare Utilization and Quality Control Peer Review Organization (PRO) Programs: Analysis and Recommendations.* Report to the Administratrive Conference of the United States. Washington, D.C.: Administrative Conference, November 8, 1988 (Reprinted in *Ohio State Law Journal* 50(1), 1989).

Kane, R.A., Kane, R.L., Kleffel, D., et al. *The PSRO and the Nursing Home: Vol. I, An Assessment of PSRO Long-Term Care Review.* R-2459/1-HCFA. Santa Monica, Calif.: The RAND Corporation, August 1979.

Lavapies v. Bowen, 687 F. Supp. 1193 (S.D. Ohio 1988).

Lohr, K.N. *Peer Review Organizations: Quality Assurance in Medicare.* P-7125. Santa Monica, Calif.: The RAND Corporation, July 1985.

McIlrath, S. Receding Tide of Physician Sanctions by Medicare PROs Triggers Debate. *American Medical News* 3: 57, April 21, 1989.

Morford, T.G., Director, Health Standards and Quality Bureau, HCFA. Testimony before the U.S. House of Representatives Committee on Government Operations, Subcommittee on Human Resources and Intergovernmental Relations, April 4, 1989a.

Morford, T.G. UpDate. Federal Efforts to Improve Peer Review Organizations. *Health Affairs* 8(2):175–178, Summer 1989b.

OIG (Office of Inspector General, Department of Health and Human Services). *The Utilization and Quality Control Peer Review Organization (PRO) Program. Quality Review Activities.* Washington, D.C.: Office of Inspector General, Office of Analysis and Inspections, August 1988a.

OIG. *The Utilization and Quality Control Peer Review Organization (PRO) Program. Sanction Activities.* Washington, D.C.: Office of Inspector General, Office of Analysis and Inspections, October 1988b.

OIG. *The Utilization and Quality Control Peer Review Organization (PRO) Program. An Exploration of Program Effectiveness.* Washington, D.C.: Office of Inspector General, Office of Analysis and Inspections, January 1989.

O'Kane, M.E. PRO Review of Medicare Health Maintenance Organizations and Competitive Medical Plans. Paper prepared for the Institute of Medicine Study to Design a Strategy for Quality Review and Assurance in Medicare, 1989.

OTA (Office of Technology Assessment). *The Quality of Medical Care. Information for Consumers.* OTA-H-386. Washington, D.C.: Government Printing Office, June 1988.

PPRC (Physician Payment Review Commission). *Annual Report to Congress, 1988.* Washington, D.C.: Physician Payment Review Commission, March 1988.

PPRC. *Annual Report to Congress, 1989.* Washington, D.C.: Physician Payment Review Commission, April 1989.

ProPAC (Prospective Payment Assessment Commission). *Medicare Prospective Payment and the American Health Care System. Report to the Congress, June 1989.* Washington, D.C.: Prospective Payment Assessment Commission, 1989.

Roper, W.L., Winkenwerder, W., Hackbarth, G.M., et al. Effectiveness in Health Care: An Initiative to Evaluate and Improve Medical Practice. *New England Journal of Medicine* 319:1197–1202, 1988.

Simborg, D.W. DRG Creep. A New Hospital Acquired Disease. *New England Journal of Medicine* 304:1602–1604, 1981.

Smith, A.H. and Mehlman, M.J. Medicare Quality Assurance Mechanisms and the Law. Paper prepared for the Institute of Medicine Study to Design a Strategy for Quality Review and Assurance in Medicare, 1989.

Vibbert, S., ed. Watchdog Criticizes HHS IG Over PRO Monetary Sanctions. *Medical Utilization Review* 17(7):1, April 4, 1989a

Vibbert, S., ed. PROs Denied 2 Percent of 1986–1988 Medicare Cases. *Medical Utilization Review* 17(9):1, May 2, 1989b.

Vibbert, S., ed. Regulatory Activity. Legal Panel Backs PRO Reform Package. *Medical Utilization Review* 17(13):5–6, June 27, 1989c.

Vibbert, S., ed. PRO Sanctions Fight Moves to Senate. *Medical Utilization Review* 17 (15):1–2, August 8, 1989d.

Vibbert, S., ed. HSQB Softpedals Controversial Pilot. *Medical Utilization Review* 17 (18):3–4, September 21, 1989e.

Vibbert, S., ed. SysteMetrics Retains SuperPRO Contract. *Medical Utilization Review* 17 (19):2–3, October 5, 1989f.

Vibbert, S., ed. Hospitals Gain Class Action Status in Federal Suit Over PRO Photocopying. *Medical Utilization Review* 17(21):1, November 2, 1989g.

Index

R